KINESIOLOGY

Fundamentals
of Motion
Description

David L. Kelley

University of Maryland

KINESIOLOGY

Fundamentals of Motion Description

Prentice-Hall, Inc.,   Englewood Cliffs, New Jersey

Printed in the United States of America
Library of Congress Catalog Card Number: 79–144098

10 9 8 7 6 5 4 3 2 1

Epigraph: From Thomas Mann, *The Magic Mountain,* trans.
H. T. Lowe-Porter (© Copyright 1952 by Alfred A. Knopf, Inc.).

0-13-516260-2

Prentice-Hall International, Inc., London
Prentice-Hall of Australia, Pty., Ltd., Sydney
Prentice-Hall of Canada Ltd, Toronto
Prentice-Hall of India Private Limited, New Delhi
Prentice-Hall of Japan, Inc., Tokyo

To my wife Ann,

and daughters,

Sarah and Elisa

Contents

Preface

The preparation of a textbook to serve as a model for organized study in any area of knowledge depends largely upon the identification and development of a unifying characteristic or theme of the subject matter that will act as a thread which courses through and binds together its various parts. In the present instance, *motion description* is the motion study characteristic which can serve this unifying function. Wherever one chooses to examine the fascinating realm of motion, or more specifically, human motion study, it becomes evident that the ability to describe motion events accurately is probably the most critical element in the student's mastery of the subject matter. It is the ability, when achieved by the student, which can provide the necessary background and vocabulary for communicating motion information to others, and encourage him to study more advanced motion problems. In this writer's experience, the lack of motion description skills is the most common and most restricting weakness encountered in students who have completed an undergraduate course in kinesiology. In most cases fundamental motion concepts have received only superficial treatment, often as a result of textbook limitations. The difficulty which arises is that the student's capacity for further growth within the subject matter is severely blunted without recourse to additional backtracking instruction to fill the vacuities. This text is offered as an attempt to present the fundamental framework of kinesiological subject matter in a manner that will eliminate the need for such backtracking and encourage continuous growth, after as well as during the formal study situations.

This book has been prepared for the undergraduate course in kinesiology which is common to physical education and physical therapy curricula. From the beginning of its preparation, a broader-than-usual perspective was sought. Because of the book's rigorous approach to and coverage of topics not usually included in previous undergraduate kinesiology textbooks, its application may well be extended to beginning graduate courses in motion analysis and biomechanics for students with limited undergraduate backgrounds in kinesiology. The topics covered and their progression offer the student a significant challenge as well as an opportunity for self-instruction. The latter advantage then may be utilized by the kinesiology teacher to bring his or her personal experiences to bear upon related topics which may not have received the desired attention in the text. Wherever possible, the book's contents were designed to carry the student beyond the usual intuitive level of understanding by combining qualitative and quantitative concepts and operations.

The book is divided into three parts, each attending to a particular approach to motion study. Part I, *Position and Motion in Time and Space*, lays the kinematic foundations upon which the two remaining sections of the text are built. Discussions of the simplest methods of studying motion with respect to reference frames are followed by progressively more complicated matters, such as time-rate functions and the classification of whole-body and body segment motions. Part II, *The Motivation and Control of Motion*, is concerned with the kinetic approach to motion study. The effects of forces and the nature of moving objects are introduced, developed, and applied. Part III, *The Anatomy of Motion*, attends to the important anatomical considerations which underly human movements. Each chapter follows the same pattern of topic presentation to provide a useful continuity from one anatomical region to the next. Frequent applications of matters covered in previous sections of the text are included. Supporting tables are to be found in the appendices.

Glancing through the text will point out that great care was exercised in the preparation of the numerous illustrations and graphs which supplement the narrative. Throughout the book, these figures have been placed to provide the reader with important conceptual assistance. They should be studied carefully as one progresses through each chapter. Whenever topics have been covered to the desired level, illustrative exercises and/or problems are suggested immediately where they connect to the narrative, rather than at the ends of chapters. In addition, numerous questions are posed to the reader to stimulate interesting discussions and lead to deeper understandings of the subjects being covered. It is hoped that these procedures can offer the immediate reinforcement and continuity required for thorough learning and avoid the searching labors of undertaking a list of problems at the end of each chapter. For the benefit of both student and teacher, each chapter includes a comprehensive reference list which should provide rewarding reading which encompasses the range from simple to complex resources.

Acknowledgements

The contributors to this book are legion, in small and large ways, ranging from my teachers, colleagues, and students, to my very generous wife and daughters who sacrificed my attentions for the sake of the book's preparation. I am indebted to **Bernard V. Kessler** for his generous counsel in presenting physical concepts; to **Donald J. Hobart** for his assistance in the preparation of the Muscle Charts and photographic models for illustrations; to **Jerome R. Noss** for his detailed criticism of the manuscript. In conclusion, a special acknowledgement is due to **Robert N. Aebersold** who was primarily responsible for the content of Chapter 12, *The Electromotive Characteristics of Muscle.*

David L. Kelley
Greenbelt, Maryland

. . . He had learned in his technical school about statistics, about supports capable of flexion, about loads, about construction as the advantageous utilization of mechanical material. It would of course be childish to think that the science of engineering, the rules of mechanics, had found application in organic nature; but just as little one might say that they had been derived from organic nature. It was simply that the mechanical laws found themselves repeated and corroborated in nature . . . The thigh-bone was a crane, in the construction of which organic nature, by the direction she had given the shaft, carried out, to a hair, the same draught-and-pressure curves (he) had had to plot in drawing an instrument serving similar purpose. . . . He enjoyed the reflection that his relation to the femur, or to organic nature generally, was now three-fold: it was lyrical, it was medical, it was *technical*. . . .

THOMAS MANN
The Magic Mountain

Position
and
Motion
in
Time
and
Space

1

Preliminary Motion Considerations

MOTION COMMUNICATIONS

The motions of life possess a most essential characteristic which makes them subject to man's curiosity. This characteristic is that motion "speaks of itself" or is innately communicative. By this, it is meant that movements of tangible objects, in a very real sense, communicate with their observers. They seem to reach out and capture the attention of the would-be observer, offering information about themselves. It makes little real difference whether or not the observer is schooled in the science of motion (mechanics); the communication nevertheless takes place, with each observer contributing to the dialogue in his own way in accordance with his own experience. The purpose of the discussion at this point is not to attach a heirarchy of values to motion cognition on the basis of past experience, but to establish that very real differences in the interpretation of the meaning of observed motions can and do exist, based upon one's experience. Thus the content of the communication varies directly with the observer's experience.

Examples of the varying content of these communications can be seen everywhere. For the ornithologist, the changing shapes of the silhouette of a distant, flying bird can immediately establish recognition and identification. The inexperienced eye probably is not aware that the bird is in view—least of all that it might be identified specifically. The soaring leap of the ballet dancer speaks not only of physical power, but of the beauty of movement in a context in which the aesthete reaps an immediate understanding. To the general observer, the side-to-side swaying in the walking gait of an individual may go unnoticed. To the orthopedist or physical therapist, it could mean the loss of function of the lateral stabilizers of the hip or the characteristic balancing accommodations of the very obese individual. The cherished memory of a motion experience can endow a still picture of a yacht at sea with conjured imaginations to close out the implied events not pictured. To the boxing fan, the lightning-like punch which produced the knockout is a thing of beauty, while to the losing fighter, it may be represented only by a blurred beginning followed by the complete loss of communication. The dialogue between man and his moving environment is one of the universal activities of life and, as indicated above, demonstrates a variety which is bounded only by his imagination.

Although the imagination is a marvelous human faculty, a thorough understanding of movement events must rest on firmer foundations. If we think of insight as the ability to look beyond the immediately apparent, we have an important clue as to how people differ in their understanding of motion phenomena. The degree to which an individual can understand the content of motion communication depends markedly on his preparation to do just that. Those who are successful in understanding motion have been alert to its occurrence, have studied its variety, and have put their minds to work as they themselves participated in movement. They have investigated the contributions of motion to life and have cultivated an acute awareness of the need for simplifying its complicated nature so that description and explanation are less complicated tasks. The message is clear: *Get involved with motion, particularly that of man, and sample much of life's true flavor!*

Motion Recognition and Identification

In order that some cognitive value can be attached to motion, it must first be recognized that it is occurring or has occurred. Motion, the entity of interest, must be defined in such a way that it can and will be recognized when it occurs. It is usually defined as the change of place or position of an object. This change of position is invariably referred to with respect to the surroundings associated with the object, thus establishing a *frame of reference*. The surroundings, including the observer, may themselves be fixed or in motion. Therefore, if an object changes its position relative to fixed or motionless surroundings, the recognition that it has taken place is relatively simple. If, however, the object moves with respect to moving surroundings, again including the observer, the task of motion recognition is more difficult. Human beings possess a remarkable ability to recognize that motion is occurring or has occurred because of their almost limitless experiences with the motions of everyday life. However, before any misconception is nurtured, it must be pointed out that humans also demonstrate a propensity toward being confused by motions, sometimes in their simplest forms.

The process of moving from place to place is recognized in part by (*1*) the characteristics of the places or positions inhabited by the object involved in the motion, (*2*) the characteristics of the motion paths followed between the successively identified positions, (*3*) the physical characteristics of the moving objects themselves, and (*4*) the characteristics of the environment which motivate and control the motion. Since there are essentially limitless varieties of these clues or evidences to support and assist the recognition, it becomes most necessary to carefully determine the *identity* of the observed motion to establish some systematic order within the complexities of motion information. This establishment of order comes about through the processes known as *classification*, where the characteristics of motion that lead to its recognition are used also to classify or establish its identity.

In some cases, classification is involved with the qualities of the motion, while in other cases, it is involved with the inherent quantities of the motion. In the former, motion is referred to as having many and highly varied aspects. A number of examples of such qualitative terms would include free, uniform, violent, curved, continuous, forced, natural, and even divine. All of these terms, many of them historically interesting, point up the importance of the observer as well as the motion information observed. These qualities play an important role in understanding what has taken place and the value to be attached to it, sometimes at the risk of a heavy dependence on one's point of view or disposition. A case in point might well be the place of expert judging in athletic competition to determine the relative quality of performance. It is usually refined and accurate, but on occasion outside influences temper its objectivity. The proper combination of carefully derived qualitative and quantitative features leads to motion identity.

The quantities of motion find their value in the classification process in *measurement* and all that the term implies regarding assumptions, accuracy, and uncertainty, whether directly or indirectly determined. Quantities involving both cause and effect, such as dimensions, forces, displacements, and time and rate functions, make the motion understandable. The quantitative features of motion serve to make the language of description more precise. This is most valuable in the establishment of motion identity because the quantities of motion may be treated mathematically. In doing so, motion description becomes more refined and less subject to misinterpretation.

The search for all accurate motion information, whether quantitative or qualitative, begins with an appeal to Kipling's Six Honest Serving Men: What, Why, When, How, Where, and Who. This questioning or curiosity springs from a basic frame of mind characterized by doubt—not the kind of doubt which immobilizes human facility, but the simple doubt that one "has all the answers." A person who does not often doubt in this manner seldom demonstrates the trait of curiosity, which is so necessary to motivate careful motion study or any other kind of careful study.

Scott makes an important point when she comments that "Man seems to think in terms of movement. A study of the art of nearly all primitive people shows that it deals largely with active participants in war, sports, or routine occupations. Seldom do we find reclining, sitting, or standing figures which are entirely passive in their attitude."[1] The early Greeks were aware of the fact that the illusion of motion could be created by first drawing a series of sequential pictures of motion positions on a wall. By running or riding rapidly past the pictures while gazing generally at them, the still pictures appeared to spring to life, depicting the motion originally conceived. These simple beginnings were obviously the simple records of attempts to describe motion in a meaningful way, employing only rudimentary knowledge of art and science. They were the precursors of the highly developed art and science of cinematography as practiced today. What transpired between these examples of the development of man's interest in motion and its description is beyond the scope of the present discussion. However, its study is a rewarding pursuit and is highly recommended to the student of kinesiology. Certainly it can be said that man has made enormous strides in his quest for an understanding of what or who has moved, when and where it moved, how it moved, and why it moved. Many of the results of that quest are contained in the discussions of motion which follow this chapter.

KINESIOLOGY AND MOTION DESCRIPTION

Centuries of study of the motions of all sorts of objects have established that the foundation science is *mechanics*. It undergirds the study of kin-

[1] M. Gladys Scott, *Analysis of Human Motion*, 2d ed. (New York: Appleton-Century-Crofts, 1963), p. 3.

esiology as it does other physical and biological sciences in a manner which is analogous to the relationship between the human form and its skeleton. For the purposes of this text, kinesiology is defined as the study of motion which is characterized by the movements of human beings and those other objects which are influenced directly by human motivation. Thus the movements of the individual as well as those of the implements he wields must be considered since they influence one another. Certainly it is as important to understand the responses of the horse as it is to understand the movement signals of the rider, the movement characteristics of the bat as well as the movements of the batter, the action of the trampoline in projecting the gymnast as well as his movements in the air. Whatever the moving object may be, human or otherwise, the description of its motion must be mechanically based.

The Mechanical Bases for Motion Description

The first considerations in motion description are *time* and *space*. We perceive these elements as useful concepts in distinguishing the differences between objects and the events associated with the objects. In mechanics, one may study motion on a space-time basis without specific concern for what is moving or the causes of the motion. This is the *kinematic* approach, where motion is described on the basis of its observed and measured space and time characteristics. One of the most difficult tasks for the student of kinesiology is to achieve a thorough grounding in understanding where motion takes place in space. Confusion is expected when complex, multi-dimensional movements such as those so easily produced by man are encountered. However, all too often the student is allowed to simply dismiss these important considerations as being beyond the scope of his interest. The result is a greatly limited understanding of motion and, therefore, a limited ability to describe it accurately. It is for these reasons that Part I of the text is organized primarily along kinematic lines, where space and time referencing are paramount.

Motion description cannot be limited to space and time concerns only. There comes a time when the nature of the moving object and the causes for its motion must be considered. This is the *kinetic* approach, where the prime concerns are with the causative actions of forces, for the word itself actually means "to set moving." The human body is often and correctly called a machine or series of machines. As such, its movements are dependent on kinetic and mechanical principles. Thus the content of Part II of the text deals primarily with kinetic and mechanical referencing in motion description.

The Anatomical Bases for Motion Description

The human body, like that of other animals, derives its vast assortment of movement abilities from its segmentally arranged skeletal structure. Individual segments work in concert with others under the motivation of muscular forces to accomplish an endless variety of tasks. Before these human motions can be understood, the nature of the human body must be mastered, particularly its musculoskeletal anatomy. Part III of the text is concerned with these structural features which set the stage for anatomical referencing in motion description.

It is important to point out that combinations of these approaches to motion description are necessary because almost all of the standard motion classification systems are inadequate in one way or another. In addition, the combination of descriptive nomenclatures and procedures spreads the burden of responsibility when descriptive systems break down, in most cases at different points and under different circumstances. When these difficulties arise, they are noted and alternative means are suggested.

From the use of the entire text, it is hoped that the reader will develop the motion analysis, description, and explanation skills which will render him literate in the investigative and educative uses of kinesiological knowledge. *Heed the call, accept the challenge, become a "people watcher," and read on!*

REFERENCES

Allport, G. W., and Vernon, P. E. *Studies in Expressive Movements.* New York: The Macmillan Company, 1933.

Billig, Harvey E., and Loewendahl, Evelyn. *Mobilization of the Human Body.* Stanford, Calif.: Stanford Press, 1949.

Birdwhistell, Ray L. *Introduction to Kinesics:* An Annotation System of Analysis of Body Motion and Gesture. Washington, D. C.: U.S. Foreign Service, 1952.

Braun, G. L. "Kinesiology: From Aristotle to the Twentieth Century." *Research Quarterly* 12 (1944): 163.

Broer, Marion R. *An Introduction to Kinesiology.* Englewood Cliffs, N.J.: Prentice-Hall, Inc., 1968.

Campbell, W. R. "Kinesiology of Swimming." *Swimming Technique* 4 (1966): 25.

Critchley, M. *The Language of Gesture.* New York: Edward Arnold, Longmans, 1939.

Edgerton, Harold E., and Killian, James R. *Flash.* Boston: Charles T. Branford Company, 1954.

Ellfeldt, L., and Metheny, E. "Movement and Meaning: Development of a General Theory." *Research Quarterly* 29 (1958): 264.

Eshkol, N., and Wachman, A. *Movement Notation:* London, Eng.: Weidenfeld and Nicolson, 1958.

Fay, Temple. "The Origin of Human Movement." *American Journal of Psychiatry* 111 (1955): 644.

Ford, Kenneth W. *Basic Physics.* Waltham, Mass.: Blaisdell Publishing Company, 1968.

Gartmann, Heinz. *Man Unlimited.* New York: Pantheon Books, Inc., 1957.

Hart, Ivor. *The Mechanical Investigations of Leonardo da Vinci.* London: Chapman & Hall, Ltd., 1935.

Hellebrandt, F. H. "Living Anatomy." *Quest* 1 (1963): 43.

Hertel, Heinrich. *Structure, Form, and Movement.* Translated and edited by M. S. Katz. New York: Reinhold Publishing Company, 1966.

Hirt, S. "What is Kinesiology?" *Physical Therapy Review* 35 (1955): 419.

Kenedi, R. M. "Biomechanics in the Modern World." *Bio-Medical Engineering* 2 (1967): 150.

Laban, Rudolf. *Principles of Dance and Movement Notation.* London: Mac-Donald & Evans, Ltd., Publishers, 1956.

Lockhart, Robert D. *Living Anatomy.* 2d ed. London: Faber & Faber Ltd., 1950.

Logan, G. A. "Movement in Art." *Quest* 2 (1964): 42.

Metheny, Eleanor. *Movement and Meaning.* New York: McGraw-Hill Book Company, 1968.

Muybridge, Eadweard. *The Human Figure in Motion.* New York: Dover Publications, Inc., 1955. (First published in 1887.)

Rasch, Philip J., and Burke, Roger K. *Kinesiology and Applied Anatomy.* 3rd ed. Philadelphia: Lea & Febiger, 1967.

Ripley, Julien A. *The Elements and Structure of the Physical Sciences.* New York: John Wiley & Sons, Inc., 1964.

Scott, M. Gladys. *Analysis of Human Motion.* 2d ed. New York: Appleton-Century-Crofts, 1963.

Smith, Hope M., ed. *Introduction to Human Movement.* Reading, Mass.: Addison-Wesley Publishing Company, 1968.

Smith, Karl U., and Smith, William M. *Perception and Motion.* Philadelphia: W. B. Saunders Company, 1962.

Van Den Berg, J. H. "The Human Body and the Significance of Human Movement." *Philosophy and Phenomenological Research* 13 (1952): 159.

Weiner, Norbert. *The Human Use of Human Beings.* Garden City, N.Y.: Doubleday & Company, Inc., 1954.

Wilt, F. "Mechanics Without Tears." *Track Technique* 28 (1967): 878.

Wooldridge, Dean E. *Mechanical Man: The Physical Bases of Intelligent Life.* New York: McGraw-Hill Book Company, 1968.

Wooten, E. P. "The Structural Base of Human Movement." *Journal of Health, Physical Education, Recreation* 36 (October 1965): 59.

2

The Spatial Characteristics of Position and Motion

Systems of motion description require the establishment of reference points about which objects may be located. Many different systems have been developed to accomplish this task in response to special motion characteristics, but all of them feature some sort of observational point of reference. The space surrounding the reference point is numerically subdivided so that positions and changes of position may be precisely identified in quantitative and directional terms. This space is characterized by three dimensions which are easily discernible through man's vision. Although most natural motion situations require three-dimensional analyses to provide accurate description, the present discussion will begin with one-dimensional situations. Discussions of two- and three-dimensional situations follow. In addition, the discussions will be limited to one coordinate system, the *Cartesian coordinate* system.

POSITION AND MOTION IN ONE DIMENSION

The choice of the reference point in space is arbitrary. All that is required of it is that it be prominently located so that its position cannot be mistaken. Probably the simplest way to represent the position of an object relative to the reference point is to draw a straight line which runs through it and extends beyond, as shown in Fig. 2-1. The line is identified by the symbol x and is called the x *coordinate line* or *axis*. The position of the object, P_1, may be noted with reference to the arbitrarily chosen point of reference, O for *origin*. Direction along the line is supplied by positive and negative scale markings, while the object's distance from O is identified by the numbers assigned to the scale. Position P_1 is seen to be located $+4$ units from O. This designation is called the coordinate of the point occupied by the object. For instance, a golf ball may come to rest exactly four feet to the right of the cup as observed from a position off the green. In this case, the cup may represent the coordinate axis origin with the scale units in feet.

Motion which is limited to one dimension along the x axis is illustrated in Fig. 2-2, where more than one position is noted. If P_1 represents the first position identified during an observational period, and if P_2 and P_3 represent subsequent positions in time, motion is apparent. The object's first change of position, $P_2 - P_1$, is seen to be negative in direction and extends from $P_1 = +4$ to $P_2 = -2$. It may be said that the coordinate of the object has received an *increment* Δx (delta x) to represent its change of position. Numerically, the object traversed a distance of six units in the negative direction, $(-2) + (-4) = -6$. At P_2 the object's motion reverses direction and ends at P_3. This final position is located at $+1$, indicating a positive increment, $\Delta x = P_3 - P_2 = 1 - (-2) = +3$. An example of such a motion could be demonstrated by a billiard ball which was set into motion at P_1. It continued uninterrupted until it struck a rail cushion at P_2, where its direction was reversed, and rolled to a stop at P_3. In general, the same motion characteristics could be demonstrated by a gymnast performing on a balance beam as she limits her movements to the beam's narrow, nearly one-dimensional path. Fig. 2-3 illustrates another motion which begins at P_1 and ends at P_3. As can be seen, it is made up of two oppositely directed segments.

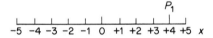

Figure 2-1. The x coordinate line with P_1 representing the position of an object relative to O in one dimension.

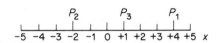

Figure 2-2. Motion in one dimension represented by sequential positions, indicating both positive and negative directions.

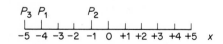

Figure 2-3

→ *Calculate Δx for each segment by employing the procedures just elaborated.*

These changes of position are called *displacements*, which demonstrate both *magnitude* (unit values) and *direction* (sign). Notice that in Figs. 2-2 and 2-3, a displacement's sign is independent of where it took place along the coordinate axis. Its sign represents only the direction of motion, and when the coordinate of P_1 is subtracted from that of P_2, both magnitude and direction are provided. It may now be seen that both position and change of position (displacement) can be illustrated along a coordinate axis.

Vector Description

Although the system for describing position and motion in one dimension is complete from the analytical standpoint as covered above, a second method of describing these elements is now introduced because of its important contributions to motion description. This method utilizes directed line segments as *vector symbols*, which may represent either position or displacement. When a quantity exhibits both magnitude and direction, it usually meets the requirements which allow it to be called a *vector quantity*. Position and displacement, as described above, are vector quantities. The directed line segments (arrows) illustrated in Fig. 2-4 indicate the magnitudes of the quantities by their lengths and the direction of the quantities by their arrowheads. Figure 2-4*a* illustrates a *position vector*, $\mathbf{d}_1$, which connects P_1 to O on the coordinate axis. The vector symbol may be substituted for the coordinate of P_1 because the magnitude and direction (-3) are both evident. Thus the position vector, $\mathbf{d}_1$, is seen to represent accurately the position of an object located at P_1.

Figure 2-4*b* illustrates a *displacement vector* between positions P_1 and P_2 to represent the motion between the two positions on the coordinate axis. It is labeled $\Delta\mathbf{d}$ rather than $\Delta\mathbf{x}$ so that it may be applied to displacements along other coordinate axes in addition to the x axis, which will be introduced later in this chapter. If positions P_1 and P_2 were represented by position vectors, the outcome would appear as shown in Fig. 2-5. The position vectors are removed from the coordinate axis only for the sake of clarity. Their numerical difference equals 4 ($d_2 - d_1 = 6 - 2 = 4$) and is obviously positive in direction, as shown by the arrowhead of the displacement vector, $\Delta\mathbf{d}$. Vector quantities are customarily denoted in boldface type, while their magnitudes and *scalar quantities* are commonly reproduced in ordinary type, as above. A scalar quantity exhibits magnitude but not direction. The final score of a football game such as $24 - 7$ illustrates two scalar quantities of differing magnitudes. Neither of the point totals for the two teams implies direction.

Since displacement was defined earlier as change of position and can be positive or negative in direction, it becomes necessary to point out that the actual *distance traversed* by an object may differ from its displacement. Figure 2-6 illustrates this situation. The motion begins at P_1, which is located at O, and ends at P_3 after changing direction at P_2. Displacement

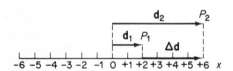

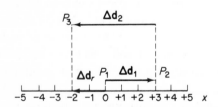

Figure 2-4. Directed line segments (arrows) indicating both magnitude and direction for (*a*) a position vector, and (*b*) a displacement vector.

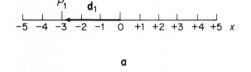

Figure 2-5. Subtracting $\mathbf{d}_1$ from $\mathbf{d}_2$ results in the displacement vector, $\Delta\mathbf{d}$.

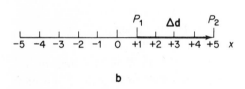

Figure 2-6. The resultant displacement vector, $\Delta\mathbf{d}_r$, is obtained by vector addition. The total distance traversed is obtained by ordinary addition of the magnitudes of the two displacement vectors, $\Delta\mathbf{d}_1$ and $\Delta\mathbf{d}_2$.

vectors $\Delta\mathbf{d}_1$ and $\Delta\mathbf{d}_2$ represent the sequential positive and negative changes of position, respectively. The net displacement is represented by the *resultant displacement vector*, $\Delta\mathbf{d}_r$, which is obtained by adding the two displacement vectors. This addition produces $\Delta d_r = 3+(-5) = -2$, or the net displacement from O, the starting position. However, the actual distance traversed, or path length, is seen to be eight units, three to the right followed by five to the left. For motion with a single dimension, distance units are added arithmetically, disregarding their signs. Displacements with opposite directions require algebraic summation. It will be seen later that differentiations between distances traversed and displacements are necessary to understand more complicated motion characteristics.

POSITION AND MOTION IN TWO DIMENSIONS

A *plane surface* is defined as a surface—real, as are table tops and walls, or hypothetically envisioned in space—such that if any two points on it are joined by a straight line, the line will be contained wholly in the surface. This surface is then described as having two dimensions, and the position of any point located on the surface may be identified by procedures similar to those just described. Figure 2-7 illustrates such a plane surface which has been subdivided into four quadrants (I, II, III, IV) bordered by perpendicular coordinate axes which intersect at O. These coordinate axes are two of the *Cartesian rectangular coordinate* axes, a third axis being necessary to describe position and motion in three dimensions. The horizontal (x) axis is the same as was used to describe positions and motions in one dimension. The vertical (y) axis provides the second dimension so that the illustration can represent a plane surface. Positive directions are seen to be to the right and above O, while the negative directions are to the left and below O. The order of coordinate presentation is alphabetical, so the x coordinate value always precedes the y coordinate value. The coordinates for P_1 are (2, 3); for P_2, $(-2, 4)$; and for P_3, $(-3, -3)$; each representing an independent position rather than positions within a motion.

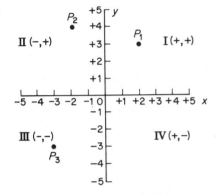

Figure 2–7. A plane, whose surface has been subdivided into four quadrants by the intersection of x and y axes, may be used to identify positions in two dimensions.

Motions in the plane can be represented by a series of positions occupied by an object, one following the other. Figure 2-8 illustrates the positions, P_1 through P_6, occupied by an object moving from the lower left quadrant through the lower right quadrant and into the upper right quadrant.

→ *Determine the coordinate identities, in sequence from* P_1 *through* P_6, *for each position represented in the figure.*

Note that the motion was limited to the plane of the page upon which it was printed. The motion may be said to have occurred in the *XY plane* because the plane receives its identity on the basis of the coordinate axes which classify its surface. The *XY* plane is commonly conceived as a vertical plane in descriptive geometry, but it may be visualized as being in any position in space. Throughout the discussions which follow, it is conceived as being vertical because of the clarity of description afforded, particularly when applied to the erect human body.

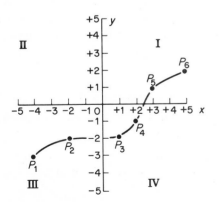

Figure 2–8. Two-dimensional motion, represented by sequentially-identified positions.

→ *Assume that you are looking through an underwater viewing window which has been marked off by* x *and* y *coordinate axes. The motion path indicated in Fig. 2-8 might well be similar to the ascent of a diver through the water after completing a practice dive.*

Vector Description

As was the case for positions and motion in one dimension, the use of vectors to describe these elements in two dimensions is valuable. Figure 2-9 illustrates vector identifications of position on the XY plane. Positions P_1, P_2, and P_3 are again represented by unrelated position vectors, $\mathbf{d}_1$, $\mathbf{d}_2$, and $\mathbf{d}_3$, respectively. Note that they connect those points on the plane to O. Their directions are indicated at least partially by their locations in the four available quadrants and by their x and y coordinate values.

Figure 2-10 illustrates the use of a displacement vector to identify motion in the plane. The change of position of an object in the XY plane from P_1 to P_2 is represented by $\mathbf{\Delta d}$, the displacement vector, and again represents the difference between the two position vectors ($\mathbf{d}_2 - \mathbf{d}_1 = \mathbf{\Delta d}$). Notice the similarities between vector applications to one- and two-dimensional situations. However, after recognizing these similarities, it becomes necessary to lay the foundations for combining vectors in two-dimensional situations before proceeding further with the elements illustrated in Fig. 2-10.

Vector Addition

When two vectors in a two-dimensional framework are added, they are geometrically connected together. This is accomplished by moving the vector to be added parallel to itself until its tail end coincides with the arrowhead end of the vector to which it is to be added. A third vector is constructed between the free ends of the two-vector pair to represent their sum. Figure 2-11 illustrates this process. Note that it is not necessary to illustrate vectors in conjunction with a coordinate system. Magnitudes and directions are still apparent. When more than two vectors are added, the same procedures are followed in any order that is convenient until all are connected in sequence, as shown in Fig. 2-12.

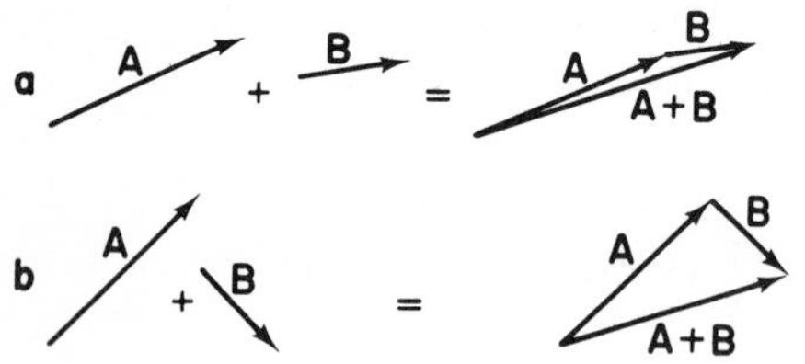

Figure 2-13 illustrates the *commutative* (reversible) nature of vector addition in that $\mathbf{A} + \mathbf{B} = \mathbf{B} + \mathbf{A}$. Figure 2-14 illustrates the *associative* nature of vector addition in that $\mathbf{A} + \mathbf{B} + \mathbf{C} = \mathbf{A} + (\mathbf{B} + \mathbf{C}) = (\mathbf{A} + \mathbf{B}) + \mathbf{C}$.

Vector Subtraction

Vector subtraction is accomplished in a similar manner with one exception. The vector to be subtracted is reversed in direction to change its sign and

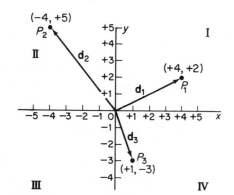

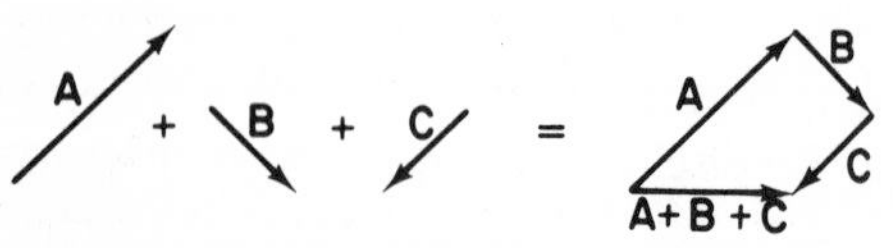

Figure 2–9. Vector identifications of positions in two dimensions in the XY plane.

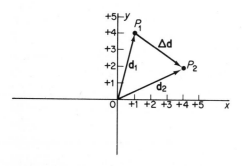

Figure 2–10. Displacement in the XY plane from P_1 to P_2.

Figure 2–11

Figure 2–12

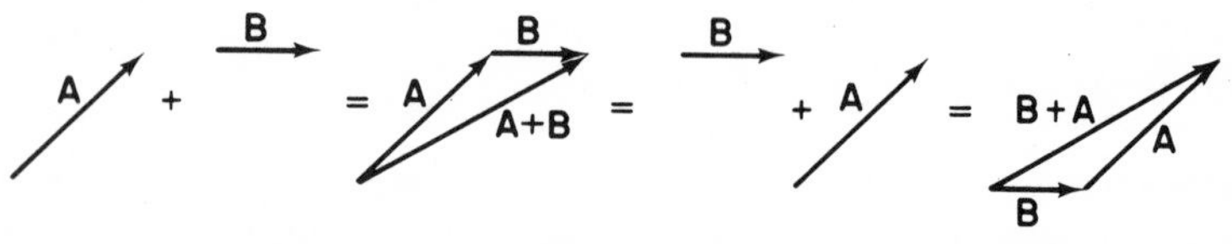

Figure 2–13

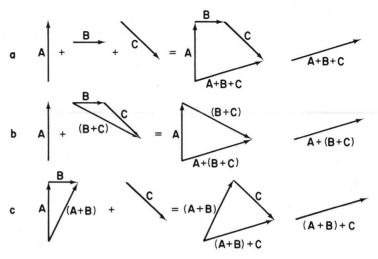

Figure 2-14

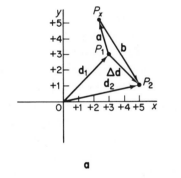

Figure 2-15

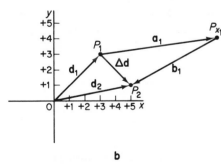

a

b

Figure 2-16. The displacements illustrated, $\Delta\mathbf{d}$ in (*a*) and (*b*), are equal vectors, although the motion path traversed in (*a*) P_1 through P_x to P_2 is much shorter than that in (*b*) P_1 through P_{x_1} to P_2.

then added as above. Figure 2-15 offers an example of vector subtraction.

It is now possible to return to Fig. 2-10, which illustrates an example of vector subtraction where position vectors $\mathbf{d}_2 - \mathbf{d}_1 = \Delta\mathbf{d}$. The displacement vector, $\Delta\mathbf{d}$, exactly represents the motion between P_1 and P_2 in the plane. It makes little difference what the shape of the path between P_1 and P_2 actually was; it simply occurred between the two positions in a given period of time. The actual path could be of any shape and still be represented by the displacement vector, $\Delta\mathbf{d}$. The displacement vector's independence from the actual motion path is illustrated in Fig. 2-16. The motion from P_1 to P_2 in the plane is shown to course through intermediate positions P_x and P_{x_1}, respectively. It can be seen that vector additions of $\mathbf{a} + \mathbf{b}$ and $\mathbf{a}_1 + \mathbf{b}_1$ both produce the same result: the displacement vector, $\Delta\mathbf{d}$. When two vectors have common magnitudes and direction, regardless of their positions in space, they are said to be *equal vectors*. Therefore, the much longer path P_1 to P_{x_1} to P_2 in Fig. 2-16*b* results in exactly the same displacement in the plane as the shorter path P_1 to P_x to P_2 in Fig. 2-16*a*. In addition, it is most important to remember that the motion is understood to proceed from P_1 to P_2 ($\mathbf{d}_1$ to $\mathbf{d}_2$) and that the equation must not be written $\Delta\mathbf{d} = \mathbf{d}_1 - \mathbf{d}_2$.

→ *To illustrate, undertake the vector subtraction $\Delta\mathbf{d} = \mathbf{d}_1 - \mathbf{d}_2$ using the position vectors $\mathbf{d}_1$ and $\mathbf{d}_2$ in Fig. 2-16. What are the outcomes in terms of magnitude and direction?*

Component Vectors

By referring again to Fig. 2-9, it will be remembered that position P_1 may be represented by its x and y coordinates ($+4$, $+2$) or by the position vector, $\mathbf{d}_1$. If the x coordinate of P_1 were also represented by a vector along the x axis from O to $+4$ and the same were true for the y coordinate along the y axis from O to $+2$, these vectors would be called the *rectangular*

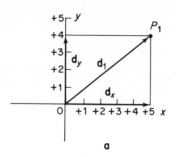

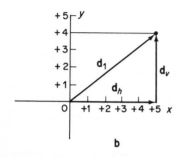

Figure 2–17. Horizontal (*x*) and vertical (*y*) component vectors of position vector, $\mathbf{d}_1$, may be constructed and their vector sum is seen to equal $\mathbf{d}_1$.

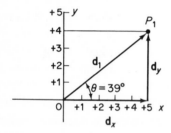

Figure 2–18. Using the scalar components of the position vector, $\mathbf{d}_1$, tangent θ may be calculated to determine the angular value of θ.

component vectors of the position vector, $\mathbf{d}_1$. Figure 2-17 illustrates the same situation with the component vectors included. Since the XY plane is commonly considered to be a vertical plane, the x component vector is often referred to as the *horizontal component*, while the y component vector is often called the *vertical component*. Because the vector sum of these component values may be substituted for the position vector, $\mathbf{d}_1$, it follows that $\mathbf{d}_h + \mathbf{d}_v = \mathbf{d}_1$. Note that in Fig. 2-17$b$, the vertical component has been moved parallel to itself until its tail coincides with the arrowhead of the horizontal component. The calculation of the magnitude of the position vector, $\mathbf{d}_1$, is accomplished through the application of the theorem of Pythagorus. In this case it reads

$$d_1^2 = d_h^2 + d_v^2 \quad \text{or} \quad d_1 = \sqrt{d_h^2 + d_v^2} =$$
$$d_1 = \sqrt{5^2 + 4^2} = d_1 = \sqrt{25 + 16} =$$
$$d_1 = \sqrt{41} = d_1 = 6.40$$

Note that these values are the magnitudes of the component vectors and are, therefore, called the *scalar components* of the vector, $\mathbf{d}_1$. The process just described is known as the *composition of vectors*, and it is often used to establish the magnitudes of position vectors which have been plotted from sequential photographic images of an object's motion with respect to a point of reference located within the photographic field.

The descriptive picture is clarified further if the exact direction of the position vector is known with respect to its x and y components. Graphically, the description would be completed by measuring the angular deviation of the position vector from either the x or y component with a protractor. To calculate this angular deviation, trigonometric functions must be employed. By referring to the trigonometric functions table and the discussion of their derivations in Appendix B, the value of the angular deviation of the position vector, $\mathbf{d}_1$, from its x axis component may be calculated since all of the sides of the triangle illustrated in Fig. 2-18 are known. The *tangent* of the angle under consideration, θ, equals the ratio of the y component, d_y (the side of the right triangle opposite the angle θ), to the x component, d_x (the side adjacent to the angle θ). Note that these are the magnitudes of the component vectors and the calculation is

$$\tan \theta = \frac{d_y}{d_x} = \frac{4}{5} = .8000$$

Therefore,

$\theta = 39°$ approximately

→ *What is the angular deviation of $\mathbf{d}_1$ from its y axis component?*

As yet, vector components have been identified only for position vectors. It follows that the same procedures may be applied to displacement vectors to yield *displacement components*. Figure 2-19 illustrates three

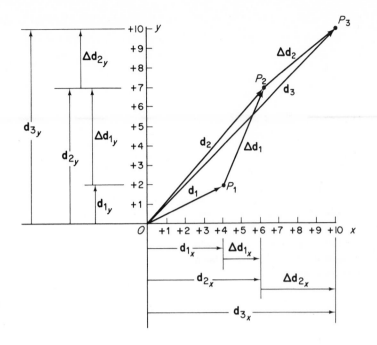

Figure 2–19. Displacement component vectors for $\Delta\mathbf{d}_1$ and $\Delta\mathbf{d}_2$ indicate changes of position relative to the x and y axes.

sequential positions in the XY plane. Position vectors, $\mathbf{d}_1$, $\mathbf{d}_2$, and $\mathbf{d}_3$ are seen to be accompanied by their x and y components along their respective axes. The displacement components, $\Delta\mathbf{d}_{1_x}$ and $\Delta\mathbf{d}_{1_y}$, may be obtained from $\mathbf{d}_{2_x}-\mathbf{d}_{1_x}$ and $\mathbf{d}_{2_y}-\mathbf{d}_{1_y}$, respectively. In a like manner $\Delta\mathbf{d}_{2_x}=\mathbf{d}_{3_x}-\mathbf{d}_{2_x}$, and $\Delta\mathbf{d}_{2_y}=\mathbf{d}_{3_y}-\mathbf{d}_{2_y}$. Thus the descriptions of the changes of position are provided by the changes of the components of the position vectors.

$\rightarrow$ *Using the scalar components of the vectors, d_1, d_2, d_3, Δd_1, and Δd_2, calculate the magnitude of each of these vectors, as listed below.*

$$d_1 = \sqrt{d_{1_x}^2+d_{1_y}^2} \qquad d_2 = \sqrt{d_{2_x}^2+d_{2_y}^2}$$

$$d_3 = \sqrt{d_{3_x}^2+d_{3_y}^2}$$

$$\Delta d_1 = \sqrt{\Delta d_{1_x}^2+\Delta d_{1_y}^2} \qquad \Delta d_2 = \sqrt{\Delta d_{2_x}^2+\Delta d_{2_y}^2}$$

Figure 2-20 illustrates elements which are similar to those in Fig. 2-19 when applied to plotting a long jumper's center of gravity for three separate positions within the jump. For each position and change of position represented, there is a horizontal and vertical component vector along the x and y axes, respectively.

Circular Motion

If an object is observed to follow a circular path about O, motion in the plane is described on the basis of the changing values of the x and y components of the position vectors, as before. The value of θ again may be

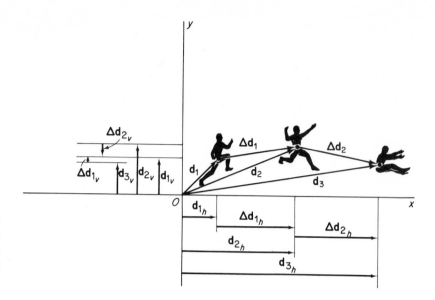

Figure 2–20. Horizontal and vertical displacement information for a movement such as the long jump may be compiled when positions throughout the jump have been recorded photographically.

found from the equation $\theta = \tan y/x$. Since the motion is circular, the magnitudes of all position vectors are equal to the radius of rotation ($\mathbf{d_1} = \mathbf{d_2}$). In Fig. 2-21, it is assumed that the counterclockwise (positive) rotation began with the object located at P_1. The motion represented between P_1 and P_2 along the circular path may be described by the displacement vector, $\mathbf{\Delta d}$, or by the difference between the angular deviations of the position vectors from the positive x axis. This is illustrated as $\Delta\theta = \theta_2 - \theta_1$ and is termed the *angular displacement* of the object as it rotates around O from P_1 to P_2.

If the choice is made to measure the magnitudes of the position vectors and the angles θ_1 and θ_2 rather than deriving them from a knowledge of the scalar components, the x component values are obtained from the equation $x = d \cos \theta$. Likewise, the y component values are obtained from the equation $y = \mathrm{d} \sin \theta$. This process of resolving the x and y components of the position vectors is known as the *resolution of vectors*. Numerous examples of the use of this process with vectors other than position and displacement vectors are to be found in later chapters.

In Fig. 2-22, a common movement of the upper extremity is illustrated in the XY plane, with O located at the center of the shoulder joint. Two points along the length of the extended limb are identified at the elbow and wrist joints. Position vectors, displacement vectors, angular deviations, and the angular displacement are identified for the two positions of the limb.

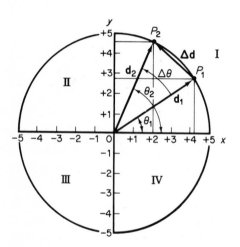

Figure 2–21. Circular motion about a center of rotation, *O*, may be represented by the angular change, $\Delta\theta$, or by the displacement vector, $\Delta\mathbf{d}$.

→ *Complete the following operations:*

  1. Identify the coordinates for the elbow and wrist joints at limb positions P_1 *and* P_2.

  2. Compute the magnitudes of the position and displacement vectors for the elbow and wrist joints, respectively, from their x and y scalar components.

  3. Compute the angular deviations, θ_1 *and* θ_2 *from the x axis and the angular displacement,* $\Delta\theta$.

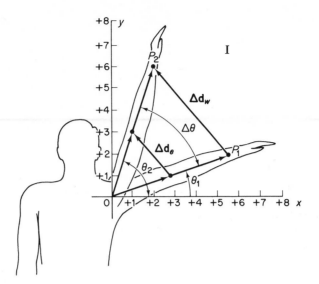

Figure 2–22. The generally circular paths traced through space by the elbow and wrist joints may be described in detail when referred to x and y coordinate information. Note the greater magnitude of wrist travel.

4. With the use of a ruler and protractor, measure the numerical values of all the vectors and angles illustrated to verify the accuracy of your computations.

5. Utilizing the measured values in operation 4, resolve the x and y scalar components from the position vectors.

Motion Path Description

By referring to Fig. 2-23, it will be recognized that the number of positions plotted throughout an observed motion is important in establishing an understanding of the shape of the motion path. In Fig. 2-23a, displacement vectors, $\Delta \mathbf{d}_1$ and $\Delta \mathbf{d}_2$, illustrate changes of position for the plotting of only three positions within an observed motion. Figure 2-23b illustrates the same observed motion with ten plotted positions rather than three. Note that the three positions, P_1, P_2, and P_3, are again identified for the sake of comparison. It is easily seen that Fig. 2-23b gives a much more detailed picture of the motion path. As the time intervals between position vectors are reduced to very small values, the movement path, as represented by the displacement vectors, will closely approximate the true path. When the time intervals between plotted positions become very small, the number of plotted positions within the observed motion becomes very large. One of the useful results of the increase in the number of plotted positions is that the displacement vectors become more and more alike in both magnitude and direction.

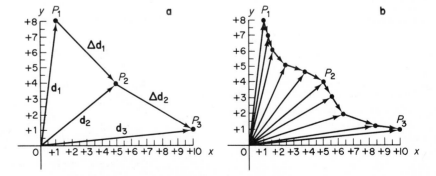

Figure 2–23. The greater the number of individual positions which can be identified within a movement, the more accurately the actual path may be described.

17　The Spatial Characteristics of Position and Motion

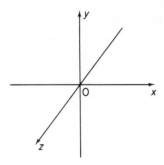

Figure 2–24. Three mutually-perpendicular axes, intersecting at *O*, may be scaled to identify position and motion in three dimensions.

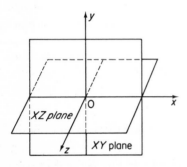

Figure 2–25. *XZ* and *XY* planes are generated by the intersection of the three coordinate axes to subdivide space into four quadrants.

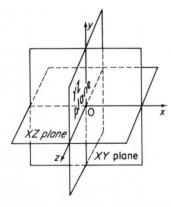

Figure 2–26. *XZ*, *XY*, and *YZ* planes are generated by the intersection of the three coordinate axes to subdivide space into eight octants.

POSITION AND MOTION IN THREE DIMENSIONS

Up to this point in the discussion, positions and motions have been limited to situations which were devoid of the depth dimension. With the addition of the *z coordinate axis*, perpendicular to both the *x* and *y* axes, as shown in Fig. 2-24, any position in space and any motion in space may be described. The arrowheads are included to indicate the positive directions for the three coordinate axes.

An interesting outcome of the addition of the *z* axis through the already described *XY* plane is the provision for the identification of two additional coordinate planes: the *XZ* plane and the *YZ* plane. Figure 2-25 shows an oblique view of the *XY* plane with the *XZ* plane added. Note that the *XZ* plane is a horizontal plane and that it is perpendicular to the vertical, *XY* plane. It can be visualized that if an object of the shape shown in Fig. 2-25 were placed into a box whose dimensions exactly received the object, the space within the box would be divided up equally into four parts: two below the *XZ* plane and two above it. These four spaces are named *space quadrants*.

Figure 2-26 illustrates another oblique view in which the third coordinate plane is added, which is the vertical, *YZ* plane. It will be seen that the three coordinate planes are mutually perpendicular, as are the three coordinate axes, and that they all intersect at *O*.

It is interesting to note that in all of the preceding figures where the *XY* plane was illustrated, our line of vision was along the *z* coordinate axis. Consequently, it follows that if our line of vision were the *x* axis, only the *YZ* plane would be apparent and viewing along the *y* axis would make the *XZ* plane apparent. As before, if the object in Fig. 2-26 were to be placed into a box whose dimensions exactly received it, the space in the box would be divided up equally into eight parts called *space octants*: four above the *XZ* plane and four below it. Also notice that each axis is perpendicular to only one of the three planes, namely, the one which does not include its symbol; that is, the *x* axis is perpendicular to the *YZ* plane, the *y* axis is perpendicular to the *XZ* plane, and the *z* axis is perpendicular to the *XY* plane.

Differing from the case for a point on a plane, the location of a point in three-dimensional space requires the assignment of three coordinate values measured from the three coordinate planes at *O* along the coordinate axes perpendicular to them. Figure 2-27 shows a point, P_1, with respect to the complete coordinate system. The point's position in space is specified, in *x*, *y*, *z* order, by (6, 3, 3) as well as by the position vector, $\mathbf{d}_1$. The magnitude of the position vector is specified by the sum of its scalar components as follows:

$$d_1 = \sqrt{d_x^2 + d_y^2 + d_z^2}$$

This equation simply represents the application of the Pythagorean theorem twice: once for d_x and d_y, followed by their resultant and d_z.

→ *Calculate the magnitude of $\mathbf{d}_1$.*

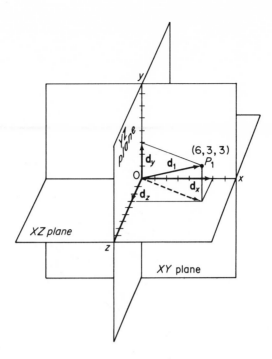

Figure 2–27. Position, P_1, in three-dimensional space resides in the space octant whose bounding edges are the positively-directed coordinate axes. Note that $\mathbf{d}_1$ is projected on the XZ plane, and although not illustrated here, it could be projected on the remaining planes as well.

Figure 2-28 illustrates an application of the above from a different viewing position. The origin of the coordinate system is located at the center of the swimmer's shoulder joint, with the center of the elevated hand being the point of interest. The coordinate values are retained from Fig. 2-27, but the limb under consideration is seen to be located in the space octant which is negative with respect to the z axis. While the coordinate specification of P_1 (6, 3, -3) is useful in identifying the space octant in which the hand is located, when the magnitude of the position vector, $\mathbf{d}_1$, is calculated, it cannot specify direction because the z component (-3) loses its negative sign when squared. Consequently, when position P_1 is represented by the magnitude of its position vector alone, the vector's angular deviations from two of the coordinate axes must be included to specify its direction exactly. The angle from the y axis to $\mathbf{d}_1$ is given the symbol θ and varies with the distance of P_1 above or below the XZ plane. The angle ϕ is measured on the XZ plane from the x axis to the projection of $\mathbf{d}_1$ on that plane. The x, z, and y component vectors are shown end to end, in series from O to P_1.

Human motion may be photographed by three motion picture cameras simultaneously for the purpose of three-dimensional analysis. The optical axes of the cameras are situated so they can represent the three coordinate axes which intersect at the center of the motion under observation. Because of the use of three mutually perpendicular optical axes, situated as in Fig. 2-29, the photographic analytical procedure is said to be *triaxial.* The images captured on film by the three cameras are independent and must be analyzed individually in their two-dimensional formats when suitably projected. The three sets of data, derived from the three independent views of the motion, may then be combined to build the three-dimensional representation.

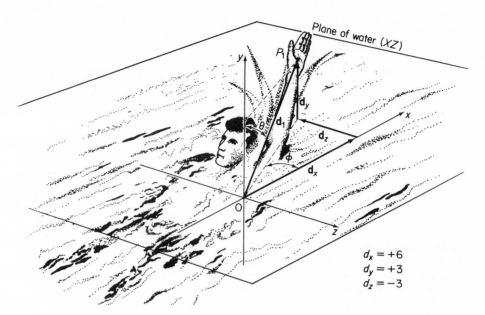

$$d_x = +6$$
$$d_y = +3$$
$$d_z = -3$$

Figure 2–28. Angles θ and ϕ in the coordinate system establish the directional characteristics of position, P_1, at the instant shown.

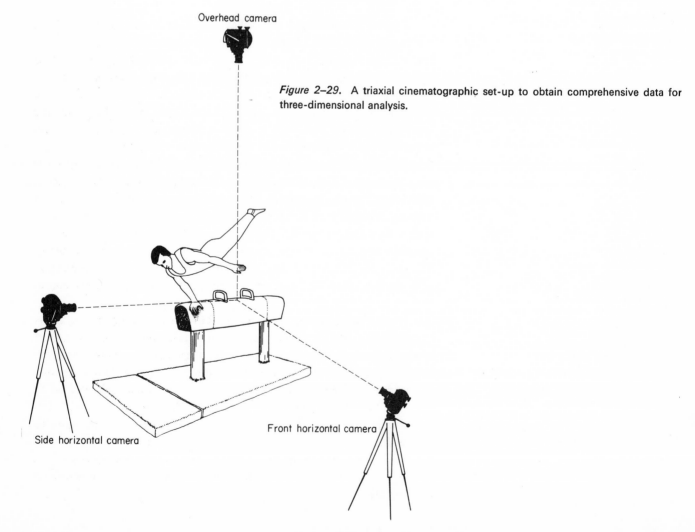

Figure 2–29. A triaxial cinematographic set-up to obtain comprehensive data for three-dimensional analysis.

Overhead camera

Side horizontal camera

Front horizontal camera

ORIENTATION OF THE HUMAN BODY IN SPACE

The discussion to this point has focused attention on objects conceived as single points. This is most convenient in that it allows for the necessary simplifications in description. When an object, as a whole, is brought into the picture, the process of establishing its orientation in space requires additional considerations. Chief among these considerations is that of identifying the space wherein the object is located with respect to the object's *outstanding physical characteristics*.

For most objects, the space occupied by and around them is usually divided into space octants by the three coordinate planes. The point of reference, *O*, is commonly placed at the object's center, with the coordinate planes receiving names which have descriptive value with respect to the object under study. In the case of the human body, these planes have been given various names which are both *spatially* and *anatomically referenced*. For example, by referring to Fig. 2-30, the *XZ* plane is often called the *horizontal* or *transverse plane*, obviously a spatially referenced term. When the space under study is visualized as a sphere, this plane is often referred to as the *equatorial plane*. The *XY* plane, since it often illustrates the front surface of an object, is called the *frontal plane*. When anatomically referenced, the term *coronal plane* is used to denote that it is parallel to the *coronal suture* of the skull. The other vertical plane, the *YZ* plane, is commonly given the name *profile plane* because it depicts the side view of an object. When applied to the human body, this plane is referred to as the *sagittal plane* because it is parallel to the *sagittal suture* of the skull.

Figure 2-30 depicts an erect, human figure in conjunction with the orientation planes and axes intersecting at his center of gravity. In the case of man, whose anatomical contours and parts can be readily identified as to directions, planes which are positioned to divide the body into halves

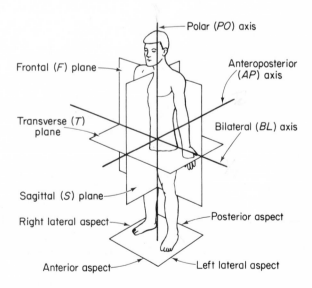

Figure 2–30. A standing figure, with its space and that surrounding it, classified by the use of orientation planes and axes.

are called *cardinal planes*. Those depicted in Fig. 2-30 are cardinal planes which result in a division of the body into front and rear halves, right and left halves, and upper and lower halves. These halves need not be symmetrical, however, as is clear in comparing upper and lower halves.

The coordinate axes, which can be seen to be generated by the intersection of combinations of planes, are given names which also assist in understanding the orientation of a body in space, especially from the standpoint of direction. They are often given names which are the same as those given to the planes just described. This practice can lead to confusion and should be avoided when applied for the purpose of orientation description. As included in this text, the axes are named so that these terms may have the widest possible application in the description of human motion. The *x* axis, since it courses from side to side, will be named the *bilateral axis*. The *y* axis, shown to be vertical in the figure, will be named the *polar axis*, indicating its lengthwise-running orientation between opposite ends of the body. The *z* axis will be called the *anteroposterior axis*, thus depicting its front-to-rear orientation in the body.

Abbreviated Notation

Because several of these terms are long and unwieldy, it may be convenient to abbreviate all of them to provide for a concise notation form to be applied later. The anteroposterior axis becomes the *AP axis*. Similarly, the abbreviations *BL* and *PO* stand for bilateral and polar, respectively. When the body is envisioned as being erect, we have two horizontal axes, the *BL* and *AP*, and one vertical axis, the *PO*. Consequently, there are two vertical planes, the *S* for sagittal and *F* for frontal, and one horizontal plane, the *T* for transverse. The terms just discussed will be used throughout the remainder of the text when referring to planes and axes for both orientation and motion description.

Orientation in Whole-Body Rotation

It was noted earlier that most quantities having both magnitude and direction are vectors. Obviously, there are quantities which exhibit both magnitude and direction which are not vectors. One example, which is most important to the discussion of orientation in space, is that of angles of rotation of objects around fixed axes. The rotation demonstrates a magnitude in the number of degrees the object rotated and discernible direction as to its being clockwise or counterclockwise. The difficulty arises with the combination of these rotations, which are seen not to follow the commutative principle of vector addition described earlier. Figure 2-31 illustrates this situation using the human body as a rigid body which rotates as a whole rather than as separate segments.

In Fig. 2-31*a*, the body is seen to have rotated around a fixed *y* axis to its left through 90 degrees from the starting position, A_1. The result of

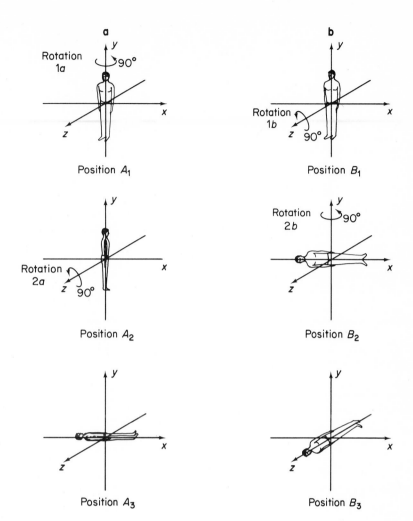

Figure 2–31. The sum of rotations 1a and 2a does not result in the same final position as the sum of rotations 1b and 2b although the rotations were started from the same initial position ($A_1 = B_1$).

this rotation (rotation 1a) is position A_2. Note how convenient the non-symmetrical, front and rear aspects of the body are for recognizing this reorientation. From position A_2, the body undergoes another rotation, rotation 2a—in this instance, about the fixed z axis. The rotation is seen to be counterclockwise in direction to result in position A_3, a position known as the *supine position*, with the head in the negative x direction. The examples shown in Fig. 2-31b simply reverse the order of the rotations given in Fig. 2-31a. The body is first rotated counterclockwise through 90 degrees around the fixed z axis (rotation 1b), producing position B_2 from position B_1. It then undergoes rotation 2b about the fixed y axis to produce the final position, position B_3. Carefully note that final positions A_3 and B_3 have quite different orientations in space and thus illustrate that rotations, except for those which are infinitesimally small, are not vector quantities.

→ *Using any objects whose different surfaces are easily differentiated, try other combinations of orientation rotations for practice and better understanding.*

REFERENCES

Abbott, Edwin A. *Flatland: A Romance of Many Dimensions*. New York: Dover Publications, Inc., 1952.

Agan, T.; Anderson, E.; Reis, I. L.; and Carson, A. M. "A Method of Measuring Postural Attitudes." *Ergonomics* 8 (1965): 207.

Barnett, Raymond. *Elementary Algebra: Structure and Use*. New York: McGraw-Hill Book Company, 1968.

"Biomechanics: Technique of Drawings of Movement and Movement Analysis." In *Medicine and Sport*, vol. 2. Proceedings of the First International Seminar on Biomechanics, Zurich, August 1967. Basel, Switzerland: S. Karger AG, 1968.

Carlsoo, S. "Kinematic Analysis of the Golf Swing." In *Medicine and Sport*, vol. 2. Proceedings of the First International Seminar on Biomechanics, Zurich, August 1967. Basel, Switzerland: S. Karger AG, 1968.

————"Commentary on Descartes and Analytic Geometry." In *The World of Mathematics*, edited by J. R. Newman, vol. 1. New York: Simon and Schuster, Inc., 1956.

Cureton, T. K. "Elementary Principles and Techniques of Cinematographic Analysis as Aids in Athletic Research." *Research Quarterly* 10 (1939): 3.

———— and Wickens, J. L. "The Center of Gravity of the Human Body in the Anterior-Posterior Plane and its Relation to Posture, Physical Fitness and Athletic Ability." *Research Quarterly* 6 (1935): 93.

Davis, R.; Wehrkamp, R.; and Smith, K. U. "Dimensional Analysis of Motion: I. Effects of Laterality and Movement Direction." *Journal of Applied Psychology* 35 (1951): 363.

Dempster, W. T. "Analysis of Two-Handed Pulls Using Free Body Diagrams." *Journal of Applied Physiology* 13 (1958): 469.

———— "Free-Body Diagrams as an Approach to the Mechanics of Human Posture and Motion." In *Biomechanical Studies of the Musculo-Skeletal System*, edited by F. G. Evans. Springfield, Ill.: Charles C. Thomas, Publisher, 1961.

deVries, H. A. "A Cinematographical Analysis of the Dolphin Swimming Stroke." *Research Quarterly* 30 (1959): 413.

Drillis, R. J. "The Use of Gliding Cyclograms in the Biomechanical Analysis of Movement." *Human Factors* 1 (1959): 2.

Eberhart, H. D., and Inman, V. T. "An Evaluation of Experimental Study of Human Locomotion." *Annals of the New York Academy of Sciences* 51 (1951): 1123.

———— and Bresler, B. "The Principal Elements in Human Locomotion." In *Human Limbs and Their Substitutes*, edited by P. E. Klopsteg and P. D. Wilson. New York: McGraw-Hill Book Company, 1954.

Elftman, H. "The Basic Pattern of Human Locomotion." *Annals of the New York Academy of Sciences* 51 (1951): 1207.

Field, Ephraim J., and Harrison, Robert J. *Anatomical Terms: Their Origin and Derivation*. 2d ed. Cambridge: W. Heffer, 1947.

Fuller, Gordon. *Analytic Geometry*. 2d ed. Reading, Mass.: Addison-Wesley Publishing Company, Inc., 1962.

Garrett, R. E.; Widule, C. J.; and Garrett, G. E. "Computer-Aided Analysis of Human Motion." *Kinesiology Review–1968*. Washington, D.C.: N.E.A., 1968.

Hellebrandt, F. A.; Tepper, R. H.; Brown, G. L.; and Elliot, M. C. "The Location of the Cardinal Anatomical Orientation Planes Passing Through the Center of Gravity in Young Adult Women." *American Journal of Physiology* 121 (1938): 465.

Howard, Ian P., and Templeton, W. B. *Human Spatial Orientation*. New York: John Wiley & Sons, Inc., 1966.

Hummel, James A. *Vector Geometry.* Reading, Mass.: Addison-Wesley Publishing Company, Inc., 1965.

Lehrman, Robert L., and Swartz, Clifford. *Foundations of Physics.* New York: Holt, Rinehart and Winston, Inc., 1965.

Murray, M. P.; Drought, A. B.; and Kory, R. C. "Walking Patterns of Normal Men." *Journal of Bone and Joint Surgery* 46-A (1964): 335.

Noss, J. "Control of Photographic Perspective in Motion Analysis." *Journal of Health, Physical Education, Recreation* 38 (September 1967): 81.

Plagenhoef, S. "Gathering Kinesiological Data Using Modern Measuring Devices." *Journal of Health, Physical Education, Recreation* 39 (1968): 81.

Race, D. E. "Cinematographic and Mechanical Analysis of External Movements Involved in Hitting a Baseball Effectively." *Research Quarterly* 32 (1961): 394.

Rock, I.; Tauber, E. S.; and Heller, D. P. "Perception of Stroboscopic Movement." *Science* 147 (1965): 1050.

Roebuck, J. A. "Kinesiology in Engineering." *Kinesiology Review—1968.* Washington, D. C.: N.E.A., 1968.

Shute, C. C. D. "The Geometry and Kinematics of the Knee Joint." *Journal of Anatomy* 90 (1956): 586.

Spitzbart, Abraham, and Bardell, Ross H. *Plane Trigonometry.* 2d ed. Reading, Mass.: Addison-Wesley Publishing Company, Inc., 1964.

Swain, Robert L. *Understanding Arithmetic*, revised by E. D. Nichols. New York: Holt, Rinehart and Winston, Inc., 1965.

Taylor, C. L., and Blaschke, A. C. "A Method for Kinematic Analysis of Motions of the Shoulder, Arm, and Hand Complex." *Annals of the New York Academy of Science* 51 (1951): 1251.

Tyson, Howell N. *Kinematics.* New York: John Wiley and Sons, Inc., 1966.

Verwiebe, F. L. "Does a Ball Curve?" *American Journal of Physics* 10 (1942): 119.

Zitzlsperger, S. "The Mechanics of the Foot Based on the Concept of the Skeleton as a Statically Indetermined Space Framework." *Clinical Orthopedics* 16 (1961): 47.

3

The Time–Rate Characteristics of Motion in Space

As one can surmise from this chapter's title, the focus of attention will be on those characteristics of motion which depend on the incorporation of time to describe the motion accurately. It will be remembered from Chapter 2 that *change of position over time* was now and then included in the discussion for the purpose of fixing the concept of time in motion *frames of reference*. Since motion and time changes are inseparable, the next weapon in the descriptive arsenal is a thorough understanding of their interactions.

AVERAGE VELOCITY

It is most convenient, when discussing two variables and their interactions, to represent the interactions graphically. This is accomplished by constructing a graph where one variable is plotted against the other. Figure 3-1 illustrates one of the simplest examples, where position is plotted against time. Position is plotted along the vertical axis or *ordinate* of the graph, while time is usually plotted along the horizontal axis or *abscissa*. The *zero* intersection point represents the point when the observation of time and position began. The interaction of the two variables is usually represented by a line drawn on the graph which connects the data points gathered from the observation of the two phenomena. As can be seen from Fig. 3-1a, change of position referred to time is plotted on the basis of $\frac{1}{2}$-second time observations. Figure 3-1b plots these observations on the x axis. Refer to both in the following discussion.

The observation began with the object located at $P_1 = +3$ on the coordinate line. Subsequent changes of position depict motion in a negative direction through P_7, at which point in time (3 sec) motion ceases and is not evident again within the observation period (4 sec). Note that at no point during the observed motion was the motion positive in direction. If it were, it would be represented by a line traced from lower left to upper right on the *position-time* graph. When the information abstracted from the graph represents matters such as *change of direction* or *no motion*, it is referred to as *qualitative information*. When it is numerical as the result of measurement and calculation, it is generally *quantitative information*. As pointed out in Chapter 1, both kinds of information are essential to accurate motion description.

When a change of position is referred to the change in time over which it occurred, *velocity* is the quantity which characterizes their interaction. Velocity is a vector quantity because it exhibits both magnitude and direction. A change of position or displacement $(P_2 - P_1)$ per time unit $(t_2 - t_1)$ describes the calculation of velocity to provide

$$\frac{P_2 - P_1}{t_2 - t_1} = \frac{\Delta d}{\Delta t} = \text{average velocity } (\bar{v})$$

Figure 3-2 illustrates a displacement vector description for the determination of average velocity in one dimension. Let us assume that the first change of position, $P_2 - P_1 = \Delta \mathbf{d}_1$, was accomplished in 2 sec and that the

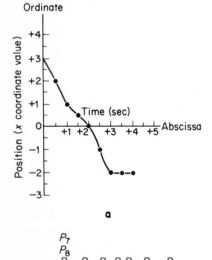

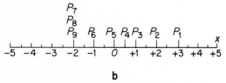

Figure 3–1. Position plotted against time. At no time was the motion positive in direction.

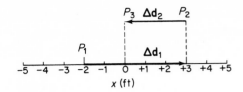

Figure 3–2

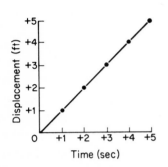

Figure 3–3. For equal displacements, equal time intervals elapse.

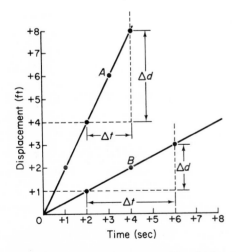

Figure 3–4. The constant velocities depicted by slopes A and B show, by comparison, a four-fold decrease in B relative to A.

second change of position, $P_3 - P_2 = \Delta\mathbf{d}_2$, required 6 sec. Velocity calculations produce

$$\bar{v}_1 = \frac{\Delta d_1}{\Delta t_1} = \frac{+5 \text{ ft}}{2 \text{ sec}} = +2.5 \text{ ft/sec}$$

$$\bar{v}_2 = \frac{\Delta d_2}{\Delta t_2} = \frac{-3 \text{ ft}}{6 \text{ sec}} = -.5 \text{ ft/sec}$$

It can be seen that, on the average, the two motions differed with respect to average velocity in both magnitude and direction, $\bar{v}_1$ indicating motion 1 to be faster and positively directed and $\bar{v}_2$ indicating motion 2 to be slower and in the negative direction. No information is available concerning the steadiness (a qualitative feature) of the velocity between P_1 and P_2 and P_2 and P_3, so these velocities must be thought of as average velocities. Average velocity then represents the average rate of change of position and is calculated on the basis of a simplification of the previous examples to be $\bar{v} = d/t$. Although nonvarying velocities are rarely present in human motion, an important distinction must be drawn between average velocity and *constant velocity*.

Constant Velocity

If velocity were nonvarying over time, the information plotted on a *displacement-time* graph would appear as in Fig. 3-3. The constant velocity is seen to be 1 ft/sec in a positive direction. For each second in time, the object moves exactly one additional foot. By the end of the period of observation, the object has moved 5 ft from the starting position and required 5 sec in the process. Note that constant velocity is plotted as a straight line, with displacement being directly proportional to time. The statement *displacement over time* signifies the calculation procedure where the displacement is divided by the time. The average velocity for any interval of time represented on the graph is the same (1 ft/sec).

Figure 3-4 illustrates two displacement lines plotted on the same graph to identify the relationship between a constant velocity and the *slope* of the displacement line on the graph. Slope A, the steeper of the two, represents the greater velocity magnitude. Each slope is calculated by dividing the displacement units by the corresponding time units to yield

$$\text{Slope } A = \frac{d_8 - d_4}{t_4 - t_2} = \frac{\Delta d}{\Delta t} = 2 \text{ ft/sec}$$

$$\text{Slope } B = \frac{d_3 - d_1}{t_6 - t_2} = \frac{\Delta d}{\Delta t} = 5 \text{ ft/sec}$$

Note that the slope of each displacement line is equal to the constant velocity it represents on the graph. It makes no difference which two intervals on the straight line are chosen for the determination of the slope; it remains the same. Satisfy this for yourself by selecting other Δd and Δt segments from the two displacement lines. It can be seen that in the case of constant velocity, the slope of the velocity line also equals the average

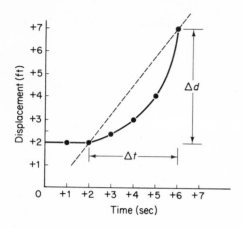

Figure 3–5. After remaining motionless for two seconds, the object progressively increases its rate of change of position as indicated by the increasing steepness of the displacement line.

velocity over any time interval. Constant velocity is not signified by a symbol as are other kinds of velocity.

Displacement Determination

When a varying (nonconstant) velocity is evident on a graph such as Fig. 3-5, the relationship between average and constant velocities becomes more subtle. The displacement line shows the object under observation to be motionless for a period of 2 sec, after which it develops an increasing positive velocity over time. Notice the general slope characteristics for the time intervals, t_2 to t_4, t_4 to t_5, and t_5 to t_6, each succeeding slope being steeper than its predecessor. The average velocities for these time intervals are seen to be .5, 1, and 3 ft/sec, respectively. The average velocity for the entire motion observed would be

$$\bar{v} = \frac{d_7 - d_2}{t_6 - t_2} = \frac{\Delta d = 5}{\Delta t = 4} = 1.25 \text{ ft/sec}$$

The constant velocity, which could produce the same outcome for the moving object as could the average velocity just calculated for varying velocity conditions, is represented by the interrupted line in Fig. 3-5. The slope of this line equals the average velocity over the same time period.

→ *Calculate its slope.*

Therefore, a constant velocity whose slope equals the average velocity over the same time period, no matter how the velocity may vary, would yield the same displacement for the moving object. This is represented by the formula $d = \bar{v}t$. To cite an example, if an object with a velocity of 20 ft/sec continues at this pace without varying for 10 sec, the displacement would equal

$$d = \bar{v}t = 20 \text{ ft/sec} \times 10 \text{ sec} = 200 \text{ ft}$$

The calculation of displacement brings up the important topic of the calculation of rates of change of position based upon displacements vs. *distances* or *path lengths*. Take, for example, the case of a runner who completes a 440-yd run on a typical running track used for track and field competition in the United States (see Fig. 3-6). The runner starts at the line marked *start* and completes one circuit of the track to arrive back at the same line. His displacement must be regarded as equaling zero since his finishing point was also his starting point. However, the actual distance traversed or path length during the circuit was 440 yd. In terms of displacement, the same result could be accomplished by running 220 yd in one direction and then returning the same 220 yd in the opposite direction. The average velocity with respect to displacement is obviously zero, while the *average speed* with respect to the total distance traversed, disregarding direction and assuming a time duration of 1 min, is

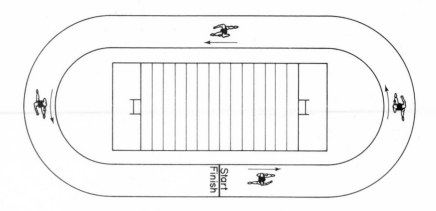

Figure 3–6. Start and finish points are identical, thus the single circuit of inconsistent direction finds the runner traversing a path length of 440 yd without demonstrating a displacement.

$$\bar{v} = \frac{440 \text{ yd}}{1 \text{ min}} = \frac{1320 \text{ ft}}{60 \text{ sec}} = 22 \text{ ft/sec}$$

Both path length and time are scalar quantities, leaving their ratio, as above, also a scalar quantity. The symbol l will be used to stand for this undirected path length unit where average speed is determined from

$$\bar{v} = \frac{\Delta l}{\Delta t}$$

Again, notice the differences in printing the vector quantity, *average velocity*, $\bar{\mathbf{v}}$, and the *scalar quantity*, $\bar{v}$, average speed.

In a race such as the 100-yd dash, the motion path is much more linear and proceeds in one direction only. Displacement and distance traversed both equal 100 yd. Therefore, average velocity and average speed for this event are equal. That is, the magnitude of the average velocity equals the average speed since a scalar quantity exhibits only magnitude. It must not be assumed, however, that the magnitudes of all average velocities are the same as the average speeds for the motions since they are scalar quantities. Remember that the calculation of velocity depends on displacement, while speed depends on path length, the characteristics of which may differ almost limitlessly. The objectives for most races are the same, that is, to traverse the required distance in the shortest possible time or, simply, to complete the traversal before any other competitor can do so. Consequently, it would appear that the runner who could make his actual path length deviate the least possible amount from the displacement between start and finish would have a distinct advantage.

When velocity is plotted on a *velocity-time* graph as in Fig. 3-7, a horizontal, straight line represents a constant velocity. The straight line illustrates that at every moment during the observation the velocity of the moving object remained the same, 4 ft/sec. Notice, in addition, that on a velocity-time graph, the straight line plotted for a constant velocity has no slope other than zero. The shaded *area under the velocity line* is seen to represent exactly the displacement during the observed motion. The vertical axis value (velocity) multiplied by the horizontal axis value (time) results in the displacement ($d = \bar{v}t$), since the area of a rectangle is obtained by calculating the product of its height and base.

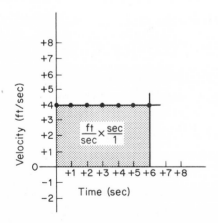

Figure 3–7. All velocity plots over time are the same, indicating a constant velocity. The shaded area under the velocity line represents exactly the displacement.

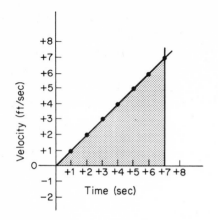

Figure 3–8. The triangular area under the uniformly-varying velocity line again represents the displacement, which is obtained by computing the product of one-half its height (velocity) and its base (time).

When a uniformly varying velocity is plotted on a velocity-time graph as in Fig. 3-8, the total displacement is again represented by the area under the velocity line. In this case, velocity varies from zero at the beginning of the observation period to 7 ft/sec at the end of the period (7 sec). The object whose velocity is plotted has obviously demonstrated *acceleration*. And, although the individual plots along the velocity line represent velocities, the slope of the line represents acceleration, as will be discussed later. The shaded area is seen to be a triangle whose area is obtained by calculating the product of one half its height (velocity) and its base (time), therefore yielding

$$d = \frac{7 \text{ ft/sec}}{2} \times 7 \text{ sec} = 24.5 \text{ ft}$$

Now that displacement has been determined, the average velocity for the plotted motion can be determined also from $\bar{v} = d/t$ to yield $\bar{v} = 24.5$ ft/7 sec = 3.5 ft/sec, or one half the velocity value plotted at the end of the observation.

→ *To take another look at the relationships between average and constant velocities, construct a velocity-time graph of 7-sec duration with a constant velocity of 3.5 ft/sec, and determine the displacement.*

In other words, the displacements produced are the same for (*1*) an object starting from rest and uniformly increasing its velocity to 7 ft/sec over 7 sec and (*2*) an object traveling at a constant velocity of 3.5 ft/sec for 7 sec. The reason for this is, of course, that they both demonstrate the same average velocity over the 7-sec observation period.

Figure 3-8 may also be used to illustrate another approach to the calculation of average velocity when the motion velocities plotted vary uniformly. The *original velocity* plotted for the observation, zero, is added to the *final velocity* plotted, 7 ft/sec, to represent the sum of the lower and upper limits of the velocities observed. When this sum is divided by 2, the result is the average velocity:

$$\bar{v} = \frac{v_o - v_f}{2}$$

where v_o = original velocity and v_f = final velocity. When the values are inserted, it becomes

$$\bar{v} = \frac{0 + 7 \text{ ft/sec}}{2} = 3.5 \text{ ft/sec}$$

If the original velocity plot showed a velocity differing from zero, but the velocity line showed the same changes over time as in Fig. 3-8, the result would appear as in Fig. 3-9. The primary outcome of interest is that the shaded area under the velocity line is larger than in Fig. 3-8. This larger area under the velocity line is seen to be partitioned into two figures, a triangle and a rectangle. Note that the triangular area in Fig. 3-9 exactly

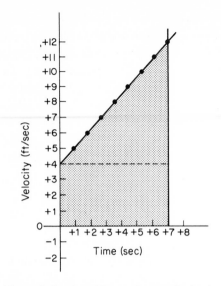

Figure 3–9. An object, whose velocity is 4 ft/sec when first observed, demonstrates the same changes over time as the object in Fig. 3–8. Displacement is represented by the trapezoidal area under the velocity line.

equals that shown in Fig. 3-8; only the scale numbers have been changed. The additional rectangular area represents exactly the increase in displacement under the conditions of an increased original velocity. The sum of the triangular area (24.5 ft) and the rectangular area (28 ft) is the total displacement (52.2 ft) under the conditions depicted in Fig. 3-9.

The average velocity for this uniformly varying motion again may be calculated as discussed above. The sum of its original and final velocities divided by 2 is seen to suffice. These values represent the two parallel sides of the shaded, *trapezoidal area* under the velocity line. When the values are inserted, the outcome is

$$\bar{v} = \frac{4 \text{ ft/sec} + 11 \text{ ft/sec}}{2} = 7.5 \text{ ft/sec}$$

When the average velocities illustrated in Figs. 3-8 and 3-9 are compared with respect to the displacements traversed under their respective conditions, it becomes apparent why so much running competition is governed by strict rules which require of all competitors a completely motionless position ($v_o = 0$) immediately prior to the starting signal. Any original velocity differing from zero would provide an unfair advantage for the runner who possesses it at the starting signal. In fact, repeated violations of this rule generally disqualify the man from further participation. The reader will, of course, recognize that other types of starting conditions are imposed in different racing environments. For example, sailing and several kinds of automobile racing initiate the competition with *running starts*, or with original velocities differing from zero. The objective is to begin the race with the highest starting velocity which is consistent with the rules governing the event.

If the velocities plotted over time do not vary uniformly, the area under the velocity line still represents the displacement, as in Fig. 3-10. Average velocity may not be calculated until the displacement for the moving object has been determined. Since the velocity did not vary uniformly, the formula, $\bar{v} = (v_o + v_f)/2$ may *not* be applied. The motion was seen to have been observed over a 10-sec period with the original velocity being 1 ft/sec and the final velocity being 10 ft/sec. The area under the line has been subdivided into ten subareas, each of which is an approximation of a trapezoid. In addition, note that each trapezoid is divided into separate triangles and rectangles. If the area of each rectangle were calculated and summed, the result would approximate the area under the line less the summed areas of the triangles. If these two sums were added, the result would equal the sum of all the trapezoid areas illustrated, from the formula $T = \frac{1}{2}(v_1 + v_2)\Delta t$, or the product of one half the sum of the two parallel sides and its base, for each trapezoid.

If the number of individual observations during the 10-sec motion period were increased to 1000, the time intervals between plots would be reduced to the small duration of $\frac{1}{100}$ sec. Under these conditions, the triangles would become tiny and each would have a long side which was very nearly a straight line. It follows that the sum of the trapezoidal areas would also benefit in its accuracy of approximating the true area under the line.

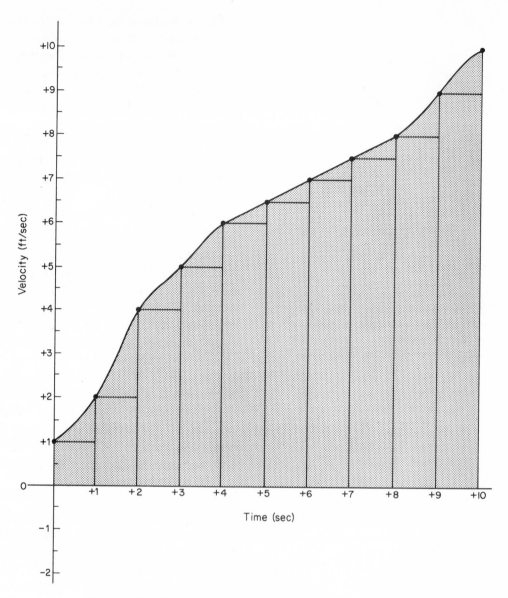

Figure 3–10. Regardless of the shape of the plotted velocity line, displacement is always represented by the area under the curve.

→ *Calculate the approximate area under the velocity line in Fig. 3-10 and then determine the approximate average velocity for the observed motion.*

It can be concluded, therefore, that the area under the velocity line, regardless of the line's shape, always equals the displacement which occurred in that time interval.

Time Determination

When the time required to traverse a known distance with a given speed is of importance, it is calculated by applying the following formula:

$t = l/\bar{v}$. To provide an example, assume that your objective in running the *mile run* is a time duration of exactly 4 min. The distance to be traversed is fixed at 5280 ft. But the average speed may vary considerably throughout the run and still allow you to reach your 4-min objective. If the average speed for the entire run were 22 ft/sec, the calculation for time would yield

$$t = \frac{l}{\bar{v}} = \frac{5280 \text{ ft}}{22 \text{ ft/sec}} = 240 \text{ sec} = 4 \text{ min}$$

Strategy applied to running events such as the mile run usually involves the careful planning of the elapsed times required for each of the quarter-mile laps. Of course, the time is read from the face of a stopwatch rather than being derived from calculation. However, if a runner who seeks to run the mile in 4 min completes the first three laps in 62, 60, and 58 sec, respectively, the characteristics of the last lap are fixed in terms of success. An average speed of 22 ft/sec is the mandatory lower limit. To achieve this, the runner must have some idea of what he must do, and if he is told that the last lap must be completed in 60 sec, he then has a means of comparing his present performance with past experience to assist him in his effort. The effort in this case is the traversal of 1320 ft in 60 sec, a pace equaling the average speed for the run in its entirety. Keep in mind the fact that although this example used average speed because of the lack of a consistent movement direction, the calculation of time using average velocity and displacement is essentially the same.

INSTANTANEOUS VELOCITY

Up to this point, the focus of attention has been on average velocity. However, numerous allusions to the velocity of an object at any *instant* or at the *end* of a given period of time were made without calling specific attention to them. These were made when the terms *original velocity*, *final velocity*, or any of the plotted velocity points on velocity-time graphs were introduced for the purpose of calculating average velocity. Although instantaneous velocities were included in several formulas in their correct form, no mention was made of their presence. The symbol for instantaneous velocity is v; to distinguish it from that of average velocity, the *bar* is omitted. The purpose of this section is to discuss instantaneous velocity in light of the previous discussion of average velocity.

It will be remembered that in the previous section, the reduction of time intervals to very small durations was introduced to assist in showing the relationship between displacement by an object and the area under the velocity line. If the same sort of reasoning were applied to time intervals on displacement-time graphs, it would be seen that as a time interval approaches zero, average velocity over that very short time span approaches the instantaneous velocity. Figure 3-11 illustrates diminishing time intervals (Δt) of $t_9 - t_3$, $t_8 - t_4$, and $t_7 - t_5$, respectively, in terms of the velocity

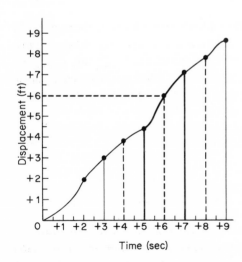

Figure 3–11. The slopes of velocity line segments more accurately approximate the slope at *t6* as their extremes approach that point on the line.

at the instant in time, t_6. Approximate average velocities for these three time intervals are

$$\text{For } t_9 - t_3: \quad \bar{v} = \frac{\Delta d}{\Delta t} = \frac{5.2 \text{ ft}}{6 \text{ sec}} = .87 \text{ ft/sec}$$

$$\text{For } t_8 - t_4: \quad \bar{v} = \frac{\Delta d}{\Delta t} = \frac{4.1 \text{ ft}}{4 \text{ sec}} = 1.03 \text{ ft/sec}$$

$$\text{For } t_7 - t_5: \quad \bar{v} = \frac{\Delta d}{\Delta t} = \frac{2.8 \text{ ft}}{2 \text{ sec}} = 1.40 \text{ ft/sec}$$

each reflecting the shape of the displacement line between its respective points.

In Fig. 3-12a, the points between t_5 and t_7 and $d_{4.4}$ and $d_{7.2}$ in Fig. 3-11 have been enlarged considerably to continue the process of reducing the time interval over which average velocity is calculated. The time interval, $t_{6.2} - t_{5.8}$, is seen to represent .4 sec. The average velocity is

$$\bar{v} = \frac{\Delta d}{\Delta t} = \frac{.85 \text{ ft}}{.4 \text{ sec}} = 2.12 \text{ ft/sec}$$

→ *Carry this process one step farther by calculating the average velocity over the time interval* $t_{6.1} - t_{5.9} = .2$ *sec.*

If this process were continued, the displacement line over infinitesimally small time intervals would approximate a straight line. When the displacement line is a straight line, it has a calculable slope which is defined as the *tangent line* to the displacement curve at that point in time. The slope of the tangent line applied to the displacement curve at point t_6 is the instantaneous velocity of the moving object at that instant during the observation.

Figure 3-12b again reduces the scale values to illustrate the segment of the displacement curve in Fig. 3-12a between $t_{5.95}$ and $t_{6.05}$. A tangent line has been constructed at $t_{6.00}$ which corresponds to $d_{5.9225}$ and $t_{6.0325}$ on the displacement and time axes, respectively. The two points could have been chosen anywhere on the tangent line for this purpose as long as they were within the scales of the graph.

→ *Complete the computation which follows:*

$$v = \text{tangent line slope at } t_{6.00} = \frac{d_{6.0500} - d_{5.9225}}{t_{6.0325} - t_{5.9500}} =$$

Instantaneous velocity, v, is therefore defined as the limit of the ratio of the increment of displacement (Δd) divided by the increment in time (Δt) as the time increment approaches zero as a limit ($\Delta t \to 0$). The formula representing this statement is as follows:

$$v = \lim_{\Delta t \to 0} \frac{\Delta d}{\Delta t}$$

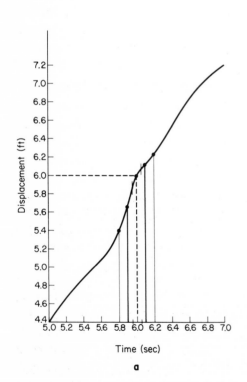

Figure 3–12a. As Δt is reduced toward zero as a limit, the displacement curve gradually approximates a straight line.

In order that the special use of the average velocity may be remembered, instantaneous velocity may also be given by

$$v = \lim_{\Delta t \to 0} \bar{v}$$

implying that, as time approaches zero as a limit, average velocity may be substituted as a close approximation for the true instantaneous velocity.

When displacement was determined with respect to the velocity-time graphs in the section covering average velocity, the formula $d = \bar{v}t$ was shown as a substitute for determining the area under the velocity line. By referring back to the graph showing a constant velocity, Fig. 3-7, it will be seen that only under conditions of a constant velocity can displacement be calculated by substituting v for $\bar{v}$ in the displacement formula shown above as $d = vt$. This may be done only under conditions of constant velocity because each instantaneous velocity plotted equals the average velocity for the entire motion under observation. In Fig. 3-8, illustrating a uniformly varying velocity, each instantaneous velocity plotted is seen to represent only one small instant in the total elapsed time rather than the total. This brings up the question of which instantaneous velocity out of the eight plotted should be chosen to be inserted into the displacement formula ($d = vt$). It will be noted that none of the velocity plots is exactly the same as the average velocity for the graph, 3.5 ft/sec. Of course, the object did, indeed, demonstrate an instantaneous velocity of 3.5 ft/sec: It occurred 3.5 sec after the motion commenced even though it is not identified by a definite plot on the line, since the velocity varied uniformly. However, if the motion illustrated in Fig. 3-10 is reviewed, the choice of the point on the velocity line where instantaneous velocity is most likely to equal the average velocity for the entire motion is most decidedly obscured by the changing slope of the velocity line over time.

Instantaneous Velocity Determination

Instantaneous velocity is a very important motion characteristic to consider when studying human motion, and the procedures for its determination follow quite closely those just described. The essential requirement for this purpose is a means of recording the motion and, at the same time, recording the elapsed time in very small fractional parts. The use of motion picture cameras to perform these combined functions is very common. The many individual pictures produced throughout the motion sequence, separated by very small intervals of time, act to simulate the approach of the time increment (Δt) to zero as a limit. Rotating mirror cameras are available which can produce framing rates up to 100 million pictures per second to examine events of phenomenally short duration.[1]

If it is assumed that the camera's film transport mechanism will produce 5000 individual pictures each second, then the increment of time

---

[1] John H. Waddell, "High-Speed Photography: The 100-Year-Old Infant," *Electro-Optical Systems Design* **2**, No. 1 (January 1970), p. 38.

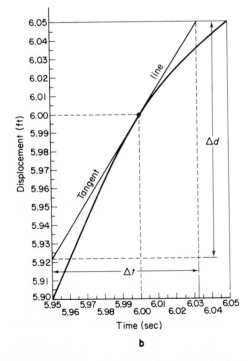

Figure 3–12b. The slope of the tangent line at t_{600} is defined as the instantaneous velocity of the moving object at that moment in time.

can be reduced to $\frac{1}{5000}$ sec. For human motion, this is a very short time interval. Depending on the movement velocities encountered, framing rates between 64 frames per second and 400 frames per second generally encompass the requirements of human motion when accompanied by suitable shutter speeds. If the instantaneous velocity is desired at a particular point in the motion, it may be obtained by calculating the average velocity for the motion which occurred in that tiny time interval whose lower and upper limits are provided by frames equally spaced before and after the point of interest. The limits of the time interval are chosen on the basis of a measurable change in the position of the object under study during the interval. If no displacement can be measured, it is obvious that no average velocity may be assigned to the interval. Because the time interval is very small, the average velocity may be offered as a reasonable substitute for the actual instantaneous velocity at that point in the motion. Additional procedures for determining instantaneous velocity are discussed in the next section, which deals with acceleration.

Since man is generally a poor judge of the velocities demonstrated by objects of various sizes at varying distances, he usually relies on mechanical contrivances to indicate instantaneous velocities. Speedometers provide velocity magnitudes for the operators of vehicles such as cycles and automobiles. Tachometers indicate the magnitudes of engine part rotation velocities. Electronic as well as mechanical devices are utilized by law enforcement agencies to detect movement behavior beyond the law. In fact, the interactions between distances traversed and elapsed time intervals play a most important role in the description of their quantitative and qualitative influences on man's behavior.

AVERAGE ACCELERATION

When an object moves in such a manner that its velocity is not constant, the motion is classified as *accelerated motion*. It will be remembered that Figs. 3-8 through 3-12 illustrated changing velocities, some of which varied uniformly and others which did not. *Positive* and *negative accelerations*, their qualitative features being *speeding up* and *slowing down*, respectively, are prime characteristics of human motion. Often, they are referred to as *acceleration* and *deceleration* for the positive and negative modes, respectively. In the study of human motion, where the changes in velocity are seldom uniform, the focus of interest is usually applied to other than constant accelerations. However, for the sake of simplicity, the discussion of acceleration will begin with constant acceleration.

Figure 3-13 illustrates a hypothetical motion situation in which positive and negative accelerations are evident as constant accelerations. The object is seen to have increased its velocity uniformly from the beginning of the observation, t_0, over the 5-sec interval to t_5. At t_5, the object abruptly stops accelerating and begins decelerating until the motion ceases altogether at t_{10}, the end of the observation period. It can be seen that the slopes of the two velocity line segments are equal in magnitude but carry opposite signs:

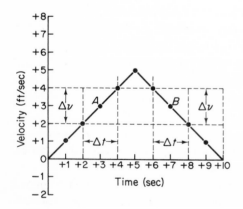

Figure 3–13. The slopes of velocity line segments *A* and *B* represent the average accelerations, *A* being positive and *B* negative.

$$\text{Slope } A = \frac{v_4 - v_2}{t_4 - t_2} = \frac{\Delta v}{\Delta t} = \frac{2 \text{ ft/sec}}{2 \text{ sec}} = 1 \text{ ft/sec/sec}$$

$$\text{Slope } B = \frac{v_2 - v_4}{t_8 - t_6} = \frac{\Delta v}{\Delta t} = \frac{-2 \text{ ft/sec}}{2 \text{ sec}} = -1 \text{ ft/sec/sec}$$

And, as was noted earlier, the slope of a uniformly varying velocity line represents acceleration. Since the change of velocity over a known time interval was divided by the duration of that interval, the acceleration must be an *average acceleration*. The formula used to represent this relationship is as follows:

$$\bar{a} = \frac{\Delta v}{\Delta t}$$

As would be expected, if an object started from rest ($v = 0$) and at first demonstrated constant positive acceleration for 5 sec, followed by 5 sec of an equal magnitude of constant negative acceleration, the object would conclude the motion at rest. However, this is not meant to imply that the object returned to its starting position at the end of the motion.

The motion plotted in Fig. 3-14 illustrates two important concepts. The first is shown as a nonvarying velocity over the first 3 sec of the observation. Acceleration is seen to equal zero, or to not exist. At t_3, the object begins to lose velocity uniformly, as shown by its slope, until t_7, where the motion ceases. The object then begins to move in the opposite direction with the same acceleration characteristics that applied to its movement in a positive direction, but in this case, the object is uniformly gaining velocity. Therefore, when an object moves in a negative direction with increasing velocity, the outcome is the same as that of an object with decreasing velocity moving in a positive direction. The result is a negative sign. The opposite also holds true for the positive sign.

The following is an example of the calculations producing the negative sign for motion in positive and negative directions, respectively. For decreasing positive velocities, for the time interval t_3 to t_5, Fig. 3-14:

$$\bar{a} = \frac{\Delta v}{\Delta t} = \frac{2 \text{ ft/sec} - 4 \text{ ft/sec}}{5 \text{ sec} - 3 \text{ sec}} = \frac{-2 \text{ ft/sec}}{2 \text{ sec}} = -1 \text{ ft/sec}^2$$

For increasing negative velocities, for the time interval t_8 to t_{10}:

$$\bar{a} = \frac{\Delta v}{\Delta t} = \frac{-3 \text{ ft/sec} - (-1 \text{ ft/sec})}{10 \text{ sec} - 8 \text{ sec}} = \frac{-2 \text{ ft/sec}}{2 \text{ sec}} = -1 \text{ ft/sec}^2$$

Note that the unit symbol ft/sec² may be used in place of ft/sec/sec to signify acceleration.

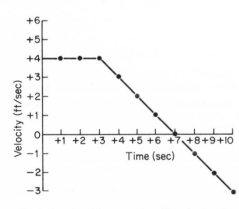

Figure 3–14. When a plotted velocity line reaches the time axis, movement has ceased. Velocity line excursions below the time axis indicate a reversal of direction of the object's motion.

→ *Now, reverse the slope of the velocity line so that it runs from* v = −4 *ft/sec at* t₃, *through* v = 0 *at* t₇, *to* v = +3 ft/sec *at* t₁₀; *and calculate the magnitude of the positive, average acceleration using the same time intervals as above.*

INSTANTANEOUS ACCELERATION

As was the case in the discussion of average and instantaneous velocities, when the time intervals over which the motion takes place approach zero as a limit, the slope of the tangent line at a point in time on a velocity-time graph is the *instantaneous acceleration*. The formula which represents this characteristic is

$$a = \lim_{\Delta t \to 0} \frac{\Delta v}{\Delta t}$$

and, as can be seen by referring again to segments A and B of Fig. 3-13, when acceleration is constant as time passes, average and instantaneous accelerations are the same at any point in time. In Fig. 3-14, this holds true even though the object is seen to reverse the direction of its movement at t_7. This does not hold true for velocities which do not vary uniformly (varying acceleration).

→ *Transform Fig. 3-12b into a velocity-time graph (by substituting velocity in ft/sec for displacement along the vertical axis) and determine the instantaneous acceleration at* t_6 *by calculating the slope of the tangent line at* t_6.

An example of the value of instantaneous acceleration is seen in a distance-running race in which two runners are about to begin their final *kicks* near the end of the race while running side by side. Quite often one runner will abruptly accelerate his pace to catch his opponent by surprise and gain an advantage which could be insurmountable. In sprint races, instantaneous acceleration plays a dominant role in providing a lead immediately following the starting signal. The sprinter who can accelerate his body to its maximal velocity in the shortest time interval has a most notable starting advantage. Although this appears to best describe the value of high average acceleration over time, it is actually the result of high instantaneous accelerations at all points in time throughout the time interval.

VELOCITY, ACCELERATION, AND TIME RELATIONSHIPS

In motion situations where average acceleration is known, final velocity (v_f) may be calculated at the end of a given period of time. This is represented by

$$v_f = \bar{a}t$$

Assume that an object demonstrated an average acceleration of 5 ft/sec/sec over a time interval of 10 sec. Further, assume that the object began its motion from rest. After 10 sec of accelerated motion, the object attained a final velocity of $v_f = 5$ ft/sec/sec $\times$ 10 sec $= 50$ ft/sec. Note that there is no information regarding how the acceleration varied from moment to moment over the 10-sec time interval. If the object did not start from rest, but was traveling at a known velocity at the start of the observation, final velocity is obtained by adding this original velocity to the product of average acceleration and time to produce

$$v_f = v_o + \bar{a}t$$

Assume that the original velocity is 20 ft/sec and that the same average acceleration and time conditions prevail as above. The velocity at the end of this accelerated motion is calculated to produce

$$v_f = v_o + \bar{a}t = 20 \text{ ft/sec} + 5 \text{ ft/sec}^2 \times 10 \text{ sec} =$$
$$20 \text{ ft/sec} + 50 \text{ ft/sec} = v_f = 70 \text{ ft/sec}$$

The formula could be written, $v_f = v_0 \pm \bar{a}t$ to indicate that the product of average acceleration and time is subtracted from the original velocity when the acceleration is negative.

The same formula may be applied to *uniformly accelerated* motion where instantaneous and average accelerations are equal at any point during the observation. In this case, a may be substituted for $\bar{a}$ in the final velocity formula. Under conditions of nonsupport, objects fall through space with constant acceleration; that is, their velocities increase by equal amounts over equal time intervals of free fall. It is therefore possible to determine a freely falling object's final velocity at the end of any period of nonsupport.

The constant acceleration which is the result of gravitational attraction on a nonsupported object is usually given as approximately 32 ft/sec/sec. This figure is rounded to the nearest whole number for the sake of calculation simplicity. If an object is released from a starting position at rest and falls for 4 sec, its final velocity is calculated by the use of the formula $v_f = gt$, where g is substituted for a to represent the gravitational constant. After 4 sec of free fall, the object is traveling at a velocity of

$$v_f = gt = 32 \text{ ft/sec}^2 \times 4 \text{ sec} = 128 \text{ ft/sec}$$

Note that this figure is also the object's instantaneous velocity at that point in time.

→ *Determine the velocities (final or instantaneous) after 1, 2, 3, and 5 sec of free fall.*

Figure 3-15 illustrates changes in time and velocity under conditions of nonsupport. Notice that these velocity values are the answers to the calculations requested above. With each succeeding second of elapsed time, the velocity increases by 32 ft/sec, or 32 ft/sec each second. Average velocity may be determined for any time interval by applying the formula $\bar{v} = (v_o + v_f)/2$. The average velocity for the time interval t_2 to t_4 is seen to be

$$\bar{v} = \frac{v_o + v_f}{2} = \frac{64 \text{ ft/sec} + 128 \text{ ft/sec}}{2} = 96 \text{ ft/sec}$$

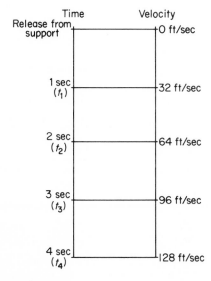

Figure 3–15

→ *Calculate all remaining average velocities from Fig. 3-15, using whole-second time intervals and their multiples.*

DISPLACEMENT, ACCELERATION, AND TIME RELATIONSHIPS

Displacement was seen to be represented by the area under the velocity line on velocity-time graphs. In the case of an object undergoing constant acceleration in free fall, displacement may be calculated if average velocity and time are known. Figure 3-16 illustrates changes in time and displacement under conditions of nonsupport. By using the formula $d = \bar{v}t$, it will be seen that the object falls 16 ft in the first second of free fall. The calculations are

$$\bar{v} = \frac{v_o + v_f}{2} = \frac{0 + 32 \text{ ft/sec}}{2} = 16 \text{ ft/sec}$$

Then

$$d = \bar{v}t = 16 \text{ ft/sec} \times 1 \text{ sec} = 16 \text{ ft}$$

Note that average velocity, when original velocity equals zero, is simply one half the value of the final velocity for the time interval. In the preceding section, it was pointed out that final velocity could be calculated from the formula $v_f = at$ when acceleration was constant. By substituting at for v_f in the displacement formula just applied, the result is

$$d = \frac{at}{2}t \quad \text{or} \quad d = \tfrac{1}{2}at^2 \quad \text{or} \quad d = \tfrac{1}{2}gt^2$$

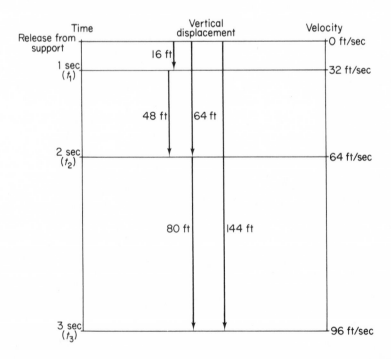

Figure 3–16. Relationships between displacement, acceleration, time, and instantaneous velocity for free fall, neglecting air friction.

Using the data available in Fig. 3-16 for the first second of fall, the calculation of displacement results in

$$d = \tfrac{1}{2}gt^2 = \tfrac{1}{2}\,32\ \text{ft/sec}^2 \times (1\ \text{sec})^2 = 16\ \text{ft/sec}^2 \times 1\ \text{sec}^2 = 16\ \text{ft}$$

→ *Calculate all remaining displacements from Fig. 3-16.*

Keep in mind that this formula may be applied only when the object's original velocity is zero. When an object has an original velocity differing from zero, displacement is calculated on the basis of an average velocity. This may be illustrated from the information in Fig. 3-16 for the displacements between t_1 and t_2. The displacement arrived at by the use of the formula $d = \tfrac{1}{2}gt^2$ would be

$$d = \tfrac{1}{2}gt^2 = 16\ \text{ft/sec}^2 \times (1\ \text{sec})^2 = 16\ \text{ft}$$

when the object actually traveled 48 ft between t_1 and t_2.

VELOCITY, ACCELERATION, AND DISPLACEMENT RELATIONSHIPS

Suppose that an object was projected exactly vertically (not a very easy thing to achieve) and that its velocity upon projection was 80 ft/sec. Gravity immediately acts to retard the motion or to decelerate the motion uniformly. The object finally comes to a complete halt, or at least stops moving upward, and falls back to earth, retracing the original path in the opposite direction. When the object returned to the original projection level, its instantaneous velocity again equaled 80 ft/sec. With this basic framework in mind, the discussion of several interesting problems follows.

The first problem may be put as follows: What velocity will a freely falling object have after falling 200 ft from a rest position? Notice that time is inherent in the problem, but not given. From the formula $v = at$, it is seen that

$$t = \frac{v}{a}$$

or, in this case,

$$t = \frac{v}{g}$$

When v/g is substituted for t in the formula $d = \tfrac{1}{2}gt^2$, the result is

$$d = \tfrac{1}{2}g\left(\frac{v}{g}\right)^2 = \frac{g}{2}\,\frac{v^2}{g^2} = \frac{gv^2}{2g^2} \quad \text{or} \quad d = \frac{v^2}{2g}$$

Using this formula to solve for velocity, the result is

$$v = \sqrt{2gd} = \sqrt{2 \times 32 \text{ ft/sec}^2 \times 200 \text{ ft}} =$$
$$\sqrt{2 \times 32 \times 200} = \sqrt{16,800} \quad \text{or} \quad v = 129.9 \text{ ft/sec}$$

The second problem may be stated as follows: If a ball was dropped from a height such that 3.5 sec were required for it to strike the earth, from what height was it dropped? Using the formula $d = \frac{1}{2}gt^2$, it follows that

$$d = \frac{1}{2}gt^2 = 16 \text{ ft/sec}^2 \times (3.5 \text{ sec})^2 = 16 \text{ ft/sec}^2 \times 12.25 \text{ sec}^2 =$$
$$d = 196 \text{ ft}$$

→ *Next, calculate the velocity with which the ball struck the earth. Notice that two formulas may be used for this purpose since both time and displacement are known; namely,* $v = gt$ *and* $v = \sqrt{2gd}$. *Which one results in the simplest calculation procedures?*

Third, to return to the original problem introduced in this section: If a ball is projected vertically and demonstrates an original or projection velocity of 80 ft/sec, how high will it rise after release? By referring back to p. 41, displacement was shown to be obtainable from the formula $d = v^2/2g$. The calculation produces

$$d = \frac{v^2}{2g} = \frac{(80 \text{ ft/sec})^2}{2 \times 32 \text{ ft/sec}^2} = \frac{6400 \text{ ft}^2/\text{sec}^2}{64 \text{ ft/sec}^2} = d = 100 \text{ ft}$$

At this point, displacement may not be determined by using the formula $d = \frac{1}{2}gt^2$ since time is still unknown. To solve for time, apply the formula $t = v/g$ to produce

$$t = \frac{v}{g} = \frac{80 \text{ ft/sec}}{32 \text{ ft/sec}^2} = 2.5 \text{ sec}$$

→ *Solve for time by using a variation of the formula* $d = \frac{1}{2}gt^2$: $t = \sqrt{2d/g}$. *Which is the easier procedure? Now that the time over which the motion took place is known, solve for displacement by using the formula* $d = \frac{1}{2}gt^2$. *Which is the simpler of the two procedures for finding the displacement?*

If the motion just described were plotted on a velocity-time graph, it would appear as in Fig. 3-17. Segments *A* and *B* represent the ball's upward and downward flights, respectively.

→ *Calculate the slopes of segments* A *and* B, *paying attention to sign, to see if they do closely approximate the acceleration and deceleration constants. Do these values represent average or instantaneous acceleration, or both?*

There is much interest in the behavior of objects falling freely through space, particularly those shaped like human beings. The growing interest in the sport of *sky diving* or *parachuting* has revived the need for a careful

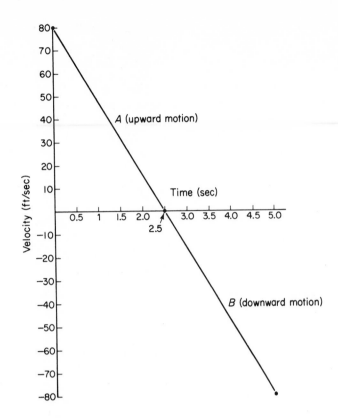

Figure 3–17. Positive and negative, vertical flight plotted on a velocity-time graph.

understanding of the control problems of free fall through the earth's atmosphere, sometimes from immense altitudes. Such elements as the atmosphere's density; the body's size, weight, shape, and clothing; and velocity all play a part in establishing that point in the fall where the body ceases to gain velocity any further. The velocity of the body at this point is called the *limiting* or, more commonly, *terminal velocity*, after which the body falls at a nearly constant rate. Additional discussions of this phenomenon, which is quite apparent to the falling individual when it occurs, are presented in Chapter 7.

REFERENCES

Bowne, M. E. "Relationship of Selected Measures of Acting Body Levers to Ball Throwing Velocities." *Research Quarterly* 31 (1960): 392.

Cureton, T. K. "Mechanics of Track Running." *Scholastic Coach* 4 (February 1935): 7.

Dern, R. J.; Levene, J. M.; and Blair, H. A. "Forces Exerted at Different Velocities in Human Arm Movements." *American Journal of Physiology* 151 (1947): 415.

Dunwoody, K. M. "Time and Motion in Physical Education." *Journal of Health and Physical Education* 10 (1939): 218.

Elbell, E. R. "Measuring Speed and Force of Charge of Football Players." *Research Quarterly* 23 (1952): 295.

Fenn, W. O. "Mechanical Energy Expenditure in Sprint Running as Measured by Moving Pictures." *American Journal of Physiology* 90 (1929): 343.

Ford, Kenneth W. *Basic Physics*. Waltham, Mass.: Blaisdell Publishing Company, 1968.

Garrett, R. E.; Widule, C. J.; and Garrett, G. E. "Computer-Aided Analysis of Human Motion." *Kinesiology Review—1968*. Washington, D.C.: N.E.A., 1968.

Goldstein, A. G. "Linear Acceleration and Apparent Distance." *Perceptual and Motor Skills* 9 (1959): 267.

Grieve, D. W., and Gear, R. J. "The Relationships Between Length of Stride, Step Frequency, Time of Swing and Speed of Walking for Children and Adults." *Ergonomics* 9 (1966): 379.

Hartson, L. D. "Analysis of Skilled Movements." *Personnel Journal* 11 (1932–3): 28.

Hellebrandt, F. A.; Hellebrandt, E. J.; and White, C. H. "Methods of Recording Movement." *American Journal of Physical Medicine* 39 (1960): 178.

Henry, F. M., and Trafton, I. R. "The Velocity Curve of Sprint Running." *Research Quarterly* 22 (1952): 409.

Hess, J. L., and Lombard, C. F. "Theoretical Investigations of Dynamic Responses of Man to High Vertical Accelerations." *Journal of Aviation Medicine* 29 (1958): 66.

Howell, A. Brazier. *Speed in Animals*. Chicago: University of Chicago Press, 1944.

Hubbard, A. W. "Homokinetics." In *Science and Medicine of Exercise and Sports*, edited by W. R. Johnson. New York: Harper & Row, Publishers, 1960.

Ikai, M. "Biomechanics of Sprint Running with Respect to the Speed Curve." In *Medicine and Sport*, vol. 2. Proceedings of the First International Seminar on Biomechanics, Zurich, August 1967. Basel, Switzerland: S. Karger AG, 1968.

Jacobson, Florence D., and Chinn, William G. *Elementary Functions*. Morristown, N. J.: Silver Burdett Company, 1968.

Johannessen, C. L., and Harder, J. A. "Sustained Swimming Speeds of Dolphins." *Science* 132 (1960): 1550.

Katz, B. "The Relation Between Force and Speed in Muscular Contraction." *Journal of Physiology* 96 (1939): 45.

King, W. H., and Irwin, L. W. "A Time and Motion Study of Competitive Backstroke Swimming Turns." *Research Quarterly* 28 (1957): 257.

King, W. H., and Scharf, R. J. "Time and Motion Analysis of Competitive Freestyle Swimming Turns." *Research Quarterly* 35 (1964): 37.

Lapp, V. W. "A Study of Hammer Velocity and the Physical Factors Involved in Hammer Throwing." *Research Quarterly* 6 (1935): 134.

Lotter, W. S. "Specificity or Generality of Speed of Systematically Related Movements." *Research Quarterly* 32 (1961): 55.

Menely, R., and Rosemier, R. A. "Effectiveness of Four Track Starting Positions on Acceleration." *Research Quarterly* 39 (1968): 161.

Nelson, R. C. "Follow-up Investigation of the Velocity of the Volleyball Spike." *Research Quarterly* 35 (1964): 83.

Owens, M. S., and Lee, H. Y. "A Determination of Velocities and Angles of Projection for the Tennis Serve." *Research Quarterly* 40 (1969): 750.

Patmor, G. "Change Your Terminal Velocity." *Parachutist* 6 (1965): 11.

Physical Science Study Committee. *Physics*. 2d ed. Boston: D. C. Heath and Company, 1965.

Pierson, W. R. and Rasch, P. J. "Strength and Speed." *Perceptual and Motor Skills* 14 (1962): 144.

Slater-Hammell, A. T. "Velocity Measurement of Fast Balls and Curve Balls." *Research Quarterly* 23 (1952): 95.

Smith, K. U.; McDermid, C. D.; and Shideman, F. E. "Analysis of the Temporal Component of Motion in Human Gait." *American Journal of Physical Medicine* 39 (1960): 142.

Steben, R. E. "A Cinematographic Study of Selective Factors in the Pole Vault." *Research Quarterly* 41 (1970): 95.

Stilley, G. D. "Approximate Theory for Terminal Velocity of a Freely Falling Body." *Journal of Spacecraft* 4 (1967): 1274.

Stock, M. "Influence of Various Track Starting Positions On Speed." *Research Quarterly* 33 (1962): 607.

Wehrkamp, R. A., and Smith K. U. "Dimensional Analysis of Motion: II. Travel-Distance Effects." *Journal of Applied Psychology* 36 (1952): 201.

White, R. A. "Effect of Hip Elevation on Starting Time of the Sprint." *Research Quarterly Supplement* 6 (1935): 128.

Whitley, J. D., and Smith, L. E. "Measurement of Strength of Adduction of the Arm in Various Positions." *Archives of Physical Medicine and Rehabilitation* 45 (1964): 326.

Zorbas, W. S., and Karpovich, P. V. "The Effect of Weight Lifting Upon the Speed of Muscular Contractions." *Research Quarterly* 22 (1951): 145.

4

Vector Descriptions of Velocity and Acceleration

Velocity and acceleration may be represented by vectors, as were position and displacement. The discussion of the uses of vectors to assist in the description of velocities and accelerations will be limited to curved motion paths. All of the vector rules which have preceded this point are valid.

AVERAGE AND INSTANTANEOUS VELOCITIES

Figure 4-1a illustrates an object moving in a curved path. Three positions are illustrated along the path and are identified by position vectors, d_1, d_2, and d_3. The instantaneous velocities of the object at those three positions along the path are identified as v_1, v_2, and v_3. Note that their directions and magnitudes vary as the object's position along the path changes. Figure 4-1b illustrates the same motion path, this time including displacement vectors between the positions along the path. If average velocities were calculated for Δd_1 and Δd_2 over equal time intervals, the average velocity vectors would exhibit the same directions as, and magnitudes proportional to, Δd_1 and Δd_2. Thus the instantaneous velocities, v_1, v_2, and v_3, in Fig. 4-1a are seen to differ in direction from the average velocity vectors between the three positions. Figure 4-1c illustrates an object rotating around an axis in the XY plane. The same elements that were included in Fig. 4-1a are included here with the addition of the symbol R, which represents the radius or rotation. Note that all of the instantaneous velocity vectors are shown to have equal magnitudes but different directions. This is meant to point up the fact that an object may demonstrate a constant speed throughout its rotation but that its velocity is not constant because the direction of its motion is always changing.

→ *Explain the relationship which exists between the radius of rotation and instantaneous velocity vectors at any point along the circular path.*

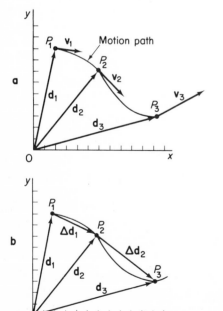

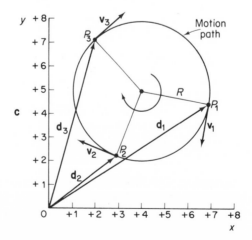

Figure 4-1. (a) Curved motion, exhibiting varying instantaneous velocity vectors tangent to the path. (b) Assuming equal Δt between positions, average velocity vectors between the positions would exhibit the same directions and proportional magnitudes as Δd_1 and Δd_2. (c) An object in clockwise rotation, demonstrating constant speed but varying velocity.

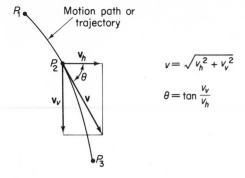

Figure 4–2. Vertical and horizontal component vectors may be constructed to indicate tendencies to move vertically as well as horizontally.

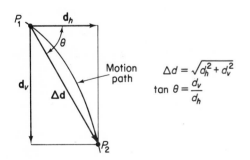

Figure 4–3. The magnitude of the vertical velocity component vector constantly changes in response to gravitational attraction, while the horizontal component is unaffected.

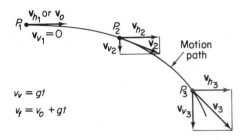

Figure 4–4. Linear displacement along a curved path is determined through the use of the Pythagorean Theorem. When the points, between which displacement is determined, are close together along the path (small Δt), the displacements closely approximate the actual path shape.

If an object is projected horizontally from a starting position which is elevated above the ground, the path of the object between its initial and final positions might appear as in Fig. 4-2. Positions P_1 and P_3 represent the initial and final positions, respectively. Position P_2 represents that point along the motion path where the object's instantaneous velocity is described by the velocity vector, $\mathbf{v}$. This velocity vector's horizontal component vector is represented by the vector $\mathbf{v}_h$ and is the result of the horizontal projection force which pushed the object into motion from its starting position. The velocity vector, $\mathbf{v}_v$, is the vertical component vector and is the result of the force of gravity operating constantly after support is released. As can be seen, the magnitude of $\mathbf{v}$ is determined by the application of the Pythagorean theorem.

Figure 4-3 illustrates a similar trajectory for a projected object. The object possesses only one velocity at the initial position, namely, the horizontal component, $\mathbf{v}_{h_1}$. At position P_2, the velocity vector, $\mathbf{v}_2$, is seen to have the same horizontal component as in the initial position. In addition, a vertical component, $\mathbf{v}_{v_2}$, is illustrated. Position P_3 again shows the same horizontal component for $\mathbf{v}_3$, plus a vertical component which has a greater magnitude than was the case for position P_2. The horizontal velocity component remains the same throughout the motion, thus allowing equal horizontal displacements to be traversed in equal intervals of time. The vertical velocity component changes throughout the motion since the constant acceleration owing to gravity causes the object's velocity to vary uniformly over time. In the language of the earlier discussion, the constant horizontal velocity component may be represented by the symbol $\mathbf{v}_o$. The varying vertical velocity component's magnitude may be continually determined from the product of g and t. Note that the instantaneous velocity vectors for the three positions in Fig. 4-3 are always of such a length (magnitude) that their horizontal velocity components are equal to $\mathbf{v}_{h_1}$, or the original velocity upon projection. Velocity vectors $\mathbf{v}_2$ and $\mathbf{v}_3$ may also be considered as final velocities and may be calculated by the use of the formula developed earlier, namely, $v_f = v_o + gt$.

Displacements

Vertical displacements in equal intervals of time follow the pattern discussed on p. 40 and may be calculated by the use of the formula $d_v = \frac{1}{2}gt^2$ The horizontal displacements over time are obtained from $d_h = \bar{v}_h t$ or $d_h = v_h t$ since the horizontal velocity component is constant. Actual displacement along the path of the moving object is obtained by the vector addition of the horizontal and vertical components, as illustrated in Fig. 4-4.

The locations of a moving object may be plotted on a graph by using the displacement components just discussed. By plotting the magnitudes of one against the other over a series of equal time intervals, the actual trajectory of the motion may be closely approximated, especially when the time intervals are reduced to very small values. The shape of the path or trajectory under these conditions of free fall is known as a *parabola* and represents the relationships between the horizontal and vertical displacement components throughout the motion. Many different parabolic trajectories are traced by human body motions and by the objects they project.

Assume that a tennis ball is stroked with a forehand drive in such a way that it is driven exactly horizontally with an original velocity of 120 ft/sec at a point exactly 4 ft above the court surface.

→ *Calculate horizontal and vertical displacement values for the ball's positions during its flight on the basis of .05-sec time increments until it strikes the court at the end of its flight. Now, prepare a graph which establishes plots of vertical over horizontal displacements using a horizontal scale of 0 to 60 ft in increments of 6 ft and a vertical scale of 0 to 4 ft in increments of 4 in. Connect the plots with a smoothly curving line and note that it represents a reasonable facsimile of the parabolic path or trajectory of the ball in flight.*

Table 4-1 provides some of the information requested.

→ *Complete the table and then plot the information as described above.*

Assuming no aerodynamics, when an object is projected into space at any angle with the horizontal other than at 90 deg, the characteristics of its flight are quite predictable. The background necessary for these predictions has already been presented. With a knowledge of the projection angle with the horizontal and the projection velocity (which, in this case, has a vertical as well as horizontal velocity component), horizontal range, height, and time of flight can be calculated. Figure 4-5 illustrates such a flight path or trajectory for a baseball thrown or projected with a velocity of 80 ft/sec at an angle with the horizontal of 40 deg. Instantaneous velocity vectors are included for each position along the path, always pointing in the direction of the path at that instant (tangent to the path). Horizontal and vertical velocity components under these conditions at the beginning of the motion are seen to be

$$v_h = v_o \cos \theta = 80 \text{ ft/sec} \times .7660 = 61.28 \text{ ft/sec}$$

$$v_v = v_o \sin \theta = 80 \text{ ft/sec} \times .6428 = 51.42 \text{ ft/sec}$$

As can be seen, the positive vertical velocity component gradually diminishes in magnitude up to the half-flight point, where it disappears. The second half of the flight sees a gradually increasing negative vertical

TABLE 4–1

t (sec)	d_v (ft ↓)	d_h (ft →)
.05	.04	6
.10		
.15		
.20		
.25		
.30		
.35		
.40		
.45		
.50		

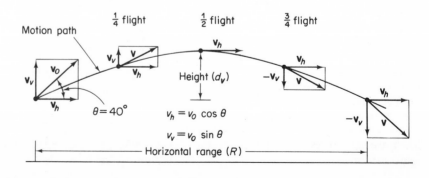

Figure 4–5. Neglecting air resistance, velocity and trajectory characteristics plotted at the beginning, $\frac{1}{4}$, $\frac{1}{2}$, and $\frac{3}{4}$, and return-to-projection levels.

velocity component. Again, the horizontal component remains unchanged throughout the flight.

On p. 41, the formula $d = v^2/2g$ was introduced to calculate the vertical displacement traveled by an object projected directly upward. Under the conditions imposed in Fig. 4-5, the original velocity of the ball, $v_o = 80$ ft/sec, must be reduced to the value of its vertical velocity component which is responsible for the vertical movement of the ball. This is accomplished as shown above and then inserted into the formula $d = v^2/2g$, producing a procedure for calculating the maximum height the object will attain above the level of release to read

$$\text{Height } (d_v) = \frac{(v_o \sin \theta)^2}{2g}$$

The maximal height is reached at the half-flight point. Note that the formula uses the projection velocity (v_o), which is reduced to the value of the vertical component and then squared. When the values are inserted, the outcome is

$$\text{Height } (d_v) = \frac{(80 \text{ ft/sec} \times .6428)^2}{2 \times 32} = \frac{2644.02}{64} = 41.31 \text{ ft}$$

Now that the maximal height is known, the time required to reach this point in space can be easily calculated. The formula $t = v/g$ is again utilized. But, again, the vertical component must be used, therefore altering the formula to read

$$t = \frac{v_v}{g} = \frac{51.42 \text{ ft/sec}}{32} = 1.61 \text{ sec}$$

Since 1.61 sec represents the time required to reach the half-flight point, doubling this value gives the time required for the entire flight where the ball has finally descended to its original projection level, that being 3.22 sec. When it is desirable to calculate total flight time directly from the projection velocity, the formula is altered to read

$$\text{Time } (T) = \frac{2v_o \sin \theta}{g}$$

→ *Use this formula to calculate total flight time again and see if it accurately corresponds to the value calculated previously.*

Since the magnitude of the horizontal velocity component does not change, the formula $d = vt$ may be used to calculate the horizontal displacement to the half-flight point. Insertion of the values produces

$$d_h = v_h t = 61.28 \text{ ft/sec} \times 1.61 \text{ sec} = d_h = 98.66 \text{ ft}$$

Doubling this figure gives the total horizontal range traversed from projection level until the return to that level, or 197.32 ft. When the projection velocity is applied to the calculation of horizontal range, the formula is modified to read

$$\text{Range } (R) = \frac{v_o^2}{g} \sin 2\theta$$

→ *Again calculate the range to satisfy your curiosity that this range formula produces essentially the same result as above.*

It can be seen, by referring again to the table of trigonometric functions in Appendix B, that the maximum sine function is 1 for a 90-deg angle. Since the sine of 2θ is employed in the range formula, maximum range is attained when the projection angle equals 45 deg, where the horizontal and vertical components are equal. All other projection angles, when air resistance is neglected, produce reduced ranges.

Under normal environmental conditions, trajectories of projected objects, particularly those which are small and therefore may be given high projection velocities, are not usually precisely parabolic in shape. Air resistance blunts their trajectories so that the second half of their flight paths are not mirror images of the first half. The objects fail to attain predicted heights and horizontal ranges, depending on such factors as weight, velocity, shape, size, and spin. Many sports implements are designed for the purpose of producing irregular trajectories. Two prominent examples are the table tennis ball and the badminton shuttlecock. For relatively massive, irregularly shaped bodies traversing very limited horizontal ranges, center of gravity paths tend to closely approximate parabolas.

MOTION RESTRICTED TO CIRCULAR PATHS

The discussion of circular motion necessitates a review of displacement. Figure 4-6a illustrates a circle with the angle θ between two radial lines measured in degrees. If the angle is meant to represent the magnitude of the circular motion of an object about an axis of rotation, the illustration is altered to that of Fig. 4-6b, which defines two positions, P_1 and P_2, and the fact that the motion proceeded in a counterclockwise direction about O. The magnitude of $\Delta\theta$ may be considered to be a fractional part of one complete revolution of the object about O. In this case, the fractional part is 45 deg/360 deg or $\frac{1}{8}$ rev. Now the straight-line displacement of the object in space between P_1 and P_2 is given as $\Delta\mathbf{d}$ if P_1 and P_2 are identified by position vectors, $\mathbf{d}_1$ and $\mathbf{d}_2$, and is a vector quantity (Fig. 4-6c). As before, it is independent of the actual circular path traced by the object, S, or *arc length*. Although the angle $\Delta\theta$ between the position vectors may represent the change in position, only very small magnitudes of rotation may be considered to be vectors.

Angular Velocity

Figure 4-6c may also be used to illustrate the *average angular velocity* of the rotating object between P_1 and P_2 if the time over which it occurred is

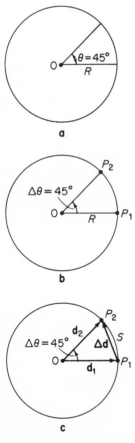

Figure 4–6. (a) Simple angular deviation between radial lines. (b) The same angular value representing an angular displacement along a circular path. (c) Vector description.

identified. If $\Delta t = 2$ sec, the average angular velocity is

$$\bar{\omega} = \frac{\Delta \theta}{\Delta t} = \frac{45°}{2 \text{ sec}} = 22.5°/\text{sec}$$

Even though large values of $\Delta \theta$ are not vector quantities, $\bar{\omega}$ is considered a vector quantity because it has a magnitude and a direction which will not be precisely specified in this discussion. Again, no information is available as to the steadiness of the object's velocity between P_1 and P_2; thus it must be considered an average velocity (using the Greek letter *omega*). The angular displacement, $\Delta \theta$, is then determined from the equation $\Delta \theta = \bar{\omega}t$. However, for rapidly rotating objects, $\Delta \theta$ in degrees of rotation becomes rather cumbersome. Human limbs may develop angular velocities of several thousand degrees per second.

A most useful solution to this problem, and others as well, is to substitute an angular unit, the *radian* (57.3 deg), for degrees. Figure 4-7 illustrates the pertinent numerical information involving the use of radian units. One complete revolution (360 deg) is seen to equal approximately 6.283 rad. The value of 2π also equals approximately 6.283. The circumference of any circle is equal to the product of 2π and its radius. Therefore the actual distance or arc length along a circular path, whose rotational interval is 1 rad, is noted to equal the value of the radius of rotation. The circumference of the circle in Fig. 4-7 is $2\pi R$, or 6.283×3 ft (radius) $= 18.849$ ft. Since the circumference is 18.849 ft and there are 6.283 rad in one complete revolution, the arc length, S, over 1 rad equals 18.849 ft $\div 6.283 = 3$ ft. The table of trigonometric functions in appendix B presents the radian values for each degree through 90 deg.

Radian measures are so commonly utilized to describe circular motion that π is included as follows:

$$180° = \tfrac{1}{2} \cdot 360° = \tfrac{1}{2} \cdot 2\pi \text{ rad} = \pi \text{ rad}$$

$$90° = \tfrac{1}{4} \cdot 360° = \tfrac{1}{4} \cdot 2\pi \text{ rad} = \frac{\pi}{2} \text{ rad}$$

$$60° = \tfrac{1}{6} \cdot 360° = \tfrac{1}{6} \cdot 2\pi \text{ rad} = \frac{\pi}{3} \text{ rad}$$

$$45° = \tfrac{1}{8} \cdot 360° = \tfrac{1}{8} \cdot 2\pi \text{ rad} = \frac{\pi}{4} \text{ rad}$$

When θ is the angular interval and $S = R$ over 1 rad, and the radian is the arbitrarily chosen angular unit, $\theta = S/R$. Note that θ is dimensionless because it is the ratio of two length measures. In addition, it follows that the arc length, S, along the circular path may be calculated from the equation $S = \theta R$, where θ is expressed in radians.

To return to angular velocity, Fig. 4-8 illustrates uniform circular motion through 90 deg or $\pi/2$ rad in a clockwise direction. Instantaneous velocity vectors for P_1 and P_2 are included as $\mathbf{v}_{\theta_1}$ and $\mathbf{v}_{\theta_2}$, respectively. Note their equal magnitudes but differing directions. With constant speed being implied, the average angular velocity over the 2-sec time interval and $\pi/2 = 1.571$ rad yields

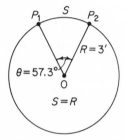

Figure 4–7. One radian equals approximately 57.3/ and the arc length over one radian in any circle is equal to the circle's radius.

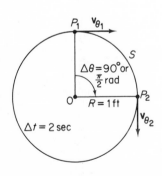

Figure 4–8. Uniform circular motion over π2 radians (90°). Average angular speed equals .725 rad/sec. The symbols used for instantaneous linear velocity vectors include the subscript, θ, to establish that they represent the linear equivalent of angular velocities.

$$\bar{\omega} = \frac{\Delta\theta}{\Delta t} = \frac{1.571 \text{ rad}}{2 \text{ sec}} = .725 \text{ rad/sec}$$

It can be seen that the equation $\bar{\omega} = \Delta\theta/\Delta t$ for average angular velocity is precisely analogous to $\bar{v} = \Delta d/\Delta t$ for average linear velocity. Since speed is constant, instantaneous velocity vectors, $\mathbf{v}_{\theta_1}$ and $\mathbf{v}_{\theta_2}$, have equal magnitudes even though they are not equal vectors. It was shown earlier that arc length $S = \theta R$ and that average angular velocity $\bar{\omega} = \Delta\theta/\Delta t$. It follows, therefore, that *average linear velocity* for rotational motion is obtained from

$$\bar{v}_\theta = \frac{S}{\Delta t} = \frac{\theta R}{\Delta t} = \bar{\omega} R$$

and since the speed is constant, $v_\theta = \omega R$, which stands for *instantaneous linear velocity* for rotational or angular motion. Because these instantaneous velocities are always directed tangent to the motion path, they are always perpendicular to the radius of the circle at that point.

→ *What are the common magnitudes for $\mathbf{v}_{\theta_1}$ and $\mathbf{v}_{\theta_2}$?*

It should be clear that the conversion of angular velocities to their linear equivalents is dependent on the radius of rotation in the same way as was the conversion of angular displacements in radians to their arc length equivalents. *Instantaneous angular velocity*, ω, is obtained, as before, by reducing the time interval over which the average angular velocity is observed to the point where Δt approaches zero as a limit. This is symbolized as would be expected:

$$\omega = \lim_{\Delta t \to 0} \frac{\Delta\theta}{\Delta t}$$

And it follows that instantaneous angular velocity may be obtained from a known instantaneous linear velocity for angular motion by the application of the equation $\omega = v/R$.

Angular Acceleration

Angular acceleration is a characteristic of all circular motion, whether of uniform speed or not. The acceleration demonstrated by objects undergoing uniform circular motion is due solely to the object's continually changing direction. Figure 4-9 illustrates a circular motion of constant speed where two velocity vectors indicate instantaneous linear velocities for angular motion at P_1 and P_2. For simplicity's sake, the angular displacement between P_1 and P_2 again equals 1 rad, or 57.3 deg. The time interval represented is 1 sec, while the radius of rotation is 3 ft. The average angular velocity, then, is 1 rad/sec; the average linear velocity is 3 ft/sec; the angular displacement is 1 rad; and the arc length is 3 ft. Since the speed is constant, instantaneous angular velocities at P_1 and P_2 equal the average angular velocity or $\omega = 1$ rad/sec. By definition,

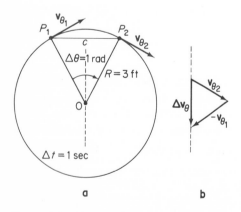

Figure 4–9. Vector subtraction indicates that the change of velocity, $\Delta\mathbf{v}_\theta$, is directed toward the center of rotation (*b*).

average angular acceleration would be represented by

$$\bar{\alpha} = \frac{\omega_2 - \omega_1}{\Delta t} = \frac{\Delta \omega}{\Delta t}$$

(using the Greek letter *alpha*). Since the speed is constant, ω_1 and ω_2 have equal magnitudes, thus suggesting that the acceleration is the result of direction changes rather than magnitude changes. If angular velocity changes during rotation, ω_1 and ω_2 would exhibit different magnitudes. In this case, average angular acceleration would be the result of changes of magnitude as well as changes of direction. Again, as Δt is reduced to zero as a limit, *instantaneous angular acceleration* may be obtained from

$$\alpha = \lim_{\Delta t \to 0} \frac{\Delta \omega}{\Delta t}$$

Angular accelerations may be positive or negative and are indicated as positive when $\Delta \omega$ is positive. When angular accelerations for circular motions show constant magnitudes, equations similar to those described earlier for linear motion may be applied to determine the following:

1. Final angular velocity: $\omega_f = \omega + \alpha t$.

2. Angular displacement when time is known: $\theta = \frac{1}{2}\alpha t^2$.

3. Angular velocity when time is not given: $\omega = \sqrt{2\alpha\theta}$.

With the speed of rotation being constant, the velocity vectors, $\mathbf{v}_{\theta_1}$ and $\mathbf{v}_{\theta_2}$ (Fig. 4-9a), both exhibit magnitudes of 3 ft/sec in their respective directions. If $\mathbf{v}_{\theta_1}$ and $\mathbf{v}_{\theta_2}$ were separated from Fig. 4-9a to be combined by vector subtraction, the resultant vector, $\Delta \mathbf{v}_\theta$, would approximate the direction of the acceleration vector. Note that $\Delta \mathbf{v}_\theta$ is approximately parallel to the line bisecting the angle θ, indicating that the direction of the acceleration under these conditions must be toward the center of rotation. If the time interval of 1 sec is reduced to approximate zero, the chord, c, would approximate the arc length, S. The instantaneous acceleration thus determined for that point on the circular path would be directed at right angles to the velocity vector (which is tangent to the path at that point) toward the center of rotation. Because this instantaneous acceleration is directed toward the center of rotation, it is designated *centripetal acceleration* and is represented by the symbol a_c. Since centripetal acceleration is always directed toward the center of rotation in uniform circular motion, there can be no acceleration component in the direction of the motion. However, when objects travel circular paths with changing speeds, they demonstrate acceleration components in the direction of the motion as well as toward the center of rotation. The continuation of the discussion of these accelerations will be deferred for a moment.

Figure 4-10 combines Figs. 4-9a and b to illustrate similarities between the vector triangle at P_2 and the space triangle, OP_1P_2. Because the speed of rotation is constant, it can be seen that the magnitude of $\Delta \mathbf{v}_\theta$ is related to the magnitudes of $\mathbf{v}_{\theta_1}$ or $\mathbf{v}_{\theta_2}$ in the same way that the chord, c,

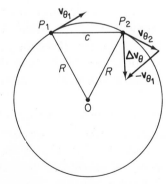

Figure 4-10. Triangles O, P_1, P_2 and $\mathbf{v}_{\theta_2}$, $\mathbf{v}_{\theta_1}$, $\mathbf{v}_\theta$ are similar, showing the relationships of $\mathbf{v}_\theta$ to $\Delta \mathbf{v}_\theta$ and c to R.

is related to the radii of rotation, R. The proportion which results is

$$\frac{\Delta v_\theta}{v_\theta} = \frac{c}{R} \quad \text{or} \quad \Delta v_\theta = \frac{v_\theta c}{R}$$

It will be remembered that acceleration is produced from

$$\bar{a} = \frac{\Delta v}{\Delta t}$$

By substitution, it follows that

$$\bar{a} = \frac{v_\theta c}{Rt} \quad \text{or} \quad \frac{v_\theta}{R} \times \frac{c}{t}$$

Now, when time is reduced to approximate zero as a limit, average acceleration is called instantaneous acceleration, which has just been identified under these conditions as centripetal acceleration. Since S and c are now equal in length, c/t is equal to S/t. And, since $S/t = v_\theta$ along the circular path, it follows that the magnitude of the centripetal acceleration is

$$a_c = \frac{v_\theta}{R} v_\theta \quad \text{or} \quad \frac{v_\theta^2}{R}$$

When angular velocities are used, the formula is

$$a_c = \omega^2 R$$

It will be remembered that v_θ and R are constant during uniform circular motion. Therefore the magnitude of the centripetal acceleration is also constant and always directed toward the center of rotation. The direction of the centripetal acceleration continually changes so that it coincides with the direction of $\Delta \mathbf{v}_\theta$, or perpendicular to the instantaneous velocity vector at any point along the path.

When an object travels along a circular path with varying speed, its instantaneous acceleration vector is at some angle with the velocity vector other than 90 deg. Under these conditions, the instantaneous acceleration vector is seen to have a component along the path as well as having one perpendicular to the path. The acceleration component along the path is in line with the instantaneous velocity vector at that point. Since this is tangent to the path, it is called the *tangential acceleration* and is represented by the symbol a_t.

Figure 4-11a illustrates the movement of a point on the rim of the wheel of a common, stationary *exercycle*. As the wheel is accelerated, its rate of rotation (angular velocity) increases. Velocity vectors for the rotational motion are included at P_1 and P_2 and indicate the direction of the tangential acceleration components at those points. Also, their magnitudes are different, indicating positive acceleration. In Fig. 4-11b, rectangular acceleration component vectors are included for the motion of

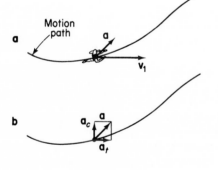

Figure 4–11. The stationary bicycle, whose wheel has undergone accelerated rotation in (a). Instantaneous accelerations are composed of the tangential and centripetal components.

the point on the rim. Note that the tangential acceleration components, $\mathbf{a}_{t_1}$ and $\mathbf{a}_{t_2}$, are in the direction of $\mathbf{v}_{\theta_1}$ and $\mathbf{v}_{\theta_2}$ (Fig. 4-11a), respectively. The centripetal acceleration components, $\mathbf{a}_{c_1}$ and $\mathbf{a}_{c_2}$, point toward the center of rotation. Tangential acceleration is, as would be expected, calculated from

$$a_t = \alpha R$$

It follows that the acceleration components, a_t and a_c, must be combined by vector addition to produce a, the instantaneous acceleration vector for the point on the rim, directed as shown in Fig. 4-11b. The tangent ϕ, for the angle between the centripetal acceleration component vector along the radius and the instantaneous acceleration vector, establishes exactly the direction of the instantaneous acceleration vector with respect to the center of rotation.

NONCIRCULAR PATHS

Human motion is often characterized by curved paths through space which are not circular. When a body part moves along such a path with varying speed, the acceleration vector will point at some angle other than 90 deg from the path at that point. Since the instantaneous velocity vector is always tangent to the path, the acceleration vector forms some angle with the velocity vector in the direction of $\Delta\mathbf{v}$. Figure 4-12a illustrates this situation. Figure 4-12b shows the acceleration vector components, $\mathbf{a}_c$ directed toward the center of an imaginary circle touching the path at the point under consideration, and $\mathbf{a}_t$ directed tangent to the imaginary circle. The change in magnitude of the velocity vector $\mathbf{v}_1$ to become $\mathbf{v}_2$ (Fig. 4-12c) over the next very short time interval is the outcome of the effect of $\mathbf{a}_t$.

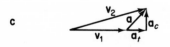

Figure 4–12. The $\mathbf{a}_t$ component is responsible for the change in velocity while $\mathbf{a}_c$ is responsible for the change in direction along the path. The combined change from $\mathbf{v}_1$ to $\mathbf{v}_2$ (including both magnitude and direction) is attributable to $\mathbf{a}$, as seen in (c).

The change in the direction of the velocity vector v_2 from that of v_1 is attributable to the effect of a_c. Their combined effects on v_1 may be claimed for a, producing v_2 from v_1 in that tiny time interval subsequent to v_1.

Objects may move along curved paths, other than circular paths, with constant speed. In this case, instantaneous acceleration is always perpendicular to the path, just as it is in uniform circular motion. But, when the path curves abruptly, the acceleration vector's magnitude increases markedly. When the path's curve varies only mildly, the magnitude of the perpendicular acceleration vector is smaller and more stable over time.

REFERENCES

American Academy of Orthopedic Surgeons. *Measuring and Recording of Joint Motion.* Chicago: The Academy, 1965.

Barnett, Raymond. *Elementary Algebra: Structure and Use.* New York: McGraw-Hill Book Company, 1968.

Cochran, Alastair, and Stobbs, John. *The Search for the Perfect Swing.* Philadelphia: J. B. Lippincott Company, 1968.

Dempster, W. T. "Free-Body Diagrams as an Approach to the Mechanics of Human Posture and Motion." In *Biomechanical Studies of the Musculo-Skeletal System*, edited by F. G. Evans. Springfield, Ill.: Charles C. Thomas, Publisher, 1961.

———— "Space Requirements of the Seated Operator: Geometrical, Kinematic, and Mechanical Aspects of the Body With Special Reference to the Limbs." WADC Technical Report 55-159. Wright-Patterson Air Force Base, Ohio: Wright Air Development Center, July 1955.

Dyson, Geoffrey H. G. *The Mechanics of Athletics.* 4th ed. London: University of London Press Ltd., 1967.

Eckert, H. M. "Angular Velocity and Range of Motion in the Vertical and Standing Broad Jumps." *Research Quarterly* 39 (1968): 937.

———— "Linear Relationships of Isometric Strength to Propulsive Force, Angular Velocity and Angular Acceleration in the Standing Broad Jump." *Research Quarterly* 35 (1964): 298.

Elftman, H. "The Basic Pattern of Human Locomotion." *Annals of the New York Academy of Sciences* 51 (1951): 1207.

Fuller, Gordon. *Analytic Geometry.* 2d ed. Reading, Mass.: Addison-Wesley Publishing Company, Inc., 1962.

Ganslen, Richard V., and Hall, Kenneth G. *The Aerodynamics of Javelin Flight.* Fayetteville, Ark.: University of Arkansas Press, 1960.

Glanville, A. D., and Kreezer, G. "The Maximum Amplitude and Velocity of Joint Movements in Normal Male Adults." *Human Biology* 9 (1937): 197.

Heusner, W. W. "Theoretical Specifications for the Racing Dive: Optimum Angle of Take-Off." *Research Quarterly* 30 (1959): 25.

Hogberg, P. "Length of Stride, Frequency, 'Flight' Period and Maximum Distance Between the Feet During Running with Different Speeds." *Arbeitsphysiologie* 14 (1952): 431.

Hopper, B. "Rotation—A Vital Factor in Athletic Technique." *Track Technique* 15 (1964): 468.

Howard, Ian P., and Templeton, W. B. *Human Spatial Orientation.* New York: John Wiley & Sons, Inc., 1966.

Hummel, James A. *Vector Geometry.* Reading, Mass.: Addison-Wesley Publishing Company, Inc., 1965.

Jones, D. E. H. "The Stability of the Bicycle." *Physics Today* 23 (April 1970): 34.

Kelly, Paul J., and Ladd, Norman E. *Geometry.* Chicago: Scott, Foresman & Company, 1965.

Lanoue, F. "Analysis of Basic Factors Involved in Fancy Diving." *Research Quarterly* 11 (1940): 102.

Lapp, V. W. "A Study of Hammer Velocity and the Physical Factors Involved in Hammer Throwing." *Research Quarterly* 6 (1935): 134.

Owens, M. S., and Lee, H. Y. "A Determination of Velocities and Angles of Projection for the Tennis Serve." *Research Quarterly* 40 (1969): 750.

Phinizy, C. "The Unbelievable Moment." *Sports Illustrated*, 23 December 1968.

Physical Science Study Committee. *Physics*. 2d ed. Boston: D. C. Heath and Company, 1965.

Plagenhoef, S. "Computer Programs for Obtaining Kinetic Data on Human Movement." *Journal of Biomechanics* 1 (1968): 221.

——— "Methods for Obtaining Kinetic Data to Analyze Human Motions." *Research Quarterly* 37 (1966): 103.

Rasch, P. J. "Relationship of Arm Strength, Weight, and Length to Speed of Arm Movement." *Research Quarterly* 25 (1954): 328.

——— and Burke, Roger K. *Kinesiology and Applied Anatomy*. 3rd ed. Philadelphia: Lea & Febiger, 1967.

Selin, C. "An Analysis of the Aerodynamics of Pitched Baseballs," *Research Quarterly* 30 (1959): 232.

Shortley, George, and Williams, Dudley. *Elements of Physics*. 4th ed. Englewood Cliffs, N.J.: Prentice-Hall, Inc., 1965.

Stroup, F. and Bushell, D. L. "Rotation, Translation, and Trajectory in Diving." *Research Quarterly* 40 (1969): 812.

Verwiebe, F. L. "Does a Ball Curve?" *American Journal of Physics* 10 (1942): 119.

5

The Classification of Whole-Body Motion

Specific considerations until now have most often been centered on the motion of particles, those infinitesimally small, idealized parts of a body or object. This was done to simplify the discussion of motion description. The kinematic concepts of position, orientation, displacement, velocity, and acceleration are complex subjects, even when applied to particles. Now, attention will be focused on the motion of whole bodies, which are made up of particles. The discussion will continue to include particles and their motions because they are often useful in the classification of the motion of an object as a whole. It will be remembered that the center of gravity may be used as if it were the most important particle of a body.[1] Its motion may be used to represent the motion of the larger object of which it is a part, a most welcome simplification.

Another idealization, like that of the particle, is the *rigid body*. A rigid body is defined as being made up of a group of particles whose positions in the body remain fixed with respect to one another. Since the positioning of the particles may not be changed, a straight line drawn between any two particles is immune to shortening, lengthening, bending, or other distortions. Although no object or body is perfectly rigid, this kind of description best fits objects made of uniform solids, such as billiard balls and ball bearings, as opposed to objects such as baseballs and tennis balls which are made of composites of materials. The human body, as a whole, certainly does not meet those idealized requirements since it may be distorted in endless ways. However, many of its individual segments may be conceived as essentially rigid bodies because they move as a whole with little observable internal reorientation of their component parts. Therefore, at least for the moment, let the discussion progress with the description of the motion of rigid bodies.

TRANSLATORY MOTION

A rigid body is said to be in *translation* when every straight line between particles of the body maintains its original orientation throughout the motion relative to some reference. In this situation, all particles demonstrate the same displacements over time, which produces equality of particle velocities and accelerations. Figure 5-1 illustrates the movements of a rigid body with respect to a coordinate frame of reference. Assume the object depicted is an ice hockey puck which slides smoothly over an icy surface and upon which two particles are identified and connected by a straight line. As can be seen, translation is depicted, respectively, as producing particle paths which are *rectilinear* (often shortened to *linear*) (Fig. 5-1*a*), curvilinear (Fig. 5-1*b*), and circular (Fig. 5-1*c*). In each case, the orientation of the straight line between the center and edge particles or points remains unchanged throughout the motion for positions P_1, P_2, and P_3. The terms *rectilinear translation*, *curvilinear translation*, and *circular*

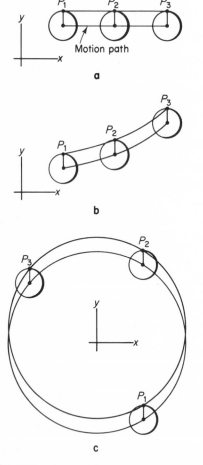

Figure 5–1. Examples of rectilinear, curvilinear and circular translations.

[1]John M. Cooper and Ruth B. Glasgow, *Kinesiology*, 2d ed. (St. Louis, Mo.: The C. V. Mosby Company, 1968), p. 150.

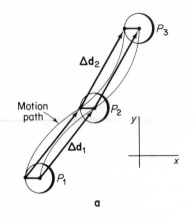

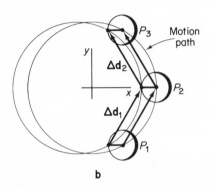

Figure 5–2. Particle displacements are parallel and equal in magnitude in (a) curvilinear translation and (b) circular translation.

translation may be applied to describe rigid-body motion, with curvilinear translation representing any curved path that is not precisely circular. It is not difficult to see that particle displacements are the same in rectilinear translation. The remaining cases of translation along curved paths are less evident and are, therefore, illustrated in Fig. 5-2. Although the particles are seen to trace curved paths through the three positions, displacement vectors constructed between successive particle positions illustrate equality over time. In summary, it can be seen that any particle of a rigid body undergoing translation may specify the motion of all other particles of the body and can, therefore, be said to represent the motion of the object as a whole. In addition, the paths mutually traced by the object's particles may be of any shape.

Translation of Animate Bodies

While rectilinear translation is relatively common for inanimate bodies, animate bodies such as man seldom move truly in such a manner. When they do so, the motion is usually externally motivated, and often the motion is controlled by a *movement guide*. Figure 5-3 illustrates both of these conditions. The body is seen to move on a conveyance (wagon) whose motion path is controlled by a movement guide, in this case the surface over which it rolls. Note that two identifiable parts of the body trace straight-line paths which are parallel and of equal length. It can be seen that the motion was externally motivated by the vigorous push applied by the other boy. Notice also that as long as the seated figure remains absolutely motionless relative to the conveyance, his entire body then demonstrates translatory motion of the rectilinear kind. If he were to move in any way from the illustrated position while moving with the wagon, his motion as a whole would deviate from pure translation. Figure 5-4*a* illustrates another example, this time with the boy sliding down a playground slide (movement guide) with the external motivation provided by gravitation. Bouncing vertically on a trampoline is a good example of rectilinear translation (Fig. 5-4*b*).

The large majority of human motion is motivated internally by muscular contractions across segment articulations. Most whole-body

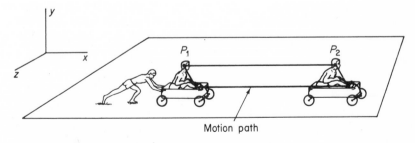

Motion path

Figure 5–3. Remaining motionless, the seated rider is carried through rectilinear translation.

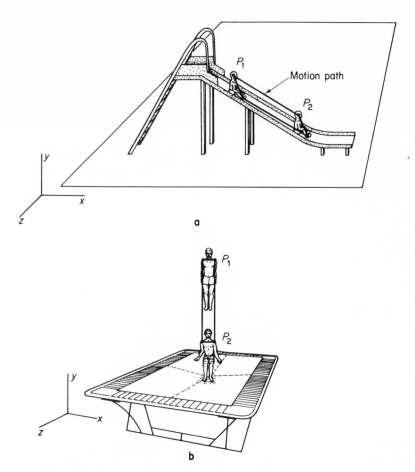

Figure 5–4. Gravitational control of rectilinear translations.

motions are made up of intricate combinations of segment movements whose identifiable parts trace paths in all directions, producing little chance for any consistent orientation of identifiable parts, and with differing velocities. Self-propelled motions such as walking and running are often classed generally as being translatory of the linear kind. In actuality, this classification is but a rough approximation since even the body's center of gravity undergoes marked side-to-side and upward and downward oscillations. Careful observation of man's muscularly motivated motions, whole-body as well as segmental, points out the difficulty he faces in producing true linear motion. Man, under his own motivation, is a producer of curved motion and is hard-pressed to demonstrate linear motion paths even with a single body segment under strict control.

Take, for example, the case when one attempts to draw a perfectly straight line on a flat, paper surface. This is a difficult movement to master, and it is seldom even remotely successful without extensive practice. Of course, if an elevated movement guide is provided such as a straight-edged ruler (the surface of the paper is also a movement guide in the plane of its surface), the task is greatly simplified with respect to the fingers or the pencil held by them. Even without the aid of a ruler, the hand can be made to move the pencil tip quite linearly, but almost never perfectly so.

→ *Using a lined pad of paper, try this simple experiment yourself. As your practice trials progress, the pencil tip's motion deviations from the transverse, printed lines on the paper will be detectable even though they grow smaller in magnitude. First, adjust your writing hand so that it touches the pad surface in a normal writing position and line up your vision from eye-to-pencil tip-to-line near one edge of the paper. Do not touch the paper with the pencil tip. Now slide your hand across the paper so that the pencil tip moves as linearly as possible with respect to the printed line in the background. Be sure to hold your head motionless! With extreme concentration and after careful practice, try actually drawing a straight line on the paper. How can you describe the resulting line? How would you explain the improvement in your movement performance as the result of the aid of a ruler? Does the speed of hand movement affect the outcome?*

At this point, it appears appropriate to mention a word or two about observation perspective. From the observational standpoint, it is most difficult to detect nonlinear motion characteristics in directions along the line of vision of the observer when the object is moving perpendicular to the line of vision. A motion may appear perfectly linear as the moving object passes by the observer from left to right but contain appreciable deviations from the straight-line path *toward* and *away from* the observer without his knowledge of its existence. The observation principle alluded to here is that motion path characteristics which are perpendicular to the line of vision of the observer are most amenable to accurate classification, while those which are oriented along or generally parallel to the line of vision may be obscured because of limited perspective. This basic principle of motion observation will be referred to a number of times as these discussions continue.

It can be concluded, therefore, that truly linear motion is rarely demonstrated by humans under conditions of continuously or periodically applied self-propulsion and under conditions devoid of movement guides. In addition, without the aid of assisting observational devices, the human eye is quite limited in the extent to which it can detect some of a moving object's motion characteristics.

Curvilinear and circular translations of the human body as a whole are generally restricted also to those situations where the body is conveyed by some external system. Generally, the system must provide for some additional means of adjusting the body's position relative to it to meet translation orientation requirements strictly. Figure 5-5*a* illustrates curvilinear translation of the human body as a whole while it is being conveyed through the use of a pulley and cable system like those employed to ford rivers or in obstacle courses for military training. Gravity performs the important functions of motivating the motion as well as maintaining the body's vertical orientation throughout the motion. The rolling pulley and cable system allows all body parts to trace the same curved paths as well as allowing the body to adjust itself constantly to the cable's changing slope to maintain the required orientation dictated by gravity. Figure 5-5*b* illustrates a similar whole-body motion of a diver springing forward and upward from a diving board while maintaining a vertical orientation throughout.

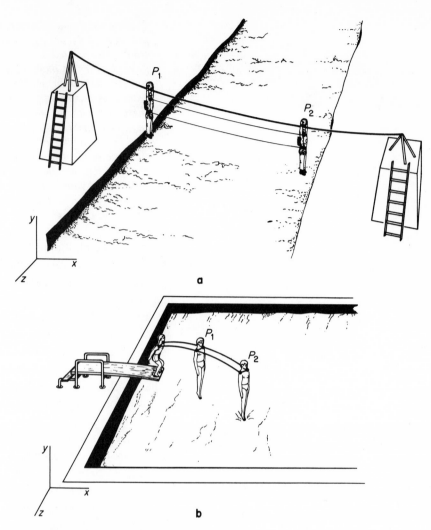

a

b

Figure 5–5. Examples of curvilinear translation.

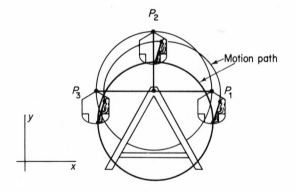

Figure 5–6. An example of circular translation. The identifiable points trace overlapping circles in space.

Figure 5-6 illustrates circular translation of the human body as a whole. It will be recognized quickly that the conveyance is a common ferris wheel whose gondolas are freely pivoted to allow continuous vertical orientation. The seated figure meets the kinematic requirements for circular translation providing no additional swinging of the gondolas takes place beyond that required for vertical orientation. In addition, the seated body must remain motionless relative to the system. It is important to note here that the orientation of the body continuously changes with respect to any radius arm of the ferris wheel which rotates about its central axis. Note also that the circular paths of the identified body parts are not *concentric circles* but are seen to intersect even though they occur in the same plane.

As was the case for rectilinear translation, curvilinear and circular translation of the human body as a whole is quite restricted. The primary reason for this is that the human body is not a rigid body, and as such, it does not easily meet the kinematic requirements for pure translation of any kind. The segmentally arranged body structure of man discriminates against simple descriptions of its motions as compared to simpler rigid bodies, but in so doing, provides for a remarkably wide range of useful motions which have rotation as their foundation.

ROTATORY MOTION

When a rigid body moves in such a manner that a straight line of stationary particles of the body does not move relative to some reference, the body is *rotating* or is in *rotation*. The straight line of stationary particles of the body serves as the axis of rotation about which all other particles revolve to trace circular paths. Although the length of the circular paths differ in proportion to their distances from the axis of rotation, angular displacements are equal over time. Figure 5-7 illustrates the rotatory motion (often referred to as *angular motion*) of a rigid body. The turntable rotates in a clockwise direction around its spindle, which represents the hypothetical straight line of motionless particles or its axis. With the turntable's base representing the reference system, all identifiable particles of the turntable rotate around the axis to trace arcs of circles.

In an attempt to illustrate the differences between circular translation and rotation, the ferris wheel will again be employed. Figure 5-8 illustrates one gondola whose ability to pivot on its frame is completely removed to render it fixed relative to the frame. Note that the gondola maintains a constant orientation relative to the radial arm which is connected to the axis of rotation. It is evident in this case that the circular paths traced by the identified parts are concentric rather than intersecting. The gondola and its rider do not maintain a constant orientation with respect to the external reference. It is obvious that the rider would have to be strapped into his seat under these conditions. This illustration also points out that an object may rotate around an axis outside its own immediate structure.

Returning once again to Fig. 5-8, at position P_1, two lines have been identified. They are the radial arm, *OA*, and the right supporting leg of the

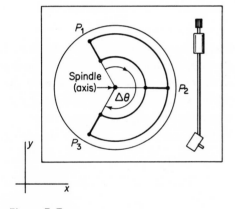

Figure 5–7

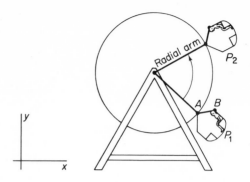

Figure 5–8

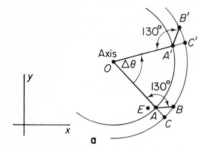

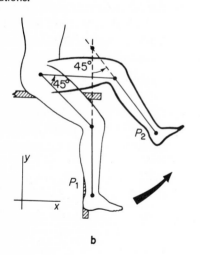

Figure 5–9. By extending *AB* and *A'B'* so that they intersect, the angle formed between them equals $\Delta\theta$. In (*b*) the same procedure allows the measurement of body segment rotations.

gondola, *AB*. In Fig. 5-9, these lines and points have been removed from the ferris wheel structure so that the rotation may be examined in greater detail. Note that the angles *OAB* and *OA'B'* are equal at 130 deg. Delta theta, $\Delta\theta$, represents the angular displacement of the wheel in its entirety during the observation. Arcs *AA'* and *BB'*, as projected on the *XY* plane, are perpendicular to the fixed axis of rotation. This plane is referred to as the *plane of rotation*. If segments *AB* and *A'B'* were extended so that they intersected at point *E*, the angle formed by their intersection would be seen to equal $\Delta\theta$.

→ *Construct these line extensions and determine if this is indeed the case.*

The importance of this relationship is that when line segments such as *AB* and *A'B'* are projected onto a plane which is perpendicular to the axis of rotation of the segments, the angle of intersection of their extensions on the plane specifies the magnitude of the rotation. Figure 5-9*b* illustrates the movement of a pair of body segments which produces motion similar to that shown in Fig. 5-9*a*. By marking and connecting two points (knee and ankle joints), the angular displacements may be determined by measuring the intersection angle.

Rotation of Animate Bodies

Human beings may demonstrate rotatory motion if some way is found to fix the axis of rotation to one position in space. This is no simple task for the whole body when it is self-propelled. One example which is often used to approximate this condition is the rapid spin or pirouette of the ice skater in which the axis of rotation is terminated at the surface of the ice. As was the case for translation, the simplest way to achieve the fixation of the axis of rotation is to have the body moved by some external device, such as a carousel, or to move the body around a fixed axis outside the body, such as the gymnast's horizontal bar.

→ *Sketch a diagram of a person sitting atop a rotating carousel as viewed from above its center. Designate a straight line between two identifiable body parts, and then explain why the body does not demonstrate circular translation.*

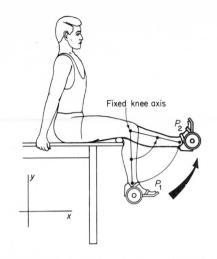

Figure 5–10. Rotation about the knee joint axis, which is essentially fixed to one position in space.

Much greater success is afforded the fixation of the axes of rotation for most of the body's segments. Most skeletal articulations are classed as *axial*, which suggests segment motions which are constrained to rotations when the axes are fixed to one position in space. Figure 5-10 illustrates an example of segment rotation. It is an example of the use of a weighted boot for purposes of muscular rehabilitation under therapeutic guidance. It can be seen that the movement is between the two largest segments of the lower extremity, the thigh and the leg. Points on the leg segment have been identified to represent particles whose paths can be noted. With the leg hanging over the edge of a table, the axis of rotation at the knee joint is essentially fixed to one position. The plane of the rotation is a *sagittal plane*, while the axis of rotation is *bilateral* (refer to Chapter 2 for the application of orientation planes and axes to the human body). As the leg swings forward and upward, the identified points trace arcs of circles in proportion to their distances from the center of rotation. It may be stated, therefore, that the leg as a whole demonstrated rotatory motion. In Part III of this text, it will be seen that a careful study of the anatomical influences on segment motion leads to a much more complex description of the motion illustrated in Fig. 5-10.

If the difficulty of axis fixation is not immediately apparent, try this simple experiment yourself. Refer to Figs. 5-11 and 5-12 in carrying out the procedures outlined below.

→ *1.   Move a table against a wall so that contact is made with the wall near an open doorway. Place a chair in the doorway so that when seated your legs will straddle the door frame. Place a large piece of construction paper against the wall so that its lower border is resting on the table top along the doorway. Attach the paper to the wall with tape. Obtain a pencil and a long piece of twine and be seated in the doorway.*

2.   Place the pencil so that it is firmly positioned at the junction between the index and second fingers of your right hand with your thumb facing toward you. Hold your fingers, hand, and wrist perfectly straight and rigid throughout the motion.

3.   Now place your right elbow on the table so that the forearm is exactly vertical in such a position that the pencil is touching the paper at its border nearest you. The point of contact of the elbow with the table must be directly below the pencil's contact point with the paper.

4.   Without rotating the forearm around its long axis and keeping the pencil horizontal throughout, move the hand forward and downward until it contacts the table top. The motion should inscribe an arc on the paper which generally appears to be circular.

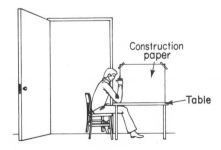

Figure 5–11

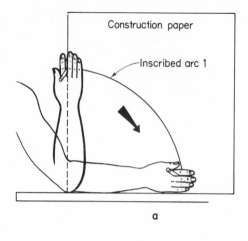
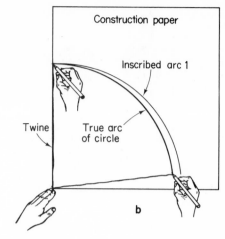

Figure 5–12

5. *Remove the table from the wall. Cut a piece of twine which is longer than the radius of the inscribed arc and tie it securely to the pencil near its tip. Using the point at the bottom of the paper directly below the beginning of the inscribed arc, fix the twine by hand so that the pencil tip again touches the starting point. Keeping the twine taut and the pencil horizontal, use the twine as a compass and inscribe a true arc of a circle through 90 deg.*

6. *Examine the two arcs carefully! If any quite obvious deviations are noted, they are most likely the result of the movement of the axis of rotation of the elbow joint during the motion as the contact point of the elbow rolled over the table top. In which direction did the elbow joint center move? Approximately how far was it displaced in that direction? How would you classify each of the pencil point's motion paths?*

This demonstration simply points out the fact that nearly all of the self-propelled motions of the body, because of axis movement through space and the problems of particle orientation, are not strictly classifiable as either translatory or rotatory. What is obvious is that most human motion is a combination of translation and rotation, a characteristic applicable to all objects whether rigid or deformable.

THE SUPERPOSITION OF TRANSLATORY AND ROTATORY MOTION

To *superpose* is to apply something upon something else. In the present case, the translatory and rotatory characteristics of the motion of a body are examined separately and one is then combined with the other. The example of the rotating forearm given above clearly showed that while the forearm rotated around its elbow axis, that axis was undergoing transla-

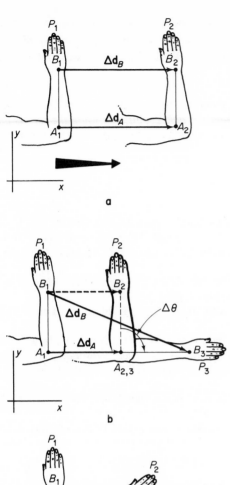

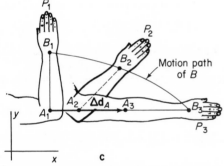

Figure 5-13. The combination of translation and rotation.

tion. For the sake of simplicity, the following discussion will again treat the motion of rigid bodies where translation is limited to rectilinear.

Figure 5-13a illustrates an arm-forearm segment combination which is considered to be rigid. Two points have been identified whose motion paths between positions P_1 and P_2 are linear and parallel. The movement illustrated for the forearm is translatory because the line connecting the two points retains its original orientation relative to the reference throughout the motion. Displacement vectors identify the proper orientation by their magnitudes. Now let point A represent the elbow axis of rotation, perpendicular to the plane of the motion. While the translation of the elbow joint takes place from A_1 to A_2, suppose the forearm rotates about A through 90 deg in a clockwise direction. As can be seen in Fig. 5-13b, when the segment arrives at P_3, its position has changed from that indicated as P_2. The displacement vectors for the two points are seen to differ in magnitude and direction. Therefore the motion of the forearm from P_1 to P_3 cannot be precisely classified as translatory or rotatory since their kinematic requirements were not met.

Among the numerous approaches to the treatment of this problem, three will be discussed. First, the forearm could be said to have undergone rectilinear translation from P_1 to P_2, as illustrated in Fig. 5-13a and b. At this point, the clockwise rotation of 90 deg about the elbow axis is undertaken to arrive at the correctly oriented position, P_3. A second solution could begin with the rotation taking place with the axis of rotation fixed in position P_1. The rotation is then followed by rectilinear translation of the forearm in its horizontal position to P_3, which is not illustrated but is easily imagined. However, if the motion from P_1 to P_3 were a functional motion of a living human being, the rotation very likely would have occurred to some extent throughout the translation from P_1 to P_3. Figure 5-13c illustrates one possible path for point B in such a situation.

The usual analytical practice is to identify the translation and then superpose the rotational effects. If some photographic technique were employed to sequentially record the limb motion, the path and time characteristics for the various identified points of the limb could be determined with high accuracy. Under these conditions, it would be found that the translations of the joint centers between body segments are almost entirely curvilinear. This should further clarify the statement made earlier that man, under his own internal motivation, is a producer of curved motion.

Steindler[2] has presented a valuable discussion of the transformation of rotatory motions into translatory motion. The reader is encouraged to pursue Steindler's discussion in the source cited in addition to that presented here. If a rod were capable of rotation about either of its ends at different times, the sequential application of these rotations could result in an outcome identical to that which could be achieved by translation alone. Figure 5-14 illustrates the procedure where a negative rotation, $-\Delta\theta_1$, about the fixed axis, $A_{1,2}$, brings about the intermediate position

[2]Arthur Steindler, *Kinesiology of the Human Body Under Normal and Pathological Conditions* (Springfield, Ill.: Charles C Thomas, Publisher, 1955), pp. 64–67.

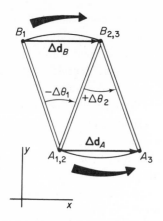

Figure 5–14. Sequential rotations about opposite ends of the rod result in motion which could have been produced by rectilinear translation alone.

$A_{1,2}B_{2,3}$. At this point in time, end $B_{2,3}$ becomes fixed, whereupon a positive rotation, $+\Delta\theta_2$, takes place to produce position $B_{2,3}A_3$. When applied to the human body, the outcomes are remarkably similar to lower limb action in ambulation.

→ *Examine a friend walking in front of you and focus your attention on the leg segment pivoting first about the ankle joint axis while the foot is on the floor and then about the knee joint while the foot is swung forward for the next heel plant.*

REFERENCES

Barnett, C. H. "The Phases of Human Gait." *Lancet* 271 (1956): 617.

Barnett, C. H.; Davies, D. V.; and MacConaill, M. A. *Synovial Joints, Their Structure and Mechanics.* Springfield, Ill.: Charles C Thomas, Publisher, 1961.

Cochran, Alastair, and Stobbs, John. *The Search for the Perfect Swing.* Philadelphia: J. B. Lippincott Company, 1968.

Cooper, John M., and Glassow, Ruth B. *Kinesiology.* 2d ed. St. Louis: The C. V. Mosby Company, 1968.

Eberhart, H. D.; Inman, V. T.; and Bresler, B. "The Principal Elements in Human Locomotion." In *Human Limbs and Their Substitutes,* edited by P. E. Klopsteg and P. D. Wilson. New York: McGraw-Hill Book Company, 1954.

Elftman, H. "The Basic Pattern of Human Locomotion." *Annals of the New York Academy of Sciences* 51 (1951): 1207.

Gowitzke, B. A. "Kinesiological and Neurophysiological Principles Applied to Gymnastics." *Kinesiology Review–1968.* Washington, D. C.: N.E.A. 1968.

Gray, James. *How Animals Move.* Cambridge: The Cambridge University Press, 1953.

Hellebrandt, F. A.; Hellebrandt, E. J.; and White, C. H. "Methods of Recording Movement." *American Journal of Physical Medicine* 39 (1960): 178.

Hicks, J. H. "The Mechanics of the Foot: I. The Joints." *Journal of Anatomy* 87 (1953): 345.

Hildebrand, Milton. "How Animals Run." *Scientific American,* May 1960, pp. 148–53.

——— "Motions of the Running Cheetah and Horses." *Journal of Mammalogy* 40 (1959): 481.

——— "Walking, Running, Jumping." *American Zoologist* 2 (1962): 151.

Hopper, B. "Rotation—A Vital Factor in Athletic Technique." *Track Technique* 15 (1964): 468.

Karpovich, P. V.; Herden, E. L.; and Asa, M. M. "Electrogoniometric Study of Joints." *U.S. Armed Forces Medical Journal* 11 (1960): 424.

Klopsteg, Paul E., and Wilson, Philip D., eds. *Human Limbs and Their Substitutes.* New York: McGraw-Hill Book Company, 1954.

Manter, J. T. "Movements of the Subtalar and Transverse Tarsal Joints." *Anatomical Record* 80 (1941): 397.

Noss, J. "Control of Photographic Perspective in Motion Analysis." *Journal of Health, Physical Education, Recreation* 38 (September 1967): 81.

Palmer, C. E. "Studies of the Center of Gravity in the Human Body." *Child Development* 15 (1944): 99.

Perry, J. "The Mechanics of Walking: A Clinical Interpretation." *Physical Therapy* 47 (1967): 778.

Rubin, G.; Von Treba, P.; and Smith, K. U. "Dimensional Analysis of Motion: III. Complexity of Movement Pattern." *Journal of Applied Psychology* 36 (1952): 272.

Salter, N. "Methods of Measurement of Muscle and Joint Function." *Journal of Bone and Joint Surgery* 37-B (1955): 474.

Shames, Irving H. *Engineering Mechanics—Statics and Dynamics.* 2d ed. Englewood Cliffs, N.J.: Prentice-Hall, Inc., 1967.

Shute, C. C. D. "The Geometry and Kinematics of the Knee Joint." *Journal of Anatomy* 90 (1956): 586.

Steindler, Arthur. *Kinesiology of the Human Body.* Springfield, Ill.: Charles C Thomas, Publisher, 1955.

Stroup, F. and Bushell, D. L. "Rotation, Translation, and Trajectory in Diving." *Research Quarterly* 40 (1969): 812.

Swearingen, J. J. "Determination of Centers of Gravity of Man." *Federal Aviation Agency Report* 62-14 (1962): 37.

Tricker, R. A. R., and Tricker, B. J. K. *The Science of Movement.* New York: American Elsevier Publishing Company, Inc., 1967.

Tyson, Howell N. *Kinematics.* New York: John Wiley and Sons, Inc., 1966.

Winter, F. W. "Mechanics of the Tuck Position in Executing the Forward Three and One-Half Somersault." *Athletic Journal* 45 (1965): 19.

Williams, Marian, and Lissner, Herbert R. *Biomechanics of Human Motion.* Philadelphia: W. B. Saunders Company, 1962.

6

The Classification of Body Segment Motion

The movements which may be performed by body segments have been named to provide a means for consistent identification. Body segment motion is restricted primarily to those special actions consistent with joint structure. The purpose here is not to examine why certain joints allow certain motions, but to introduce the basic, anatomically referenced movement nomenclature which has been developed; pointing out the many difficulties, inadequacies, and special circumstances under which the terminology is applied. It is notable that the segments of the human body may produce such complicated movement combinations that one would expect description nomenclatures of commensurate complexity.

BODY SEGMENTS

For the purposes of this text, the human body will be divided into *eight* functional movement segments or components. These segments are easily identified (Fig. 6-1) from the standpoint of both anatomy and motion. Six of the eight segments come in pairs, with the remaining single segments located *axially* with respect to the body as a whole. The *appendicular* segments, those most easily recognized as appendages, include the *pair of feet*, the *pair of legs*, the *pair of thighs*, and the *pairs of hands, forearms, and arms*. The *axial* segments are the *trunk* and, finally, the *head-neck*.

Simple observations of the movement of man's body segments point up the fact that they differ with respect to their degree of compliance with the requirements for being classified as rigid bodies. Four segments meet these requirements rather accurately because they contain only one bone.

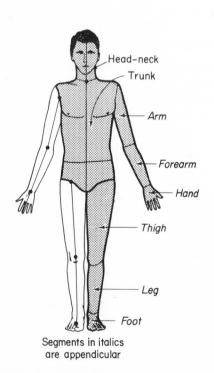

Segments in italics
are appendicular

Figure 6-1. The segments of the human body.

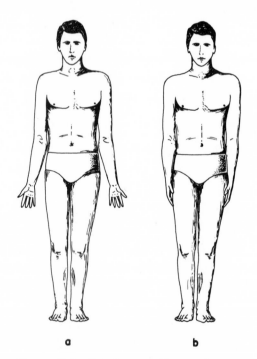

Figure 6-2. Standing positions: (*a*) the anatomical position; (*b*) the fundamental position.

70

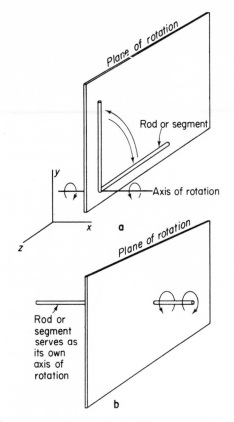

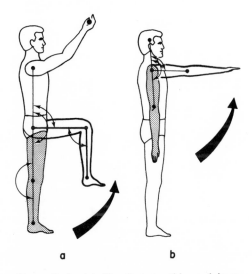

Figure 6–3. Primary modes of rotation of body segments.

Figure 6–4. (a) Simultaneous hip and knee flexion from the anatomical position. (b) Shoulder flexion, showing the reduction of the angle between arm and head-neck segments.

They are the arm and thigh segments, containing the *humerus* and *femur* bones, respectively. Two others, the leg and forearm segments, each contain two bones but differ considerably in the amount of motion available between the bone pairs. The foot and hand segments are made up of numerous bones and their articulations. Therefore they do not meet rigid-body requirements with much strictness. The trunk and head-neck segments are notable for their abilities to be deformed in many ways.

The conventional plan for establishing a coherent movement nomenclature is first to establish a reference system from which the individual movements may be classified. The reference used for this purpose is a standardized body position known as the standing *anatomical position.* As can be seen in Fig. 6-2, this position is described as being that of a standing or erect body which is extended with the feet together, the arms at the sides of the body with the palms of the hands facing forward. This position is very similar to what is known as the *fundamental standing position,*[1] which offers only one alteration from the former—that being the position of the hands facing toward the sides of the thighs. The anatomical position then becomes the anatomical reference for the qualitative classification of body segment motion. Each segment movement class will be described as well as those movements residing within each class as they typically occur.

BODY SEGMENT MOVEMENT CLASSES

There are *six* primary segment movement classes. All but one of these classes, *circumduction,* clearly depend on rotatory motion. They do so in one of the two following ways. The first kind of rotation requires the segment to rotate around an axis at one of its two ends with the plane of rotation traced through space by the segment itself. Figure 6-3*a* illustrates that procedure using rods to simulate segment action. The second kind of rotation occurs around the *longitudinal axis* of the segment, as illustrated in Fig. 6-3*b*. In both cases the axis of rotation is perpendicular to the plane of rotation, but in neither case is the axis of rotation restricted in its position in space, even though each movement will at first be defined as originating from the anatomical position. These rotations may, of course, occur simultaneously.

FLEXION: Flexion refers to bending and is, therefore, not restricted to the operation of a single joint. It is generally a movement in which two adjacent segments change their positions relative to one another so that the angle formed between them is made to decrease in magnitude. One or both of the segments may move to accomplish this change, although it is customary to identify which of the segments moves predominantly on the other. In this way, it is possible to establish which segment's movement is least restricted in the action. The movement is then specified as to the segment intersection or joint in which the movement occurs. Figure 6-4*a*

[1]Katharine F. Wells, *Kinesiology,* 4th ed. (Philadelphia: W. B. Saunders Company, 1966), p. 9.

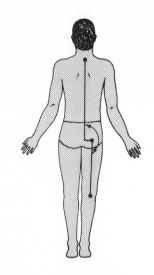

illustrates flexion movements at the knee and hip joints, with each starting from the anatomical reference position. It can be seen in Fig. 6-4*b* that shoulder flexion is illustrated in a side view. This view was chosen so that the head-neck segment could act as the adjacent member of the segment pair. From this view, the decreasing angular magnitude is quite evident, while from other views it is usually not nearly so evident.

Several other kinds of flexion have been identified to meet special descriptive needs. These flexions arise from the need to establish the directional characteristics of the movement. Illustrated in Fig. 6-5 are *lateral flexion*, *radial flexion*, *ulnar flexion*, *dorsal flexion* (*dorsiflexion*), and *plantar flexion*. In Fig. 6-5*a*, the trunk segment is seen to move to decrease the angle between it and the right thigh. Figure 6-5*b* illustrates opposite movements between the hand and forearm segments. Radial flexion refers to the movement of the thumb side of the hand toward the side of the forearm segment where the *radius bone* resides. Ulnar flexion, as would be expected, refers to the opposite side of the hand's movement toward the forearm where the *ulna bone* resides. These designations hold their validity of description with the upper extremity in any position relative

Trunk lateral flexion

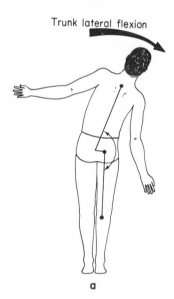

a

Figure 6–5. Special flexions of the trunk, wrist and ankle joints.

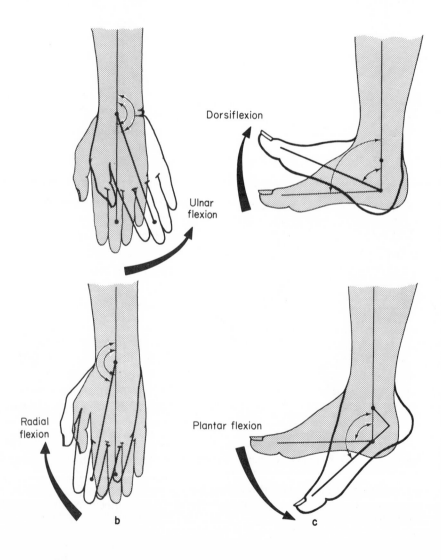

Dorsiflexion

Ulnar flexion

Radial flexion

Plantar flexion

b

c

to the body, as will be covered in detail later in this chapter. Figure 6-5c illustrates special flexions at the ankle joint. They begin from a position which is at right angles with the leg segment in which the foot segment leads the movement with its *dorsal* (upper) *surface* or *plantar* (lower) *surface*. These surfaces then designate the movement sense or direction. Note that dorsal flexion could qualify as a simple flexion movement because it results in a reduction of the angle formed by the leg and foot segments. Plantar flexion represents a special case in which the usual classification requirements are waived in favor of the anatomically referenced term, *plantar*. It will be seen that the plantar flexion movement meets more precisely the requirements for the movement class which follows, *extension*.

EXTENSION: *Extension* refers to lengthening or stretching to a greater length and is generally defined as the return from flexion. In this situation the angle formed between segments is increased. By visualizing the opposites of the movements illustrated in Fig. 6-4, extension movements become apparent. When the moving segments return to the anatomical position, extension is said to be complete. As mentioned above, plantar flexion is, strictly speaking, ankle extension in returning from dorsal flexion to the anatomical position. As will be clearly evident as this discussion continues, the term *flexion* appears to be favored under many others conditions. Figure 6-5a illustrates, at least in part, that not all returns from flexion are called extension. The return from lateral flexion to the right is simply referred to as lateral flexion in the opposite direction or to the left. The remaining parts of Fig. 6-5 also show that the identification of direction is an overriding motivation in the establishment of these movement terms.

It should be made clear at the outset that rigid segment movements such as flexion and extension are, in almost all cases, referred to the joints involved rather than the segments themselves. Occasionally terms such as thigh flexion or forearm extension are used to identify the freer moving segment. This practice should be avoided or used most carefully because in those contexts they imply a bending and stretching of the segments mentioned. This is, of course, not likely to arise very often in rigid segments.

Figure 6-6 illustrates that flexions and extensions may occur within a single segment which is internally flexible. The starting position shown is one of *trunk flexion*, which is the result of the summation of multiple movements in the *vertebral column*. The extension shown is a return to the anatomical position with the increase in the angle illustrated from intersecting lines within the segment itself. Other flexible segments such as the hands, feet, and head-neck also exhibit this tendency toward internal flexion-extension as well as twisting. The many special terms which are applied to specific joint movements within and between segments are discussed in Part III of the text.

It may be stated generally that while flexions tend to shorten segment combinations and flexible segments, extensions function to lengthen them and bring their long axes into alignment. Walking and running are examples of the alternation of shortening and lengthening functions of the

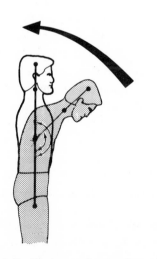

Figure 6–6. Flexion and extension within a flexible body segment.

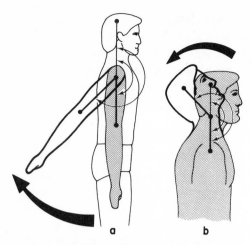

Figure 6–7. Hyperextension of the shoulder joint and head-neck segment.

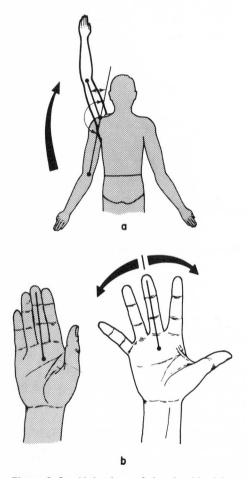

Figure 6–8. Abductions of the shoulder joint and the fingers. Abduction, once begun, maintains that designation even though the segment may finally move back toward the midline of the body, as in (*a*).

lower extremities—shortening when rapid motion is needed and lengthening as a preparation for firm support.

A modification of extension is *hyperextension*. When extension movements are carried beyond the anatomical reference position, the additional extension receives the prefix *hyper*, meaning to exceed. Figure 6-7*a* illustrates hyperextension at the shoulder joint. Flexible segments may also exhibit hyperextension, as illustrated in Fig. 6-7*b*.

ABDUCTION: *Abduction* refers to the movement of a body segment *away* from the midline of the body or body part to which it is attached. Figure 6-8 illustrates abductions at the shoulder joint and the fingers of the hand. Note that in Fig. 6-8*b*, the second finger is designated as the midline part from which the other fingers move away. The hand segment, including the fingers, may perform many intricate movements which do not always conform to the format just described. Although the abduction movements in Fig. 6-8*b* originate at the *metacarpophalangeal joints*, the movement term is applied to the fingers. In the case of shoulder abduction, once the movement of abduction begins, it continues to maintain that designation even after it begins to move inward toward the midline again (Fig. 6-8*a*).

A variation of abduction is that which occurs with a segment or segment combination in a position parallel to the surface upon which the vertically erect body stands. As the segments in Fig. 6-9 illustrate, *transverse abduction* is a movement away from the midline of the body. The use of the word *transverse* here differs from the usual designation of *horizontal abduction*. They are one and the same, where the former designation is preferred because it does not limit its plausible use when the body as a whole is not oriented vertically in space. This situation will be discussed further in a subsequent section of this chapter.

ADDUCTION: *Adduction*, as would be expected, refers to the movement of a body segment or segment combination *toward* the midline of the body or body part to which it is attached. It can be visualized as the return from abduction in the same way extension was the return from flexion. Adduction may continue past the anatomical reference position and still maintain that designation. An example would be the drawing of the arm to and past the midline of the body, a commonly encountered movement of daily living. *Transverse adduction* is a variation of simple adduction which is opposite to that of transverse abduction. Figures 6-8 and 6-9 may be used to visualize this returning action at the shoulder and hip joints, respectively.

ROTATION: When a body segment rotates around its longitudinal axis, the motion is known as *rotation*. This will be recognized as the second of the two kinds of rotatory motion exhibited by body segments discussed earlier. In flexible segments such as the trunk, the rotation is actually a twisting which results from the actions of many individual parts. Rather than applying the name of the joint or joints involved, rotations usually carry the name of the segment. Again, much attention is paid to the

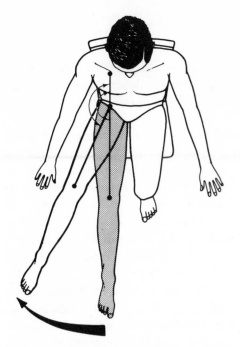

Figure 6–9. Transverse abduction of the hip joint.

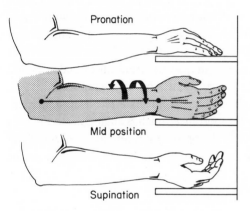

Figure 6–11. Pronation and supination of the forearm.

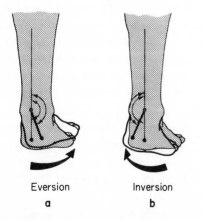

Figure 6–12. Eversion and inversion of the foot.

direction of the rotation relative to the anatomical position. Figure 6-10 illustrates head-neck rotation, arm rotation, and thigh rotation. The rotation shown in Fig. 6-10a is typical of that demonstrated by axial segments. Direction is designated as being to the left or to the right. That which is illustrated is *rotation to the left*. Figure 6-10b illustrates arm *outward rotation*. Figure 6-10c illustrates thigh *inward rotation*.

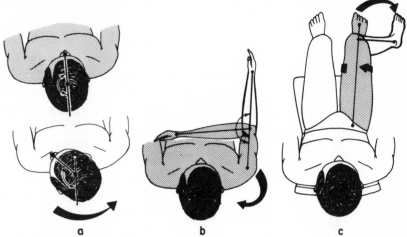

Figure 6–10. (a) Head-neck rotation to the left; (b) Arm outward rotation; (c) Thigh inward rotation.

Two very special terms are applied to the rotations available to the hand and forearm segments. From the anatomical position, inward rotation of the forearm (the hand is carried along) is designated *pronation*. The return to the reference position, outward rotation of the forearm, is given the name *supination*. Figure 6-11 illustrates these two segment movements. The rotation of the foot about its longitudinal axis receives special movement terms which are seldom if ever applied elsewhere. The first is the rotation of the foot which lifts its lateral border to turn the sole or plantar surface outward. As illustrated in Fig. 6-12, the movement is called *eversion*. *Inversion* lifts the medial border of the foot to turn the sole inward. Eversion and inversion cannot take place without some abduction and adduction occurring, respectively. When these movement combinations take place, they are often referred to as pronation in the former case and supination in the latter case.[2]

→ *Try these movements and the combinations of actions will be quite obvious.*

Rotation is also applied to the movements of skeletal parts which are not designated as segments. For instance, the trunk segment contains the shoulder and pelvic girdles. When a specific bony landmark is established as the point whose motion specifies the direction of rotation, the terms

[2]Wilhelmine G. Wright, *Muscle Function* (New York: Hafner Publishing Company, 1962), pp. 91–95.

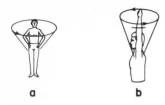

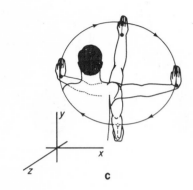

Figure 6–13. Circumductions.

upward rotation and *downward rotation* come into being. Since these are not segment motions, their detailed coverage will be deferred to Part III of the text where specific attention is paid to the structures of motion.

CIRCUMDUCTION: *Circumduction* is a special movement term which implies drawing around. When a segment is moved so that its free end traces a circle in space, the segment itself describes the outline of a cone. Most body segments or segment combinations can be made to demonstrate circumduction to some extent. Figure 6-13 illustrates circumduction for the trunk and arm segments. In Fig. 6-13*a*, the base of the cone is upward with the apex situated in the area of the hips. Figure 6-13*b* illustrates two circumduction movements with the forearm and hand segments carried along with the arm. One is vertically oriented above shoulder level and is of a *narrow-based* kind. The other example is produced in front of the shoulder and is of a *wide-based* kind. Beyond these two designations of base dimensions, no consistent quantitative terminology exists. In addition, no consistent designation of direction is available. To provide a solution to the latter problem, the assumption is made that the direction of circumduction is either clockwise or counterclockwise. The frame of reference is centered on the line of vision originating at the apex and terminating at the base of the cone. Figure 6-13*b* illustrates examples of each within that reference frame. It also illustrates that circumduction movements may produce excellent examples of segment, circular translation.

The kinesiology student is encouraged to spend an extended period of time in the observation and demonstration-upon-command of the segment movements just described. Their immediate recall upon demonstration, and vice versa, is of an importance which is analogous to the time savings which accrue as a result of the *overlearning* applied to spelling and multiplication tables early in one's schooling. To be correct is to be expected. To be quickly correct is to have gained the advantage of the truly skilled.

THE DESCRIPTION OF SEGMENT POSITIONS

Since motion is described on the basis of changing positions, and those positions are described in quantitative terms relative to some reference, it is now time to approach the description of the positions of the human body in a somewhat similar manner. This approach immediately establishes a need for a differentiation between motion and position descriptions. It will be remembered that all of the movements illustrated thus far in this chapter have been simulated by the use of sequential images (positions) which imply the motion which occurred between them. In every case, a starting position was evident from which the movement progressed through the subsequent images (positions), assisted by the application of arrows to establish the direction or sense of the movement. The illustrations then functioned to portray body motion.

An illustration of a body position should portray no movement at all.

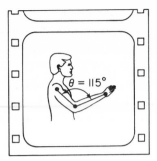

Figure 6–14

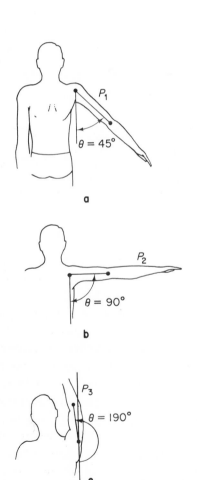

Figure 6–15. Quantitative position information to specify the motion between them.

The anatomical position serves as a good example. When it was described on p. 71, absolutely no allusion was made as to the movements required to attain the position. The anatomical position simply represents a fixed position whose characteristics may be described without regard to motion of any sort. Any method of body position description must recognize this *absence* of motion. This is difficult to achieve completely because of the practice of using movement terminology for position description. Although this is so, these terms *do not necessarily* specify the actual movements which were used to reach the positions under study. Figure 6-14 illustrates an example: one frame from a series of frames which was obtained with the aid of a motion picture camera. The assumption here is that a movement of the right, upper extremity was photographed. The movement itself is irrelevant at this time. What *is* important is that this single exposure has fixed the motion at one instant in time, giving a detailed, clearly defined image of a position of the arm-forearm combination. If the preceding and following frames are not available for study, there is very little or no information concerning the movement which was photographed. The task then is to describe the position illustrated in that single frame so that any sequential composite of individually described positions would specify the movement of which the positions are a part.

Let our attention be focused upon the elbow joint in Fig. 6-14 for the sake of simplicity. In addition, and for the purpose of position description, let the term *elbow* stand for the elbow joint. Moreover, let the same convention apply to all other joints under position consideration. Two relationships are then identified. The *qualitative relationship* between the two segments is identified as a *position of elbow flexion* or, alternatively, a *flexed position*. Both descriptions are correct, with the latter exceeding the former in speech usage and facility. For this reason, it is incorporated here as the procedure of choice. Neither procedure implies in any way that the position was attained as the result of an elbow flexion movement. It is entirely possible that the movement which was photographed was one of elbow extension. Next, the *quantitative relationship* between the two segments is identified as the angle subtended by the segments—in this case, 115 deg.

Figure 6-15*a* illustrates another position, which shows the shoulder to be in an abducted position, 45 deg. Note that the angle is measured from a line constructed through the joint center which simulates the segment's place in the anatomical position. Figure 6-15*b* and *c* illustrates additional positions of shoulder abduction, that is, 90 and 190 deg, respectively. It is now clear that the sequence of positions (*a, b, c*) specifies a shoulder abduction movement through

$$(P_2 - P_1) + (P_3 - P_2) = (90° - 45°) + (190° - 90°) = 45° + 100° = 145°$$

Some movement terms are used far more often than others in position description. Flexion appears to be a favorite, just as it was in movement description. Extension and adduction are examples which are used rather sparingly in position description. Occasionally, a position will be referred

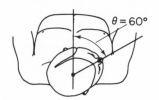

Figure 6–16. Head-neck position—rotated to the right; 60°.

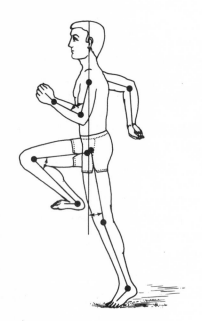

Figure 6–17

to as a position of *full extension* or, simply, *fully extended*. It can be seen in Fig. 6-15 that the elbow joint was maintained fully extended throughout. The anatomical position demonstrates forearm and hand segments which are *fully supinated*. When rotation terms are used in position description, it is customary, as it was in movement description, to apply position terminology to the segments themselves rather than to the joints. The position illustrated in Fig. 6-16 shows the head-neck segment *rotated to the right*, 60 deg.

→ *To provide some practice in position description, describe the positions illustrated in Fig. 6-17 for the right and left ankle, knee, hip, shoulder, elbow, and wrist joints, noting the qualitative and approximate quantitative features. Some of the positions are identified in Table 6-1, but test yourself on each before referring to the table.*

When all observable joint positions have been identified, their aggregate then represents the position of the body as a whole at that instant.

TABLE 6–1

Joint	Ankle	Knee	Hip	Shoulder	Elbow	Wrist	Body Side
Position	Dorsiflexed	Flexed					Left
Approx. angle		50°					
Position	Plantar-flexed		Hyperex-tended		Flexed		Right
Approx. angle			15°		75°		

SPATIAL ORIENTATION OF SEGMENT MOVEMENTS

A typical anatomical approach to body movement is "...the body is always considered erect, the arms by the sides.... The student must use this convention from the outset and think of the subject erect irrespective of its actual position during dissection."[3] This practice is most convenient in terms of the dissection of a lifeless, motionless cadaver. From the standpoint of studying the motion of living human beings, this convention is extremely limiting. The human body spends much of its time in positions other than the anatomical position. In addition, any motion description procedure which is limited to only one reference system is indeed restrictive. Not only must a motion description procedure function in terms of an anatomical reference position, it must also function simultaneously in terms of some spatial reference. The discussion which follows examines both of these functions, integrated so that under most circumstances, few conflicts arise.

[3]R. D. Lockhart, G. F. Hamilton, and F. W. Fyfe, *Anatomy of the Human Body* (Philadelphia: J. B. Lippincott Company, 1959), pp. 1–2.

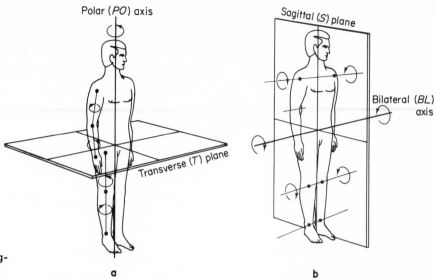

Figure 6–18. Spatial orientation of body segment rotations.

a   b

TABLE 6–2

Movement	Orientation	
	Plane	Axis
Abduction		
Adduction		
Dorsiflexion		
Eversion		
Extension		
Flexion		
Hyperextension	S	BL
Inversion		
Inward rotation	T	PO
Lateral flexion		
Outward rotation		
Plantar flexion		
Pronation		
Radial flexion	F	AP
Supination		
Transverse abduction		
Transverse adduction		
Ulnar flexion		

The longitudinal axes of the segments of the body in the standing anatomical position are seen in Fig. 6-18 to be vertically oriented with respect to the supporting surface with the exception of the foot segments whose longitudinal axes are approximately parallel to that surface. The vertically oriented, longitudinal axes are seen to be parallel to the polar (*PO*) axis of the body as a whole. The horizontally oriented, longitudinal axes of the feet show themselves to be parallel to the anteroposterior (*AP*) axis of the whole body.[4] The planes of segment rotations around the vertically oriented, longitudinal axes in Fig. 6-18a are seen to lie parallel to the transverse (*T*) plane of the body as a whole. The plane of foot segment rotation about its horizontally oriented, longitudinal axis is seen to lie approximately parallel to the frontal (*F*) plane of the whole body. Note that the arrows, which again indicate segment rotations, are used to demonstrate the planes of those rotations.

With the body in the standing anatomical position, most of the primary joint axes of the body are horizontally oriented relative to the supporting surface. Figure 6-18b illustrates this fact for several joints. In addition, they can be seen to lie parallel to the bilateral (*BL*) axis of the body as a whole. The planes of segment movements about these axes are again illustrated with the use of arrows, all of which lie parallel to the sagittal (*S*) plane of the body as a whole.

Movements whose planes of rotation lie parallel to the transverse plane of the body as a whole are said to have a *transverse orientation*. Likewise, segments may also move so that they have *frontal* or *sagittal orientations*. Table 6-2 summarizes the movements discussed in the first section of this chapter relative to their orientation to the standing anatomical position. Keep in mind that the movements included in the table may be identified as such from any viewing position around the erect body.

[4]The reader should refer again to the original discussion of body orientation planes and axes provided in Chapter 2.

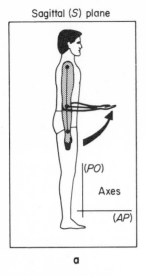

Sagittal (S) plane

(PO)

Axes

(AP)

a

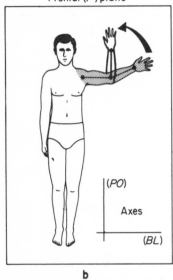

Frontal (F) plane

(PO)

Axes

(BL)

b

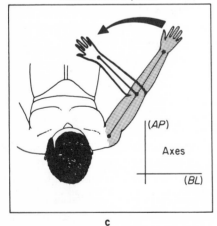

Transverse (T) plane

(AP)

Axes

(BL)

c

Figure 6–19. Elbow flexions that are sagittally, frontally, and transversely oriented.

→ *Complete the table. Choose a partner to demonstrate those movements while you change your position of observation and this will be made clearly evident.*

Since the orientation planes and axes just discussed *move with the body* as it changes its position in space, the segment movements that you have just practiced identifying continue to remain the same.

→ *To establish this fact, again ask your partner to simulate the standing anatomical position with the body lying on its back, face upward, the supine position. Again classify segment movements and notice that their classifications are independent of whole-body orientation in space as long as the anatomical position is simulated.*

When segment movements occur from starting positions other than those which simulate the anatomical position, their anatomically referenced names continue to be used as before. That is, elbow flexion is recognized as such irrespective of the position of the upper extremity in space. The same cannot be claimed for the planes and axes of rotation involved in the movements. Their orientations may change, as is illustrated in Fig. 6-19. It can be seen that elbow flexion need not always be performed parallel to the sagittal plane of the body because the elbow axis of rotation is not restricted to bilateral orientations. Note that the planes of rotation for the three flexions are mutually perpendicular. Figure 6-19*a* illustrates elbow flexion in the sagittal plane. Figure 6-19*b* and *c* illustrate elbow flexions in the frontal and transverse planes, respectively.

To complete the description of orientation with respect to the planes and axes of rotation, the axis of rotation is added. Referring again to Fig. 6-19, it will be seen that mutually perpendicular axes are illustrated as would be expected: the bilateral, anteroposterior, and polar axes. Consequently, the movements depicted in Fig. 6-19 are all given the same anatomically referenced designation of elbow flexion, but each requires a separate and different orientation designation. The addition of their orientations offers much more detail to the description, which markedly reduces the number of possible locations around the body in which the movement can be performed. Again, the use of the abbreviations established earlier can be applied to simplify the movement identifications to this point and are as follows:

1. Elbow flexion: *S, BL*
2. Elbow flexion: *F, AP*
3. Elbow flexion: *T, PO*

Experience has shown that a certain percentage of students finds it easier to identify the axis of rotation before doing so for the plane of rotation. In this case, the plane and axis abbreviations should be reversed in order of presentation. Since the abbreviations for planes and axes differ as to the number of letters used, there should be no confusion in interpretation.

Figure 6-20 illustrates two additional movements. Note that these movements arise from whole-body positions which differ markedly from

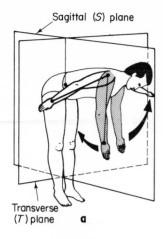

Sagittal (S) plane

Transverse (T) plane **a**

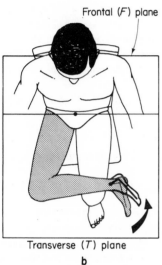

Frontal (F) plane

Transverse (T) plane

b

Figure 6–20. Movements whose orientations are based upon a reference system fixed within the trunk segment.

the anatomical position, yet they bear the same orientations. It can be seen that the orientation of the segment movements is referred to that of the trunk segment. Since the trunk is the largest axial segment of the body and generally acts as the seat of the body's center of gravity, it can serve nicely as the central reference segment for the orientation of segment motion when the body is in complicated positions.

Irregular Movements

It is not difficult to demonstrate segment movements whose planes and axes of rotation do not run precisely parallel to the orientation planes and axes of the body discussed above. Figure 6-21*a* illustrates one example which is known as abduction of the shoulder joint in the plane of the *scapula*. The plane of the motion is oriented about midway between the body's sagittal and frontal planes. Its axis of rotation is oriented horizontally, between the body's bilateral and anteroposterior axes. In fact, much human movement is oriented diagonally to cut across the traditional orientation planes, as in Fig. 6-21*b*. For a general discussion of such diagonal movements, the reader is referred to Logan and McKinney.[5]

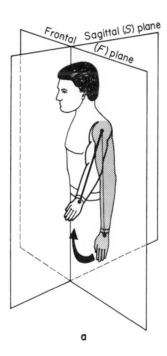

Frontal (F) plane   Sagittal (S) plane

a

Figure 6–21. Oblique movements.

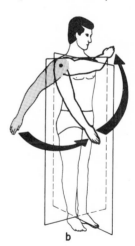

b

Technical approaches to the description of movements as complex as this require the quantitative application of spherical coordinate values and in some cases may lead to the development of entirely new motion nomenclatures.[6] The treatment of these matters is beyond the scope of this text.

[5]Gene A. Logan and Wayne C. McKinney, *Kinesiology* (Dubuque, Iowa: William C. Brown Company, Publishers, 1970), p. 46.

[6]J. A. Roebuck, Jr., "Kinesiology in Engineering," *Kinesiology Review 1968* **1** (1968), 5.

REFERENCES

Adrian, M. J. "An Introduction to Electrogoniometry." *Kinesiology Review–1968* Washington, D.C.: N.E.A., 1968.

Ahlback, S., and Lindahl, O. "Sagittal Mobility of the Hip Joint." *Acta Orthopaedica Scandinavica* 34 (1964): 310.

American Academy of Orthopedic Surgeons. *Measuring and Recording of Joint Motion.* Chicago: The Academy, 1965.

Barnett, C. H. "Further Observations Upon the Axis of Rotation at the Human Ankle Joint." *Journal of Anatomy* 87 (1953): 449.

———— Davies, D. V.; and MacConaill, M. A. *Synovial Joints, Their Structure and Mechanics.* Springfield, Ill.: Charles C Thomas, Publisher, 1961.

Barnett, C. H., and Napier, J. R. "The Axis of Rotation of the Ankle Joint in Man: Its Influence Upon the Form of the Talus and the Mobility of the Fibula." *Journal of Anatomy* 86 (1952): 1.

Cureton, T. K., and Wickens, J. L. "The Center of Gravity of the Human Body in the Anterior-Posterior Plane and its Relation to Posture, Physical Fitness and Athletic Ability." *Research Quarterly* 6 (1935): 93.

Darcus, H. D., and Salter, N. "The Amplitude of Pronation and Supination with the Elbow Flexed to a Right Angle." *Journal of Anatomy* 87 (1953): 169.

Defibaugh, J. J. "Measurement of Head Motion, Part I: A Review of Methods of Measuring Joint Motion." *Physical Therapy* 44 (1964): 157.

Duvall, Ellen Neall. *Kinesiology: The Anatomy of Motion.* Englewood Cliffs, N.J.: Prentice-Hall, Inc., 1959.

Elftman, H., and Manter, J. T. "The Axis of the Human Foot." *Science* 80 (1934): 484.

Eshkol, N., and Wachman, A. *Movement Notation.* London: Weidenfeld and Nicolson, 1958.

Field, Ephraim J., and Harrison, Robert J. *Anatomical Terms: Their Origin and Derivation.* 2d ed. Cambridge: W. Heffer, 1947.

Gollnick, P. D., and Karpovich, P. V. "Electrogniometric Study of Locomotion and of Some Athletic Movements." *Research Quarterly* 35 (1964): 357.

Hellebrandt, F. A.; Hellebrandt, E. J.; and White C. H. "Methods of Recording Movement." *American Journal of Physical Medicine* 39 (1960): 178.

Hellebrandt, F. A.; Tepper, R. H.; Brown, G. L.; and Elliot, M. C. "The Location of the Cardinal Anatomical Orientation Planes Passing Through the Center of Gravity in Young Adult Women." *American Journal of Physiology* 121 (1938): 465.

Hirt, S. P. "Joint Measurement." *American Journal of Occupational Therapy* 1 (1947): 209.

———— Fries, C.; and Hellebrandt, F. A. "Center of Gravity of the Human Body." *Archives of Physical Therapy* 29 (1944): 280.

Jones, R. L. "The Functional Significance of the Declination of the Axis of the Subtalar Joint." *Anatomical Record* 93 (1945): 151.

Karpovich, P. V.; Herden, E. L.; and Asa, M. M. "Electrogoniometric Study of Joints." *U.S. Armed Forces Medical Journal* 11 (1960): 424.

Levens, A. S.; Berkeley, C. E.; and Inman, V. T. "Transverse Rotation of the Segments of the Lower Extremity in Locomotion." *Journal of Bone and Joint Surgery* 30-A (1948): 859.

Logan, Gene A., and McKinney, Wayne C. *Kinesiology.* Dubuque, Iowa: Wm. C Brown Company, Publishers, 1970.

MacConaill, M. A., and Basmajian, J. V. *Muscles and Movement: A Basis for Human Kinesiology.* Baltimore: The Williams & Wilkins Company, 1969.

Mathews, D. K.; Shaw, V.; and Woods, J. B. "Hip Flexibility of Elementary School Boys as Related to Body Segments." *Research Quarterly* 30 (1959): 297.

Moore, M. L. "The Measurement of Joint Motion: Part I. Introductory Review of the Literature." *Physical Therapy Review* 29 (1949): 195.

Murray, M. P.; Sepic, S. B.; and Barnard, E. J. "Patterns of Sagittal Rotation of the Upper Limbs in Walking: A Study of Normal Men During Free and Fast Speed Walking." *Physical Therapy* 47 (1967): 272.

Muybridge, Eadweard, *The Human Figure in Motion.* New York: Dover Publications, Inc., 1955. (First published in 1887.)

Ramsey, R. W.; Norris, A. H.; LeVore, N. W.; Shock, N. W.; Street, S.; Bower, J.; Miller, M. R.; Rosser, R.; and Szumski, A. "An Analysis of Alternating Movements of the Human Arm." *Federation Proceedings* 19 (1960): 254.

Ray, R. D.; Johnson, R. J.; and Jameson, R. M. "The Rotation of the Forearm." *Journal of Bone and Joint Surgery* 35-A (1951): 993.

Roebuck, J. A. "Kinesiology in Engineering." *Kinesiology Review–1968.* Washington, D.C.: N.E.A., 1968.

Saha, A. K. "Zero Position of the Glenohumeral Joint: Its Recognition and Clinical Importance." *Annals of the Royal College of Surgeons of England* 22 (1958): 223.

Salter, N., and Darcus, H. D. "The Amplitude of Forearm and of Humeral Rotation." *Journal of Anatomy* 87 (1953): 407.

Schenker, A. W. "Finger Joint Motion: A New, Rapid, Accurate Method of Measurement." *Military Medicine* 131 (1966): 22.

Scott, M. Gladys. *Analysis of Human Motion.* 2d ed. New York: Appleton-Century-Crofts, 1963.

Steindler, Arthur. *Kinesiology of the Human Body.* Springfield, Ill.: Charles C. Thomas, Publisher, 1955.

Taylor, C. L., and Blaschke, A. C. "A Method for Kinematic Analysis of Motions of the Shoulder, Arm and Hand Complex." *Annals of the New York Academy of Science* 51 (1951): 1251.

Troup, J. D.; Hood, C. A.; and Chapman, A. E. "Measurements of the Sagittal Mobility of the Lumbar Spine and Hips." *Annals of Physical Medicine* 9 (1968): 308.

Wells, Katharine F. *Kinesiology.* 4th ed. Philadelphia: W. B. Saunders Company, 1966.

West, C. C. "Measurement of Joint Motion." *Archives of Physical Medicine* 26 (1945): 414.

Williams, Marian, and Lissner, Herbert R. *Biomechanics of Human Motion.* Philadelphia: W. B. Saunders Company, 1962.

Williams, P. O. "The Assessment of Mobility in Joints," *Lancet* 2 (1952): 169.

Wooten, E. P. "The Structural Base of Human Movement." *Journal of Health, Physical Education, Recreation* 36 (October 1965): 59.

Wright, Wilhelmine G. *Muscle Function.* New York: Hafner Publishing Company, 1962.

Zitzlsperger, S. "The Mechanics of the Foot Based on the Concept of the Skeleton as a Statically Indetermined Space Framework." *Clinical Orthopedics* 16 (1961): 47.

The Motivation and Control of Motion

7

An Introduction to Forces

Starting with this chapter, the focus of attention will shift from the description of motion without regard to how it was made to come about to the consideration of how the value of motion description may be improved by studying the causes of that motion. This is not meant to imply that no mention of these causes was to be found in the preceding chapters. Numerous examples were used without calling any particular attention to their motivating properties as such. Also, it was not intended that the causes of motion should be disguised in any way. Their detailed discussion has simply been deferred until a basic system of motion description and analysis could be introduced as a foundation from which to proceed. As before, the discussions will progress from general principles to their applications to the movement of the human body.

Two of the most ubiquitous causes of motion, and also the most significant for the study of human movement, are *gravitation* and *muscular contraction*. The results of their actions are an unrelenting part of every moment of our lives. Gravitation *acts* to motivate motion when certain conditions are in effect, such as that of nonsupport. This could be stated in another way by substituting the word *forces* for *acts* to say that gravitation *forces* unsupported objects to move. From this substitution comes the realization that motion is the result of the application of forces. In addition, forces may act to control and prevent motion, a combination of functions which is so essential to life in general that it is difficult to think in terms which require an understanding of what results in the *absence* of force. And yet it is precisely that frame of reference which led to some of the most important scientific discoveries in our quest to understand motion.

Man appears to understand how forces function to produce motion because he continually meets with notable success when he uses them. His intuition tells him that forces exhibit themselves as *pushes* and *pulls*. Certainly, we know when we must apply a push or a pull to achieve a desired outcome. Therefore, if we carefully examine the influences of objects on one another, we are struck with the fact that they *interact* in such a way that the outcome specifies the forces involved as pushes or pulls. Sometimes these forces occur without any physical contact occurring between interacting objects. Magnets may *attract* or *repel* each other depending on the orientation of their poles without any actual contact. Muscles contract to pull on bony levers of the skeleton which may transfer the forces externally as either pushes or pulls.

Forces are so much a part of human experience that man creates analogies in other aspects of his life which describe similar reactions between bodies. For example, two individuals may exhibit personalities which are *attractive* and consequently draw them closer together. Conversely, others may find traits in their associates with whom they must interact that are *repulsive*. Our language is filled with terms which describe forceful human interactions that clearly establish our intuitive grasp of the motivating characteristics of forces.

Another clearly understood characteristic of forces is that they are directional in nature. Decisions as to the correct way to *apply* a force are based on directional matters. The gymnast knows when a pulling force is required to move his body closer to the horizontal bar. He also knows when he must push against the vaulting horse to move his body away from that piece of equipment during a vault. These circumstances denote opposite directions with respect to the movements which result as well as the forces which produced them. Obviously, forces are directional in nature, and in combination with magnitudes, they may be classified as vector quantities.

Experience also makes it clear that forces exhibit magnitudes as well as direction. Again, it is the outcome of a force application which often makes this clear. Small individuals are usually disadvantaged when compared to larger persons in attempts to move massive objects. They cannot apply enough force, no matter how well placed or directed the force may be, to compete with the larger and stronger individual. Man has always been fortunate to recognize this relationship between large animals and himself. By utilizing the animal's ability to exert forces of great magnitudes in conjunction with the animal's apparent willingness to do so, early man significantly improved his standard of living. The addition of man's intellect in guiding or directing these great forces renders them useful. The addition of magnitude to direction in force description establishes it as a vector quantity which may be manipulated in the same way as the vector quantities which have been discussed previously. Like those other vector quantities, their usefulness is markedly improved by identifying a point of application. In addition, the combination of point of application and direction of the force vector establishes its *action line* or its location with respect to the object upon which it acts.[1] More will be said concerning this important force characteristic in a later section, but it is clear that man would have met with little success in his marshalling of animal power if he had not discovered the proper means of directing and applying the animal's forces.

Weight

When a person weighs himself on a weight scale, he is measuring the force with which his body interacts with the earth. This interaction (attraction) is said to be directed toward the center of the earth. The magnitude of the force is read from the face of the scale and can be specified in units of *pounds* and fractional parts of pounds. Figure 7-1 illustrates this situation for a child, with the force vector applied to his center of gravity. Note that the action line of the force vector is in evidence relative to the segments of the body and that probable outcomes of the force application may be inferred from inspection. The magnitude of the force is given since there is no scale from which the force vector's magnitude may be obtained. The

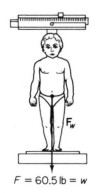

$F = 60.5 \text{ lb} = w$

Figure 7–1. Weight, a vector quantity.

[1]Marian Williams and Herbert R. Lissner, *Biomechanics of Human Motion* (Philadelphia: W. B. Saunders Company, 1962), p. 9.

usual symbol denoting a force vector is **F**, and the force with which the child is attracted to the earth is then referred to as the child's *weight*, **w**. Therefore, weight is a vector quantity.

MASS, A SCALAR QUANTITY

The kinematic concepts of position, displacement, velocity, and acceleration were often described in terms of idealized points or particles for the sake of simplicity. Now that forces have been added to the descriptive picture, it again becomes necessary to consider objects as whole bodies. These whole objects exhibit a characteristic known as *mass*. The concept of a body's mass must be understood before the discussion of forces may continue. In the section just completed, it was pointed out that there is a notable relationship between the forces applied to a massive object and its tendency to move. Larger and stronger individuals were said to have distinct advantages for motivating massive objects when compared to smaller individuals. Somehow, mass and force act as the criterion quantities which control the motivation of motion.

Mass is a scalar quantity since it exhibits no directional characteristics and is said to be the quantity of matter which a body contains. Hence, a massive object exhibits the *property* of a large mass, m, meaning that it contains a large quantity of matter. If two objects were placed on opposite sides of a weight balance, and the balance arm was noted to remain in a horizontal position, as in Fig. 7-2, the quantities of substance in each object would be the same. Therefore, the objects are said to have masses of equal magnitude. The force vectors F_1 and F_2 signify that gravitation exerts equal downward forces on the objects which establishes their equal weights. Since the mass equivalence of the two objects was obtained through procedures like those used for weighing objects, which depend on gravitational attraction, these masses are referred to as *gravitational masses*.

In an earlier section, it was noted that gravity forces objects to fall through space in a predictable manner. The constant acceleration exhibited by the falling object, g, was used to represent the outcome of gravitational attraction on the object. If the objects in Fig. 7-2 were free to fall, they would both exhibit that acceleration. It is obvious, therefore, that mass and weight are uniquely related in some way. That relationship is represented by the equation $m = w/g$. Using this equation to calculate the masses in Fig. 7-2, it follows that

$$m = \frac{w}{g} = \frac{16\,\text{lb}}{32\,\text{ft/sec}^2} = .5\,\text{slug}$$

The *slug* is the unit which is conveniently substituted for the complicated ratio of weight to acceleration units. It follows that if a 16-lb quantity of a substance has a mass of .5 slug, then one slug mass equals 32 lb. To state this in another way which may assist in clarifying the relationship, a mass which accelerates at the rate of 1 ft/sec each second as the result of 1 lb of applied force is called a slug. Since gravitation produces an acceleration

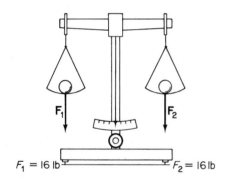

Figure 7–2. Equal gravitational masses.

$F_1 = 16\,\text{lb}$ $F_2 = 16\,\text{lb}$

of 32 ft/sec each second, its force must be 32 times as great as the 1-lb force which produces the smaller acceleration. Now, since the weight of an object is the result of gravitational attraction almost entirely, it is found to be proportional to the mass of the object as is shown by the equation $w = mg$.

FORCE, WEIGHT, MASS, AND ACCELERATION RELATIONSHIPS

Using the equation just introduced, $w = mg$, it is now necessary to clarify several relationships which are essential to an understanding of motion motivation. Four concepts have been touched upon thus far: force, mass, weight, and acceleration. All of the relationships to be discussed are easily within the experience of most people and, surprisingly, are better understood in practical ways than most of us would expect.

Weight is a force and increases or decreases in magnitude in proportion to like changes in mass. It is, therefore, easily understood that massive or heavy objects are difficult to set in motion. Acceleration is a property of motion which was discussed in some detail with respect to gravitation's influence on unsupported objects. The force of gravity (weight) causes those objects to be accelerated in the direction of the force, or toward the earth. Neglecting air resistance, objects of any mass are accelerated in the same manner. The interactions of all of these relationships are summarized by the equation $w = mg$. Since weight is a force, F may be substituted for w in the equation and, similarly, a for g, so that the equation may apply to any acceleration and not just that attributable to gravitation. The equation then reads

$$F = ma$$

Since mass is a scalar quantity and can impose no directional effects, the acceleration vector, **a**, exhibits the same direction as the force vector, **F**, which produces it. The magnitude of the acceleration is proportional to the magnitude of the force. When an object is acted upon by a force whose magnitude is sufficient to move the object, it is accelerated in the direction of the force, and the greater the force applied, the more the object will be accelerated. These relationships describe what happens when a body *is acted upon* by a force and carries the axiomatic name of the *law of acceleration*, or *Newton's second law of motion* to commemorate its originator, Sir Isaac Newton. This principle of motion provides us with the ability to describe forces in quantitative terms, one of the most important abilities in motion description and study.

Figure 7-3 illustrates an example of the application of this principle. Assume that the total weight of the shell, its oarsmen, and oars equals 400 lb. Suppose that in traversing the first 300 ft of the racecourse, the shell's velocity increases from rest to 15 ft/sec in 30 sec. The magnitude of the average acceleration is

$$\bar{a} = \frac{\Delta v}{\Delta t} = \frac{15 \text{ ft/sec}}{30 \text{ sec}} = .5 \text{ ft/sec}^2$$

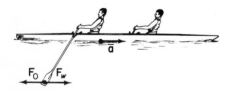

Figure 7–3. Propulsive forces applied to the water result in the shell's forward movement and acceleration.

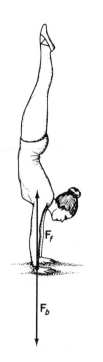

Figure 7–4. Equal and opposite forces resulting from the interaction of the gymnast's body and the floor.

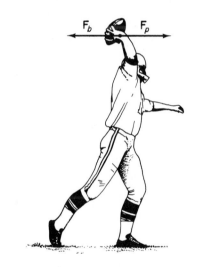

Figure 7–5

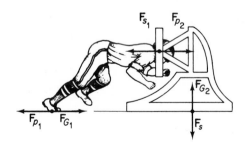

Figure 7–6. Force interactions between three different objects: the player, the earth, and the blocking sled.

The mass of the combined objects is

$$m = \frac{w}{g} = \frac{400 \text{ lb}}{32 \text{ ft/sec}^2} = 12.5 \text{ slugs}$$

It is clear that the propulsive forces of the oars actually were applied intermittently throughout the movement. The magnitude of a continuously acting force which would produce the same outcome over that time interval must be

$$F = m\bar{a} = 12.5 \text{ slugs} \times .5 \text{ ft/sec}^2 = 6.25 \text{ lb}$$

This effective force is the result of the many interactions of the oars being applied to the water. Note that the force vector, $\mathbf{F}_w$, indicates the correct direction (that which is the same as the acceleration) of the motivating force and is the result of the water's reaction to the oars passing through it to push the shell forward.

The example just cited directs our attention once again to the fact that forces are the result of the interaction of material objects and that an object, by itself, will encounter no forces, nor can it bring any to bear. When objects do interact in such a way to exert forces, the forces are of equal magnitude, occur simultaneously, and are applied in opposite directions. This principle has been designated the *law of reaction*, or *Newton's third law of motion*.

In addition to the example contained in Fig. 7-3, numerous others may be given. Figure 7-4 illustrates a gymnast performing a hand balance. Her body exerts a force, $\mathbf{F}_b$, equal to the weight of her body on the floor, and the floor simultaneously presses, $\mathbf{F}_f$, upward in equal measure against her body. Since $\mathbf{F}_b$ and $\mathbf{F}_f$ oppose each other to the same degree, neither the gymnast nor the floor demonstrate accelerations once equilibrium has been established since the net force is zero. Figure 7-5 illustrates a football player passing a football with the force vectors identified. Force $\mathbf{F}_p$ represents the force of the player's body applied to the ball, while $\mathbf{F}_b$ represents the ball's reaction force to the applied force.

Figure 7-6 illustrates another football player pushing against a blocking sled. Force pairs are given for the primary interactions. The player's body interacts with the ground as well as the sled, while the sled interacts with the ground and the player. If the blocking sled were to remain unmoved by the player's actions against it, the system would be in equilibrium with any net force being equal to zero. If the frictional resistance between the sled and the surface of the ground is overcome, the net force which motivates the sled to move or accelerate must equal the product of the sled's mass and acceleration in accordance with $F = ma$. This applies to the athlete as well should his cleats fail to support his effort against the sled.

Inertia

In addition to frictional resistance, applied forces are met with another kind of opposition which is innate to the object itself, namely, *inertia*.

Inertia is defined as the property of an object or body to resist changes in its condition. That is, if an object is still, it tends to remain still; or if moving, it tends to continue moving with uniform velocity in a straight line. It will be remembered that a body demonstrating the condition of being still is said to be at rest, where $v = 0$. When a body is at rest, it tends to remain at rest until acted upon by some external force which is capable of moving it or overcoming its *static equilibrium*. A similar situation applies to moving objects. They tend to continue moving as before until acted upon by an external force to overcome their *dynamic equilibrium*. When summarized, these relationships explain what may happen when forces *do not act* upon a body so that it is left to itself alone. As an axiom of motion, it is given the name, the *law of inertia*, or *Newton's first law of motion*. Since there are no known situations in which forces do not act, this law really implies that applied forces may cancel one another to result in no net force. Because objects react to applied forces of sufficient magnitude to move them by accelerating, and larger objects are less reactive to a given force than smaller objects, inertia and mass are seen to be intimately related. In fact, the relationship is that inertia is proportional to mass. Because of this proportionality, when motion is the result of forces other than the force of gravity, m, in the equation $F = ma$, is referred to as *inertial mass*.

To progress further in the discussion of the effects of applied forces, it becomes necessary to incorporate once again the concept of time. Average acceleration was defined earlier as $\Delta v / \Delta t$. It follows that the change in velocity of a body over time is proportional to the force applied. Figure 7-7 illustrates a notably hypothetical situation in which a disc is made to slide over a flat, frictionless surface under the influence of continuously applied forces of different magnitudes. Alongside the surface is a distance scale in 3-ft increments to indicate the amount of disc travel. Assume that the first force to be continuously applied over a 3-sec observation period was exactly 2 lb. Also, let the mass of the disc equal .25 slug. With the motivating force and object mass given, $F = m\bar{a}$ is applied in the form $\bar{a} = F/m$ to solve for the average acceleration:

$$\bar{a} = \frac{F}{m} = \frac{2 \text{ lb}}{.25 \text{ slug}} = 8 \text{ ft/sec}^2$$

With average acceleration known, disc velocity at the end of 3 sec, v_f, may be calculated from the equation $v_f = \bar{a}t$:

$$v_f = \bar{a}t = 8 \text{ ft/sec}^2 \times 3 \text{ sec} = 24 \text{ ft/sec}$$

The change in velocity, Δv, as the result of the applied force was $v_f - v_o$ = 24 ft/sec. The application of a force of doubled magnitude, 4 lb, results in a change in velocity of 48 ft/sec, in this case producing an acceleration of

$$\bar{a} = \frac{\Delta v}{\Delta t} = \frac{48 \text{ ft/sec}}{3 \text{ sec}} = 16 \text{ ft/sec}^2$$

→ *Calculate the outcome using* $\bar{a} = F/m$. *Are they equal?*

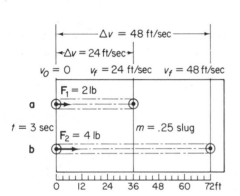

Figure 7–7. Movements in response to continuously-applied forces of different magnitudes, neglecting friction.

The resulting acceleration is proportional to the applied force, with a doubled force producing a doubled acceleration. As would be expected, displacement is also seen to double under these conditions of continuously applied forces as follows:

1. $d = \frac{1}{2}at^2 = \dfrac{8 \text{ ft/sec}^2}{2} (3 \text{ sec})^2 = 36 \text{ ft}$

2. $d = \frac{1}{2}at^2 = \dfrac{16 \text{ ft/sec}^2}{2} (3 \text{ sec})^2 = 72 \text{ ft}$

→ *Calculate displacements under these conditions using average velocity and* $d = \bar{v}t$. *Are the results the same? Calculate the acceleration, final velocity, and displacement for the same disc under the same conditions with the continuously applied force increased to 8 lb.*

The equation $a = F/m$ shows acceleration to be inversely proportional to mass. This certainly appears reasonable from the discussion of the direct proportionality between mass and inertia. Using the same circumstances as shown in Fig. 7-7, Fig. 7-8 illustrates the results of applying the same force to objects of unequal mass, and, therefore, unequal inertia. With the applied force of 5 lb operating continuously for 3 sec on a 2-slug mass,

$$\bar{a} = \frac{F}{m} = \frac{5 \text{ lb}}{2 \text{ slugs}} = 2.5 \text{ ft/sec}^2$$

Thus the displacement which resulted is

$$d = \frac{1}{2}at^2 = 1.25 \text{ ft/sec}^2 \times (3 \text{ sec})^2 = 11.25 \text{ ft}$$

→ *Calculate the outcomes for the doubled mass.*

It is now possible to see that the tendency to resist (inertia), being proportional to the inertial mass of the disc, reduced the acceleration and resulting displacement by one half.

The outcomes depicted in Fig. 7-8 suggest a means for determining inertial mass from a knowledge of acceleration. If a *criterion object* of a known mass is acted upon by a known force, a predictable acceleration will result, the *criterion acceleration*. With this set of specifications at hand, the application of an identical force on an unknown mass will produce an acceleration, *measured acceleration*, which is either smaller than, larger than, or equal to that developed by the *criterion mass*. If the measured acceleration is less than that for the criterion mass, the unknown mass is of greater magnitude than the criterion mass. The exact opposite would apply as well. The proportion used to calculate the unknown inertial mass is based upon the inverse proportionality between mass and acceleration, $m = F/a$, to produce

$$\frac{m}{m_{\text{ct}}} = \frac{a_{\text{ct}}}{a_m} \qquad \text{or} \qquad m = m_{\text{ct}}\left(\frac{a_{\text{ct}}}{a_m}\right)$$

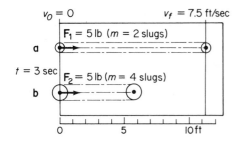

$v_O = 0 \qquad\qquad v_f = 7.5 \text{ ft/sec}$

$F_1 = 5 \text{ lb } (m = 2 \text{ slugs})$

a

$t = 3 \text{ sec}$ $F_2 = 5 \text{ lb } (m = 4 \text{ slugs})$

b

0   5   10 ft

Figure 7–8. Under equal applied-force conditions, the doubled mass results in halved acceleration and displacement.

which reads "the unknown mass is to the criterion mass as the criterion acceleration is to the measured acceleration."

→ *Although these outcomes are obvious from the examination of Fig. 7-8, complete the necessary calculations using the 2-slug mass as the criterion mass to derive the unknown mass (4 slugs).*

Resistive Forces

It is now time to consider how objects move under conditions which could be classified as being normal when compared to those requiring the assumption of frictionless conditions. If a force is applied in opposition to a moving object, the object's motion will be decelerated and will soon come to a halt. Many kinds of opposing forces are constantly at work, such as air resistance and friction. Muscular contractions often act as opposing forces to decelerate body segment motions depending on how and when the forces are applied. More will be said about muscular resistances in a later section. The problem now is to determine some of the characteristics and outcomes of opposing or impeding forces as they are applied to moving objects.

When a body moves through a fluid medium such as water or air, the resistance of the fluid to the movement is related to the velocity of the body. This is not the case for objects sliding over smooth surfaces where the resistive force applied to the moving object is generally constant regardless of the velocity. In a fluid, the resistance varies approximately with the square of the instantaneous velocity of the body and must carry the negative sign in accordance with the negative acceleration which it produces. As the swimmer in Fig. 7-9 glides through the water, his progress is resisted by a continually decreasing amount since his velocity continually decreases. As he pushes against the wall, his velocity is high, as is the magnitude of the water resistance which is applied to his body in a direction exactly opposite to the motion. As he nears the end of his glide, while his velocity may have decreased by a factor of 10, the water resistance has undergone a 100-fold reduction. This tends to explain why the gliding movement persists in inching forward for a prolonged period of time before coming to a complete halt.

In Chapter 4, the sport of sky diving was discussed. It was pointed out that the continual action of the force of gravity increases the velocity of fall to a point beyond which no more acceleration is allowed. This point is reached when the air resistance exactly equals the weight of the falling body. Since these two forces are then equal in magnitude and oppositely directed, a dynamic equilibrium is attained. It has been shown that for an object of irregular shape, like that of a human body, the magnitude of the air resistance is approximately equal to

$$F_R = .01(v_{mph})^2$$

with the resistance expressed in pounds and the velocity expressed in miles per hour.[2]

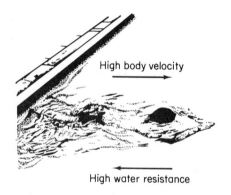

High body velocity

High water resistance

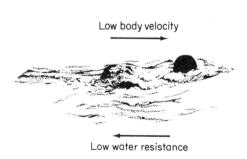

Low body velocity

Low water resistance

Figure 7–9. The water acts to impede the swimmer's glide to a marked degree when his velocity is high and to a continually lesser degree as his velocity subsides.

[2] R. H. Carleton and H. H. Williams, *Physics For the New Age* (Philadelphia: J. B. Lippincott Company, 1947), p. 85.

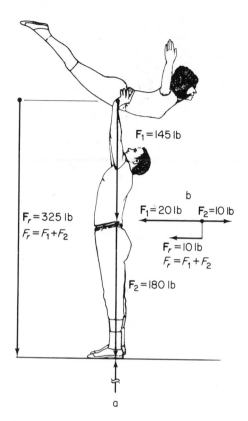

$F_1 = 145$ lb

$F_r = 325$ lb
$F_r = F_1 + F_2$

b

$F_1 = 20$ lb $F_2 = 10$ lb

$F_r = 10$ lb
$F_r = F_1 + F_2$

$F_2 = 180$ lb

a

Figure 7–10

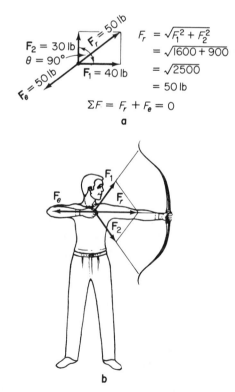

$F_2 = 30$ lb
$\theta = 90°$
$F_r = 50$ lb
$F_e = 50$ lb
$F_1 = 40$ lb

$F_r = \sqrt{F_1^2 + F_2^2}$
$= \sqrt{1600 + 900}$
$= \sqrt{2500}$
$= 50$ lb

$\Sigma F = F_r + F_e = 0$

a

b

Figure 7–11. (a) Composition of two forces acting at right angles to one another. $\mathbf{F}_e$, the equilibrant, is the force which can exactly counter the resultant force, $\mathbf{F}_r$.

→ *Thus, after attaining a velocity of 50 mph, what resistance would the falling body experience? What resistance force would accrue with a doubled velocity of 100 mph? Experiments have shown that about 12 or more sec and 1600 or more ft of fall are required to reach a terminal velocity of about 120–150 mph for objects shaped like humans. Using the 120-mph velocity, what was the approximate weight of the falling body? What general effect would a greater body weight have upon the terminal velocity?*

Earlier in this chapter, it was mentioned that forces, being vector quantities, could be manipulated as position, displacement, velocity, and acceleration vectors were manipulated in previous sections of the text. Since the law of reaction makes it clear that forces cannot exist without object interactions, and when one considers the endless array of objects which populate our world, it becomes clear that systems of forces may exist which range from the very simple to the very complex. The purpose of the following section is to discuss several ways in which force interactions may be analyzed and thus make their effects more meaningful in both quantitative and qualitative terms.

THE COMPOSITION OF FORCES

When two or more forces act on an object at the same point and at the same time, they are called *concurrent forces*. When two concurrent forces are applied to an object with the same direction and action line, as in Fig. 7-10a, their net result may be obtained by computing their sum ΣF. In this case, the sum results from a simple arithmetic addition. The net effect produced by the two performers in the pyramid is a downward-directed force, the *resultant force*, $\mathbf{F}_r$, or the sum of the similarly directed, individual forces. If the carried performer weighs 145 lb and her bearer weighs 180 lb, their combined effect on the supporting floor is 325 lb. With the floor reacting in equal measure and in direct opposition to support the pyramid, the forces are exactly counterbalanced and no motion results. Thus we may say that static equilibrium is apparent since the algebraic sum of the applied forces is zero. Figure 7-10b illustrates another example of forces in opposition, this time of unequal magnitudes and with horizontal action lines. The resultant force is such that the outcome of their concurrent application would result in the object being accelerated to the left to a degree consistent with $F_r = ma$. The motion is then said to be the result of *unbalanced forces*.

Concurrent forces may act on an object at any angle between 0 and 180 deg. The sum of these forces is obtained by vector addition, as was the case for all previous situations. To begin with the simplest example, let two forces be applied to an object at 90 deg to one another in the same plane (Fig. 7-11). The resultant force, $\mathbf{F}_r$, may be construed as being able to produce exactly the same outcome, if it were applied alone, as would the two concurrent forces, $\mathbf{F}_1$ and $\mathbf{F}_2$, combined as shown. The single force which is able to counteract exactly the resultant of the two concurrent forces is called the *equilibrant*, $\mathbf{F}_e$.

→ *In Fig. 7-10a, what force acts as the equilibrant?*

Equilibrant force action is demonstrated by the archer in holding the bow string just prior to release in Fig. 7-11*b*. The equilibrant force is applied to the bow string by the archer's right hand to exactly counteract the resultant of the concurrent forces applied to the hand through the bow string as a result of the bending of the bow. When his fingers release the taut string, an unbalanced force condition results to accelerate the arrow in the direction of $\mathbf{F}_r$.

→ *Calculate the direction of $\mathbf{F}_r$ in Fig. 7-11a as being the angle formed between it and $\mathbf{F}_1$.*

When concurrent forces act upon an object at an angle other than 90 deg, the determination of the net result is more difficult. The example given here, and illustrated in Fig. 7-12, shows two forces acting at 80 deg from one another. By applying a form of the *law of cosines*, the resultant force is calculable. Since the two concurrent forces are of equal magnitude, the resultant force would be expected to act in a direction which bisected the angle between $\mathbf{F}_1$ and $\mathbf{F}_2$. Applying the *law of sines* to compute the angle between $\mathbf{F}_r$ and $\mathbf{F}_1$,

$$\sin \phi = \frac{F_1}{F_r} \sin \theta$$

$$= \frac{30}{45.96} .9848$$

$$= .6420$$

Referring to the trigonometric functions table, a sine function of .6420 is seen to be very close to a 40 deg angle. It follows that the angle β also equals 40 deg.

Muscular forces may be applied as concurrent forces, and very often they are not directed perpendicular to each other. Figure 7-13 illustrates an example of the *triceps brachii* muscle acting across the posterior aspect of the elbow joint. It is seen to be made up of two visible portions which apply forces at 60 deg to one another.

→ *Calculate the magnitude of the result of their concurrent action and the angle with which it acts with respect to $\mathbf{F}_2$. How might an equilibrant force be applied?*

THE RESOLUTION OF FORCES

From the foregoing it becomes clear that two concurrent forces may be composed to result in a single force which could be substituted for them and produce the same outcome. It would seem reasonable, conversely, to

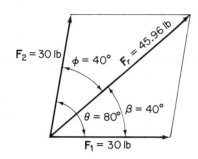

$$F_r = \sqrt{F_1^2 + F_2^2 + 2F_1F_2 \cos \theta}$$

$$= \sqrt{30^2 + 30^2 + 2(30 \times 30) \times \cos 80°}$$

$$= \sqrt{1800 + 1800 \times .1736}$$

$$= \sqrt{2112.48}$$

$$= 45.96 \text{ lb}$$

Figure 7-12. Concurrent forces acting at an angle less than 90° to one another.

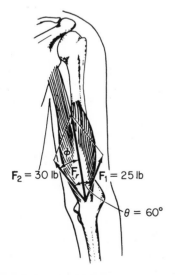

Figure 7-13. Muscular concurrent forces.

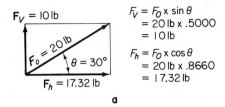

$$F_v = F_o \times \sin \theta$$
$$= 20 \text{ lb} \times .5000$$
$$= 10 \text{ lb}$$

$$F_h = F_o \times \cos \theta$$
$$= 20 \text{ lb} \times .8660$$
$$= 17.32 \text{ lb}$$

a

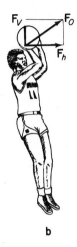

b

Figure 7–14. Resolution of forces.

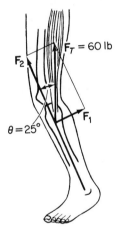

Figure 7–15. Resolving a muscle force into its components.

expect that any applied force could be resolved into at least two concurrent forces. However, it is not customary to refer to these resolved forces as concurrent forces. They are termed *component forces*, which, of course, is consistent with the vector description terminology introduced earlier. Figure 7-14*a* illustrates a simple example of resolution to determine the magnitudes of two rectangular component forces when a force of known magnitude and direction is applied.

The known or original force, F_o, has a magnitude of 20 lb and is directed at an angle of 30 deg with the horizontal. The rectangular component forces, F_h for horizontal force component and F_v for vertical force component, are resolved with respect to the parallelogram. It may be concluded, therefore, that if such an original force were applied to an object with the intent of moving it horizontally, only a part of the force, the horizontal component, would be effective in bringing about that result. Figure 7-14*b* shows a basketball player shooting a jump shot. The horizontal force component is responsible for the ball's horizontal travel, while the vertical force component is responsible for the ball's rise to a greater height than that at release.

If a muscle applied a force, F_T (tension), directed along its length, to a bone, resolution into rectangular component forces would help describe the resulting bone movement. Figure 7-15 depicts a hypothetical situation in which a muscle force is applied to a bone at an angle of 25 deg and with a magnitude of 60 lb.

→ *Calculate the magnitudes of component forces, F_1 and F_2, and describe their tendencies to move the bone.*

The coverage of muscular forces and resulting skeletal movements will be attended to in greater detail in subsequent discussions.

REFERENCES

Alley, L. E. "An Analysis of Water Resistance and Propulsion in Swimming the Crawl Stroke." *Research Quarterly* 23 (1952): 253.

Anderson, T. McClurg. *Human Kinetics and Analysing Body Movements.* London: William Heinemann Medical Books, Ltd., 1951.

Blader, F. B. "The Analysis of Movements and Forces in the Sprint Start." In *Medicine and Sport*, vol. 2. Proceedings of the First International Seminar of Biomechanics, Zurich, August 1967. Basel, Switzerland: S. Karger AG, 1968.

Brining, T. R. "Measuring Air Resistance in Running." *Athletic Journal* 11 (1941): 32.

Buchthal, F. "Factors Determining Tension Development in Skeletal Muscle." *Acta Physiologica Scandinavica* 8 (1944): 38.

Bunn, John W. *Scientific Principles of Coaching.* Englewood Cliffs, N.J.: Prentice-Hall, Inc., 1959.

Counsilman, James E. "Forces in Swimming Two Types of Crawl Strokes." *Research Quarterly* 26 (1955): 127.

——— *The Science of Swimming.* Englewood Cliffs, N.J.: Prentice-Hall, Inc., 1968.

Cureton, T. K. "Mechanics of the High Jump." *Scholastic Coach* 4 (1935): 9.

———— "Mechanics and Kinesiology of the Crawl Flutter Kick." *Research Quarterly* 1 (1930): 87.

———— "Mechanics of the Shot Put." *Scholastic Coach* 4 (1935): 7.

deVries, H. A. "A Cinematographical Analysis of the Dolphin Swimming Stroke." *Research Quarterly* 30 (1959): 413.

Dyson, Geoffrey H. G. *The Mechanics of Athletics.* 4th ed. London: University of London Press Ltd., 1967.

Eaves, G. "Biomechanical Problems in Swimming and Diving." In *Medicine and Sport*, vol. 2. Basel, Switzerland: S. Karger AG, 1968.

Egstrom, G. H.; Logan, G. A.; and Wallis, E. L. "Acquisition of Throwing Skill Involving Projectiles of Varying Weights." *Research Quarterly* 31 (1960): 420.

Elbell, E. R. "Measuring Speed and Force of Charge of Football Players." *Research Quarterly* 23 (1952): 295.

Fenn, W. O. "Frictional and Kinetic Factors in the Work of Sprint Runners." *American Journal of Physiology* 92 (1930): 583.

Ford, Kenneth W. *Basic Physics.* Waltham, Mass.: Blaisdell Publishing Company, 1968.

Fox, M. G., and Young, O. G. "Placement of the Gravity Line in Antero-posterior Posture." *Research Quarterly* 25 (1954): 277.

Ganslen, R. V. "Do Athletes Defy the Law of Gravity?" *Sports College News*, October 1955.

Gaughran, G. R. L., and Dempster, W. T. "Force Analyses of Horizontal Two-Handed Pushes and Pulls in the Sagittal Plane." *Human Biology* 26 (1956): 67.

Gray, J. "Aquatic Locomotion," *Nature* 164 (1949): 1073.

Grombach, J. V. "The Gravity Factor in World Athletics." *Amateur Athlete* 31 (1960): 24.

Heiskanen, W. A. "The Earth's Gravity." *Scientific American*, September 1955.

Henry, F. M. "Force-Time Characteristics of the Sprint Start." *Research Quarterly* 23 (1952): 301.

Henry, F. M., and Whitley, J. D. "Relationships Between Individual Differences in Strength, Speed, and Mass in Arm Movement." *Research Quarterly* 31 (1960): 24.

Hill, A. V. "The Air-Resistance to a Runner." *Proceedings of the Royal Society* 102-B (1928): 380.

Jammer, Max. *Concepts of Force: A Study in the Foundations of Dynamics.* New York: Harper & Row, Publishers, 1957.

———— *Concepts of Mass in Classical and Modern Physics.* New York: Harper & Row, Publishers, 1961.

Johannessen, C. L., and Harder, J. A. "Sustained Swimming Speeds of Dolphins." *Science* 132 (1960): 1550.

Lehrman, Robert L., and Swartz, Clifford. *Foundations of Physics.* New York: Holt, Rinehart and Winston, Inc., 1965.

Little, A. D., and Lehmkuhl, D. "Elbow Extension Force." *Physical Therapy* 46 (1966): 7.

Lissner, H. R. "Introduction to Biomechanics." *Archives of Physical Medicine and Rehabilitation* 46 (1965): 2.

Magel, J. R. "Propelling Force Measured During Tethered Swimming in the Four Competitive Swimming Styles." *Research Quarterly* 41 (1970): 68.

Manter, J. T. "Distribution of Compression Forces in the Joints of the Human Foot." *Anatomical Record* 96 (1946): 313.

Margaria, R., and Cavagna, G. A. "Human Locomotion in Subgravity." *Aerospace Medicine* 35 (1964): 1140.

May, W. W. "Relative Isometric Force of the Hip Abductor and Adductor Muscles." *Physical Therapy* 48 (1968): 845.

Owens, J. A. "Effect of Variations in Hand and Foot Spacing on Movement Time and on Force Charge." *Research Quarterly* 31 (1960): 66.

Patmor, G. "Change Your Terminal Velocity." *Parachutist* 6 (1965): 11.

Payne, A. H. "The Use of Force Platforms for the Study of Physical Activity." In *Medicine and Sport*, vol. 2. Proceedings of the First International Seminar in Biomechanics, Zurich, August 1967. Basel, Switzerland: S. Karger AG, 1968.

Rasch, Philip J., and Burke, Roger K. *Kinesiology and Applied Anatomy*. 3rd ed. Philadelphia: Lea & Febiger, 1967.

Smith, J. W. "The Act of Standing." *Acta Orthopedica Scandinavica* 23 (1953): 159.

Stilley, G. D. "Approximate Theory for Terminal Velocity of a Freely Falling Body." *Journal of Spacecraft* 4 (1967): 1274.

Whitley, J. D., and Smith, L. E. "Velocity Curves and Static Strength-Action Correlations in Relation to the Mass Moved by the Arm." *Research Quarterly* 34 (1963): 379.

Williams, Marian, and Lissner, Herbert R. *Biomechanics of Human Motion*. Philadelphia: W. B. Saunders Company, 1962.

8

Forces
and
Curved
Motion

Our concerns with forces to this point have been with situations where straight-line motions were generally the outcomes. The principles elaborated in Chapter 7 need not be limited to straight-line motion. Our pursuit of the contributions of forces in this chapter will be focused primarily on curved motion situations. To begin these studies, it is necessary to return to the law of inertia once again. Newton apparently stated this principle first to establish frames of reference within which his second law was valid. As noted earlier, an object in equilibrium persists in its static or dynamic condition until acted upon by some external force. Thus a reference frame *devoid* of interaction and, consequently, *devoid* of forces could be envisioned.

It will be remembered that when an elevated object is pushed horizontally into motion, its horizontal velocity component remains constant. The object, within limits, traverses equal horizontal distances in equal increments of time. This outcome of a constant horizontal velocity is very much like the situation devoid of forces mentioned above. Figure 8-1 illustrates these conditions with respect to vertical and horizontal movement scales, with the original velocity ($\mathbf{v}_o = \mathbf{v}_{h_1}$) the result of the horizontal force, $\mathbf{F}_h$. No horizontally directed force is applied to the object after the first push ($\mathbf{F}_h$) is applied. However, the motion is seen not to conform to a straight-line path, indicating the continuous application of a force across the path of motion.

The vertical motion of the projected object shows the result of gravity, $\mathbf{F}_g$, continuously acting to curve the motion path. Since the object traverses increasing vertical distances over equal increments of time, the motion is accelerated. The force of gravity maintains the same magnitude and direction with respect to space throughout the motion. However, its

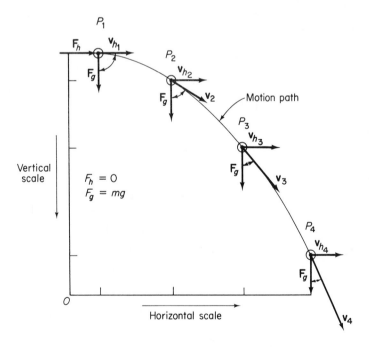

Figure 8–1. Gravity acts continually across the path of motion to curve it downward.

action line, relative to the instantaneous velocity vectors, continuously changes to make the angle between them decrease in magnitude. Only at position P_1 is the action line of $\mathbf{F}_g$ perpendicular to the motion path. Under these conditions, it is evident that the vertical and horizontal motions are independent of each other. It appears reasonable to conclude that for curved motion to take place, some deflecting force must be continuously applied to the moving object across its motion path.

The second law of motion implies that if an acceleration is exhibited by a moving object, a force must exist which produces it. In the foregoing discussion, the horizontal motion was not accelerated but rather exhibited constant velocity. Thus, after the pushing force, $\mathbf{F}_h$, was applied and released, no additional horizontal force acted. The vertical motion was constantly accelerated downward, which specifies the constant downward-directed force which produces it. In addition to increasing the downward velocity of the object, gravity tends to pull the path of motion in line with its own direction. The longer the object falls unobstructed, the closer the direction of the velocity vector, $\mathbf{v}$, approaches that of $\mathbf{F}_g$. The special case of the uniform circular motion serves as an appropriate condition for continuing this line of thought.

CIRCULAR MOTION

In uniform circular motion, the speed of the moving object is constant, while its direction is continuously changing to attend precisely to the circular path. This is a condition of accelerated motion with constant speed without a straight-line motion path as an outcome. Therefore, according to the law of inertia, interaction must be in evidence to result in a force application. The acceleration which is responsible for the continuation of a circular path traversal is the centripetal acceleration, a_c. Under these circumstances, the equation $F = ma$ may be modified to include the centripetal acceleration to read $F = ma_c$. Since the force has the same direction as the acceleration it produces, the result is a force continually directed toward the center of rotation, the centripetal force, F_c. The force equation may be altered again to include the center-directed force to read $F_c = ma_c$.

Figure 8-2 illustrates a somewhat contrived example of the effects of a continuously acting, inward-urging force applied to a gymnast's body while executing one half of a giant swing on a horizontal bar. In actuality, this movement is not uniform in terms of path or speed. However, it will serve our purposes here since it does not deviate to a completely invalidating degree from uniform circular motion. Centripetal force vectors indicate their path-controlling functions through the body to the supporting horizontal bar. Instantaneous velocity vectors at each position illustrated are seen to be perpendicular to those of centripetal force. Hence, the curved motion is again the result of a continuously acting force across the motion path. Since there is no tangential acceleration component, a_t, to

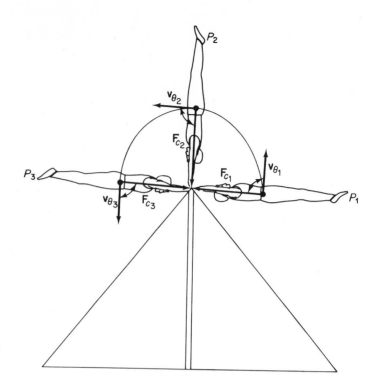

Figure 8–2. Centripetal force, acting to constrain the gymnast's body to a circular path about the bar.

affect a change in speed, the acceleration is due entirely to the centripetal force and its resulting centripetal acceleration.

To provide an example of the calculation of the magnitude of the centripetal force, assume the gymnast weighs exactly 160 lb and that his center of gravity lies 2.5 ft from the bar. In addition, let the constant angular velocity, ω, equal 3 rad/sec. Since centripetal acceleration may be obtained from $a_c = \omega^2 R$, the equation $F_c = ma_c$ may be altered to read

$$F_c = m\omega^2 R$$

With 160 lb equaling a mass of 5 slugs, centripetal force is

$$
\begin{aligned}
F_c &= m\omega^2 R \\
&= 5 \text{ slugs} \times (3 \text{ rad/sec})^2 \times 2.5 \text{ ft} \\
&= 5 \times 9 \times 2.5 \\
&= 112.5 \text{ lb}
\end{aligned}
$$

Using the linear equivalent of the angular velocity, v_θ, for any of the positions depicted, the equation becomes

$$F_c = \frac{mv_\theta^2}{R}$$

Since the linear equivalent velocity is obtained from the equation $v_\theta = \omega R$, the product of 3 rad/sec and the 2.5-ft radius of rotation is 7.5 ft/sec. The outcome is identical to the above, or

$$F_c = \frac{5 \text{ slugs} \times (7.5 \text{ ft/sec})^2}{2.5 \text{ ft}}$$

$$= \frac{5 \times 56.25}{2.5}$$

$$= 112.5 \text{ lb}$$

From the former equation, $F_c = m\omega^2 R$, it can be seen that the centripetal force varies in proportion to the mass of the moving object so that a doubling of the mass results in a doubled force. When the angular velocity is doubled, centripetal force increases four times because it is a function of the square of the velocity. Last, the centripetal force varies in proportion with the radius of rotation so that increases in the radius instigate similar increases in the force, all other things being equal.

→ *Can you see any potential advantages for gymnasts of differing body weights and heights in terms of centripetal force and acceleration in a task such as the giant swing?*

If the gymnast were to release his grasp of the bar at P_2 (Fig. 8-3a), his body would tend for an instant to return to a state of dynamic equili-

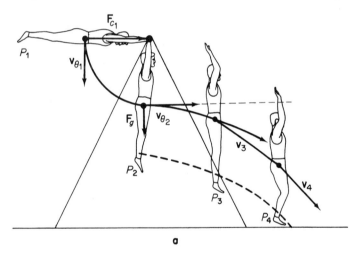

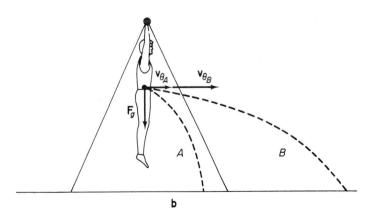

Figure 8–3. Curved motion paths after the dissolution of the centripetal force.

brium and translate in a straight line tangent to the circular path as the result of v_{θ_2}. Actually, under the immediate influence of the force of gravity upon release of the bar (dissolution of $\mathbf{F}_c$), the gymnast's body would tend to translate along a parabolic path like any projectile (interrupted lines). Depending on the magnitude of v_θ at the moment of release, the parabolic path may vary from one which is quite steep (curve A, Fig. 8-3b), indicating a small v_θ magnitude, to one which curves less sharply, indicating a large v_θ magnitude (curve B). In both cases, the downward force of gravity, acting across the motion path, produces a curving tendency which is opposite in direction to that of the centripetal force during the uniform circular motion. A circumstance of real concern to anyone releasing from a swinging movement in such a manner is the tendency for the freely falling body not to conform to pure translation. Most beginners soon learn the importance of the proper positioning and timing of the release to avoid concurrent translation and rotation which could result in the embarrassing and often dangerous outcome of landing on one's back.

CENTRIFUGAL TENDENCY

The question arises as to why an object in sharply curved motion tends to move away from the path on a tangent when the controlling, centripetal force is abolished. When a discus thrower whirls around in the discus ring in preparation for release, he is abundantly aware of the fact that he must pull inward on the discus to counteract a seeming tendency for the discus to pull outward on his body. He perceives this outward-pulling tendency because he is accelerating nearly circularly himself. It appears to the thrower that the discus is acting in opposition to his applied force, the centripetal force, with an equal and oppositely directed force in accordance with the law of reaction. But this is not the case really. He must pull inward on the discus to overcome its tendency to move in a straight line (an inertial tendency) and thus constrain it to the unnatural, curved path. When the discus is released, the centripetal force is abolished, allowing the implement to travel along its natural, straight-line path. The force which was perceived by the accelerating thrower as an outward-urging force has been given the name *centrifugal force*. This force, although of practical significance in movement situations, is not a true force in a real sense. It is a fictitious construct which is used to make the law of acceleration apply in accelerated frames of reference. It should not be conceived as producing the tangent path motion upon release from centripetal restriction.

The force-like tendencies experienced by individuals in curved motion, particularly at high velocity, are countered in several ways. The counteraction is necessary because real centripetal forces are not usually applied to moving bodies in such a way to distribute their effects evenly over the body. The force application usually occurs at the base of support. For instance, when a runner moves around a sharply curved track, centri-

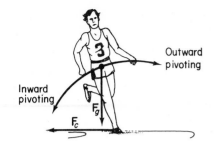

Figure 8-4. The pivoting tendencies in running around curves.

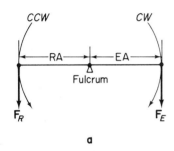

a

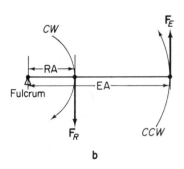

b

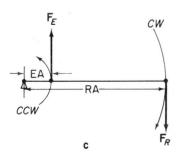

c

Figure 8-5. Lever systems: (a) 1st class; (b) 2nd class; (c) 3rd class.

petal forces in the form of friction act to turn the motion of the lowest part of the body but have little effect above. The rest of the runner's body continues straight ahead, which pivots it outward around the point of contact with the track. One way of reducing this pivoting tendency is to reduce the velocity of travel. Since this tends to be inconsistent with the time criteria underlying running competition, the runner usually chooses to lean toward the inside of the curve where the force of gravity may assist in counteracting the outward-pivoting tendency. Gravity provides an inward-pivoting tendency, as is shown in Fig. 8-4. This maneuver is a common sight in motorcycle racing, where leaning into curves is even more in evidence—so much so, in fact, that the rider uses his inside leg as a brace for the cycle in the event that friction breaks down, abolishing the centripetal action to allow gravity to topple the rider and cycle inward.

A third means of counteraction is to "bank" (tilt) the curve surface so that it faces somewhat inward rather than directly upward. The degree of banking depends on the velocities expected during use. From an anatomical point of view, the muscles of the thighs which apply internal resistance forces to counteract the outward pivoting are often severely taxed and occasionally are injured when they cannot meet the challenge. When one examines the continual development of greater and greater human velocities in racing competition, it would appear reasonable to begin to bank track curves in a manner consistent with the increasing velocities. This practice could also lessen the stabilizing demands placed upon the musculatures of the lower extremities and, conceivably, reduce the chances of muscular injury. Indoor tracks, with their short radii of curvatures, are generally banked for this reason.

ROTATION AND LEVERAGE

The usual outcome of applying forces off center is to produce pivoting or rotation. To begin with the simplest situations, let the discussion now attend to the effects of applying forces to objects which are limited to rotate around some fixed point. A rigid bar or rod which is pivoted around a fixed point is called a *lever*. Actually, a lever need not be limited to barlike objects. Most objects may be used as levers under favorable conditions. The axis about which the lever pivots is called the *fulcrum* and is generally thought to provide a supporting function. When a *lever system* is sketched, the forces acting upon it are included as vectors to indicate direction, action line, magnitude, and point of application. Figure 8-5 illustrates three classes of levers depending on the relative positions of the forces and the fulcrum. Note that the fulcrum symbol used is a small triangle which represents a clearly defined edge point about which the pivoting takes place. The force vectors have been identified as to function, that is, whether they act as a motivating or *effort force*, F_E, or a *resistance force*, F_R. Also note that all force vectors are applied at right angles to the lever.

The distance along the lever to the applied forces specifies the *lever arms*. The *effort arm*, EA, extends from the fulcrum to the effort force,

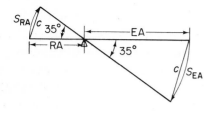

Figure 8-6

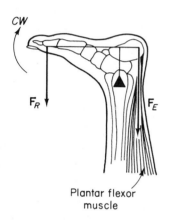

Figure 8-7. Foot and leg segments demonstrating a first-class lever arrangement to produce clockwise rotation of the foot at the ankle joint.

while the *resistance arm*, RA, is the distance between the fulcrum and the resistance force. It can be seen in Fig. 8-6 that the effort arm shows the same relationship to the arc through which it rotates, S_{EA}, as does the resistance arm to its arc of rotation, S_{RA}. Since this relationship exists, it is customary to include the lever arm distances or lengths in calculations of lever action rather than the arc lengths. The condition of equilibrium is met when the product of the effort force and the effort arm equals the product of the resistance force and the resistance arm:

$$F_E EA = F_R RA$$

This relationship holds true only when the applied forces act at right angles to the lever and is termed the *law of moments*. We shall return to this relationship after each lever class has been examined separately.

First-Class Lever

The first-class lever has its fulcrum placed between the two forces which act to pivot the lever. Practical devices of this configuration are the see-saw, balance scale, crowbar, and scissors. If the fulcrum is placed near the resistance force, thus lengthening the effort arm and shortening the resistance arm, the first-class lever may be used to apply great forces, as in the case of the crowbar. When the fulcrum is centered between the two forces, the action is generally in the service of balance.

First-class levers exist in the musculoskeletal system of the body, with the bones acting as the rigid bars upon which muscle forces are applied. Unfortunately, the situation of gaining the advantage of a large effort-to-resistance arm ratio, as with the crowbar, is not available. In fact, the exact opposite is the usual case in most musculoskeletal lever systems. Figure 8-7 illustrates the pertinent information for the first-class lever system at the ankle joint with the leg segment in an inverted, vertical position. As the muscle acts to rotate the foot segment in a clockwise direction, the weight of the resistance arm part of the foot resists that action. Note that the effort arm is considerably shorter than the resistance arm, indicating a rather limited ability to apply force through the lever system.

Second-Class Lever

The second-class lever is seen (Fig. 8-5) to exhibit always a favorable effort-to-resistance arm ratio in that the effort arm is always of greater length than the resistance arm. Probably the most useful of all practical devices of this configuration is the wheelbarrow. It allows the user to apply very great forces to act against formidable resistances. The question arises as to whether or not any second-class levers are truly represented in the human body. The movement of rising onto the toes in the standing position is often offered as a convenient example, although it is strongly disclaimed in some quarters. Needless to say, if there were any in the body, their small numbers would suggest that the human body is not designed to apply great forces through its lever arrangements.

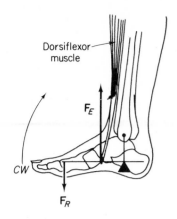

Figure 8–8. Active dorsiflexion of the unsupported ankle joint illustrates a third-class lever arrangement.

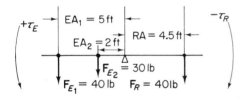

Figure 8–9. When positive and negative torques are equal, a balanced system ensues.

Third-Class Lever

The third-class lever is always burdened by a poor effort-to-resistance arm ratio. The shovel is an example of a lever of this class when the hand nearest the spade end applies the effort force. Only when the effort force is applied near the point of application of the resistance force does this configuration tend to overcome its basic force application disadvantage. However, by applying the effort force near the fulcrum, the advantages of increased range of motion and velocity of motion result. This class of lever abounds in the human body to the point where one must conclude that, from a design standpoint, great force application abilities were sacrificed in favor of increased range and velocity of motion as well as compactness of design. Figure 8-8 illustrates one of the many third-class lever systems in the body. The foot segment is unsupported from below, and again the weight of the resistance arm part of the foot acts to oppose the action of the muscle in dorsiflexion of the ankle joint.

Law of Moments

The tendency of a lever to rotate about a center of rotation or fulcrum is related to both the magnitude of the applied force and the perpendicular distance between the point of application of the force and the fulcrum. The product of the values of these lever elements is termed the *moment* or *torque* of the force and represents the lever's tendency to rotate in response to the applied force. This product is expressed in pound·foot units, with the Greek letter tau, τ, standing for torque. When viewing such a system, it is customary to refer to the counterclockwise rotation tendency as positive and the clockwise rotation tendency as negative. Therefore, and as noted earlier, equilibrium in a rotational sense is met when the sum of positive and negative torques equals zero. Thus the product of effort force and effort arm specifies the *effort torque*, $\tau_E = F_E \text{EA}$; and $\tau_R = F_R \text{RA}$ specifies the *resistance torque*; when they are equal and opposite, $\Sigma \tau = 0$.

Figure 8-9 illustrates a first-class lever system in which the lever arms are of equal length. Assume that the lever is precisely balanced ($\Sigma \tau = 0$) in the illustrated position before any additional forces are applied and that counterclockwise torque is identified as being the effort torque. It can be seen that the sum of positive torques is

$$\Sigma \tau_E = F_{E_1}\text{EA}_1 + F_{E_2}\text{EA}_2 = 120 \text{ lb·ft} + 60 \text{ lb·ft}$$
$$= +180 \text{ lb·ft}$$

while the negative torque is

$$\Sigma \tau_R = F_R \text{RA} = 40 \text{ lb} \times 4.5 \text{ ft} = -180 \text{ lb·ft}$$

Therefore the sum of positive and negative torques is zero and the system is seen to be in equilibrium.

The law of moments applies to each of the three lever classes, and when solving for an unknown quantity, it is desirable to sketch the system in

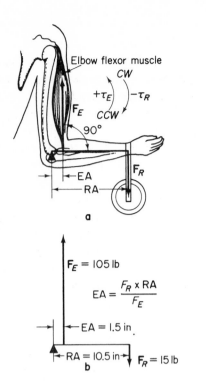

$$F_E = 105 \text{ lb}$$

$$EA = \frac{F_R \times RA}{F_E}$$

EA = 1.5 in.

RA = 10.5 in. $F_R = 15$ lb

b

Figure 8–10. A balanced third-class lever arrangement in (*a*) qualitative terms, and (*b*) quantitative terms.

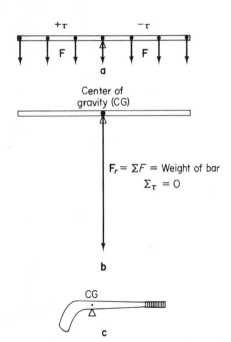

Figure 8–11

diagram form so that the elements of the system are quite clear. Take, for example, the problem of determining an anatomical effort arm length when the three other quantities are known and the system is in equilibrium. Assume the structures involved are an arm-forearm pair in a flexed position, 90 deg, in which the forces acting across the elbow joint are arranged into a third-class lever system. Figure 8-10 illustrates this situation in two ways. Figure 8-10*a* is a qualitative illustration which gives much of the anatomical detail without representing any quantitative information. From it, the third-class lever configuration is evident, as are the torque directions. In Fig. 8-10*b*, a simple line diagram of the system is given, including the quantitative information. We shall disregard the weight of the forearm segment at this point and place the resistance force 10.5 in. from the fulcrum. Note that $\mathbf{F}_E$ has seven times the magnitude of $\mathbf{F}_R$, and because the system is in equilibrium, we would expect RA to be seven times the length of EA.

→ *Is this the case? Satisfy your curiosity that $\Sigma \tau = 0$. What is the effect of the poor effort-to-resistance arm ratio?*

→ *For practice, use the diagram in Fig. 8-10b as a model for solving the following problems. How much flexor muscle force, F_E, is required for a woman to hold her forearm segment perfectly still in its horizontal position if F_R is supplied by a handbag weighing 10 lb which is hung by a strap over her forearm 8 in. from the joint center? Now, suppose she has held the handbag in this position for some time and is becoming fatigued. Which way should she slide the handbag's strap to lessen the demand on the elbow flexor muscles? What flexor force would be required if the handbag applied its force 3 in. from the joint center? What has happened to the poor effort-to-resistance arm ratio of the third-class lever system? Try your hand at solving for other elements of the lever system and do so within other lever classes.*

None of the situations discussed thus far have taken into account the torque-producing effects of the body segment itself. To do this, an introduction to the concept of the center of gravity must first be undertaken. In Fig. 8-9, we saw three forces acting on the lever, all of which had parallel action lines. The torques exerted by these parallel forces were seen to result in a condition of equilibrium. It was noted that the lever itself was perfectly balanced over the fulcrum before the other forces were added. Figure 8-11*a* shows a balanced, symmetrical rigid bar with force vectors equally distributed on either side of the fulcrum to indicate that each of its constituent parts exerts equal downward forces in response to gravitational attraction. The net effect or resultant of the individual forces in Fig. 8-11*b* is a single force, $\Sigma \mathbf{F}$, equal to the weight of the bar. The action line of this resultant force, $\mathbf{F}_r$, intersects with the bar at its center of gravity. This is the only point along the bar's length where all torques will be canceled if a fulcrum is placed there as a support. Thus, as indicated earlier, the center of gravity, CG, is that point in an object where all the weight of its body may be considered to be centered.

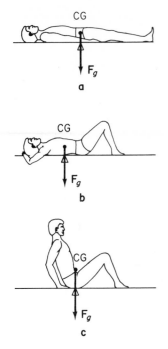

Figure 8–12. Center of gravity locations for varying positions.

Figure 8–13. The forearm-hand combination exerts a resistance torque of 31.5 lb·in. by itself (*a* and *b*), and with additional weight (*c*).

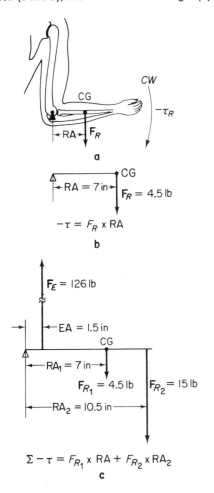

With objects which are not symmetrically shaped, the center of gravity will be found to be located nearer the greater concentration of weight than the lesser concentration, as illustrated with the hockey stick in Fig. 8-11*c*. The center of gravity or *balance point* is an important consideration in the use of sports implements such as javelins, baseball bats, firearms, and rackets, to name a few. With flexible objects such as the human body, the center of gravity moves in response to the changes in shape experienced by the body by changing the positions of body segments relative to one another. Figure 8-12 illustrates examples of the location of the center of gravity for different body positions. Note that the CG may be located outside the body when hip flexion is prominently in evidence.

Returning again to lever action, the incorporation of the rotating effect of the anatomical lever itself provides a greater accuracy in determining rotational outcomes. Since the entire weight of a body segment may be considered as centered or concentrated at its CG, the rotating tendencies may be calculated with the resistance arm measured to this point. Figure 8-13*a* illustrates the same situation as that in Fig. 8-10, but no additional forces are applied. Assuming that the forearm-hand combination weighs 4.5 lb and that its CG is 7 in. from the joint center, negative torque may be determined for the segment combination alone. Figure 8-13*b* provides the quantitative information to indicate that the segment combination, by itself, produces a negative (clockwise) torque of 31.5 lb·in. Figure 8-13*c* illustrates the necessary information to allow the calculation of the flexor force required to hold the forearm-hand segment combination in the horizontal position with the addition of the external 15-lb weight.

First, the sum of the negative torques must be computed (189 lb·in.). This is the magnitude of negative torque, which must be exactly counterbalanced in the positive direction by the flexor muscle working with an effort arm of 1.5 in. Once again employing the law of moments where positive and negative torques are equal,

$$+\tau_E = -\tau_R$$
$$F_E \times 1.5 \text{ in.} = 189 \text{ lb·in.}$$

Solving for the effort force,

$$F_E = \frac{189 \text{ lb·in.}}{1.5 \text{ in.}}$$
$$= 126 \text{ lb}$$

The cost of the poor effort-to-resistance arm ratio is again in evidence when 126 lb of force are required to balance an object whose total weight is 19.5 lb. It is noteworthy to point out that this is the predominant situation encountered throughout man's musculoskeletal system. Fortunately, with relatively light body segments to be moved, the musculature is generally up to the task.

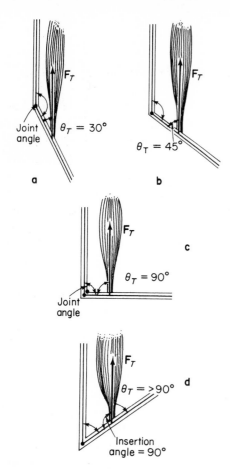

Figure 8–14. The tension angle, θ_T, is dependent generally upon the joint angle.

Figure 8–15. The insertion angle and tension angle, θ_T, are one and the same in (a), (b), and (c). In (d), they are seen to differ in magnitude and position relative to $\mathbf{F}_T$.

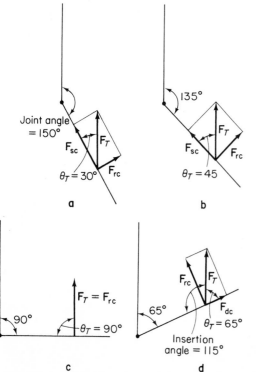

Muscular Force Components

We have been concerned with parallel force situations in which all of the applied forces were directed at right angles to the lever under study. However, muscles apply their forces to bony levers at angles differing from 90 deg far more often than they do at 90 deg. Figure 8-14 illustrates the changing angular relationship between muscular tension and the axis of the bone to which the muscle is attached as the bone is carried through a flexion movement. When the joint is only slightly flexed, the angle formed between the *tension vector*, $\mathbf{F}_T$, and the bone's axis—the *tension angle*, θ_T—is quite small. As flexion progresses, the angle proportionately increases to 90 deg (Fig. 8-14c) and decreases as the joint angle becomes smaller than 90 deg (Fig. 8-14d).

As noted in Chapter 7, when a force is applied at an angle differing from 90 deg, the motion which results can be described on the basis of the rectangular components of the force. Referring back to Fig. 7-15, it is seen that one force component is directed along the axis of the bone, while the other is directed at right angles to the bone. In Fig. 8-15, these force components are included with the latter, given the name, *rotary component*, $\mathbf{F}_{rc}$, because its effect is purely rotational. The component directed lengthwise along the bone axis is called the *stabilizing component*, $\mathbf{F}_{sc}$, because its effect is to pull the bone toward the joint center, which would oppose a tendency for the joint to be separated by some external force (Fig. 8-15a and b). When $\theta_T = 90$ deg (Fig. 8-15c), all of the muscular force is rotatory and $\mathbf{F}_T = \mathbf{F}_{rc}$. When the insertion angle exceeds 90 deg, the component along the bone is termed the *dislocating component*, $\mathbf{F}_{dc}$, because its direction reveals its tendency to pull the bone out of its articulation.

The rotatory component, with a tension angle of 30 deg, is considerably smaller than the stabilizing component. As the tension angle increases (joint angle decreases) to 45 deg, the rotary and stabilizing components are of equal magnitude. As the joint angle is reduced to a point where the insertion angle exceeds 90 deg, the rotary component diminishes in magnitude and the dislocating component comes into being. In all cases, when stabilizing or dislocating components are decreasing in magnitude, rotatory components are increasing and vice versa. Dislocating component forces can be felt occasionally when a joint is carried to the limits of flexion and then externally forced to go beyond those limits.

→ *Flex your elbow joint until you can carry it no further muscularly. Use your other arm to apply an external force in the direction of flexion to sharply carry the joint past its active limits. A noticeable discomfort can be detected on the back of the elbow joint as the result of the dislocating component's force being transferred from the bone to the joint capsule and triceps brachii tendon.*

Most women will not experience this sensation because their elbow joint ranges of flexion motion are not as muscularly limited as those of men.

In light of the background gained from the earlier discussions of

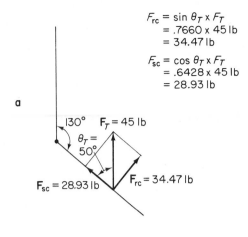

$$F_{rc} = \sin \theta_T \times F_T$$
$$= .7660 \times 45 \text{ lb}$$
$$= 34.47 \text{ lb}$$

$$F_{sc} = \cos \theta_T \times F_T$$
$$= .6428 \times 45 \text{ lb}$$
$$= 28.93 \text{ lb}$$

a

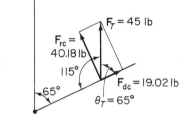

$$F_{rc} = \sin \theta_T \times F_T$$
$$= .9063 \times 45 \text{ lb}$$
$$= 40.18 \text{ lb}$$

$$F_{dc} = \cos \theta_T \times F_T$$
$$= .4226 \times 45 \text{ lb}$$
$$= 19.02 \text{ lb}$$

b

Figure 8-16

TABLE 8-1

	Tension Angle (deg)				Insertion Angle (deg)
	10	30	45	80	110
$F_T = 80$ lb					
F_{rc}					
F_{sc} or F_{dc}					

force component resolutions, it is now time to provide quantitative examples in which muscle forces are involved. Figure 8-16a provides the pertinent information for a beginning, simplified example. With a 45-lb force applied to the bone at a tension angle of 50 deg, only 34.47 lb are available to rotate the bone in the joint. Nearly 29 lb are available for stabilization. Figure 8-16b is given to illustrate the calculation of the dislocating component when the insertion angle exceeds 90 deg. With a 115-deg insertion angle, the angle at which the muscle pulls on the bone is $\theta_T = 65$ deg. Under these circumstances, 40.18 lb are available for rotation, while a force of 19.02 lb acts to pull the bone away from its articulation.

→ *To provide some additional practice, complete Table 8-1 by providing the component forces in each cell under the five conditions for a muscle tension force of 80 lb.*

It is now time to examine the action of a muscle or muscle group to work against an externally applied resistance force when the effective tension angle is less than 90 deg. Under these conditions it is as necessary to determine the angle at which the external force acts upon the lever as it is to know the muscle tension angle. Figure 8-17 illustrates such a compound system of forces. The joint angle is such that both the muscle and resistance forces act at 30 deg with the bony lever. The resistance force is $F_R = 20$ lb and acts through a resistance arm of 8 in. This represents the combined weights of the segments and external force at their center of gravity. The muscle tension force is applied through an effort arm of 2 in. and represents our unknown quantity.

A 20-lb force, F_R, acting at 30 deg with the lever may be resolved into two rectangular component forces: $F_{Rrc} = 10$ lb, the rotatory component of the resistance force, and $F_{Rdc} = 17.32$ lb, the dislocating component of the resistance force. Referring to Fig. 8-17b, the lever has been positioned in a horizontal position for the purposes of clarity. Applying the law of moments ($\Sigma \tau = 0$), the rotatory component of the resistance force is seen to produce a negative torque equaling

$$-\tau_R = F_{Rrc} \times RA$$
$$= 10 \text{ lb} \times 8 \text{ in.}$$
$$= 80 \text{ lb} \cdot \text{in.}$$

To balance the negative torque, an equal amount of positive torque must be applied through an effort arm, EA = 2 in. To determine the magnitude of the perpendicular force (F_{rc}) required,

$$F_{rc} \times EA = 80 \text{ lb} \cdot \text{in.}$$
$$F_{rc} = \frac{80 \text{ lb} \cdot \text{in.}}{2 \text{ in.}}$$
$$= 40 \text{ lb}$$

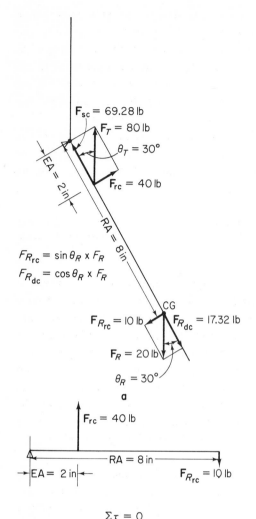

$F_{sc} = 69.28$ lb
$F_T = 80$ lb
$\theta_T = 30°$
$F_{rc} = 40$ lb
EA = 2 in.
RA = 8 in.

$F_{R_{rc}} = \sin \theta_R \times F_R$
$F_{R_{dc}} = \cos \theta_R \times F_R$

CG
$F_{R_{rc}} = 10$ lb $\quad F_{R_{dc}} = 17.32$ lb
$F_R = 20$ lb
$\theta_R = 30°$

a

$F_{rc} = 40$ lb

RA = 8 in
EA = 2 in
$F_{R_{rc}} = 10$ lb

$$\Sigma \tau = 0$$
$$+\tau = -\tau$$
$$F_{rc} \times EA = F_{R_{rc}} \times RA$$

b

Figure 8–17. A compound problem using muscle and resistance force components.

The final step is to calculate the muscle tension force acting at 30 deg with the bony lever which will produce a rotatory component of 40 lb:

$$F_T = \frac{F_{rc}}{\sin \theta_T} = \frac{40 \text{ lb}}{.5} = 80 \text{ lb}$$

In this situation, a muscle force of 80 lb acting through a lever arm of 2 in. at 30 deg will supply just enough positive torque to balance the oppositely directed torque of the resistance forces.

True Effort Arm

It is now time to investigate why we have had to be so concerned with rotatory, stabilizing, and dislocating components. Leverage changes are brought about when nonperpendicular forces are applied to lever systems. As the tension angle increases or decreases, the perpendicular distance (effort arm) over which the muscle force is applied is effectively increased or decreased, respectively. Therefore, the *true effort arm* of a lever system is defined as the perpendicular distance from the action line of the applied force to the joint center or fulcrum of the system. Figure 8-18a illustrates a muscle force acting upon a bony lever at a 30-deg tension angle, with the true effort arm included. In Fig. 8-18b, the triangle thus formed is simply turned over so that its hypotenuse (EA) is in a more easily recognized position. The true effort arm then becomes the vertical side of the triangle, opposite the tension angle, $\theta_T = 30$ deg. From the calculations included, it is clear that the true effort arm is exactly half the length of the anatomical effort arm. When the torque created under these conditions is computed, the true effort arm must be incorporated rather than the anatomical effort arm. Solving for the effort torque,

$$+\tau_E = F_T \times \text{true EA}$$
$$= 80 \text{ lb} \times 1 \text{ in.}$$
$$= 80 \text{ lb} \cdot \text{in.}$$

By referring to the previous problem with identical effort circumstances, it will be seen that effort torques resulting from the different approaches are identical, where

$$+\tau_E = F_{rc} \times EA = +\tau_E = F_T \times \text{true EA}$$
$$40 \text{ lb} \times 2 \text{ in.} = 80 \text{ lb} \times 1 \text{ in.}$$
$$80 \text{ lb} \cdot \text{in.} = 80 \text{ lb} \cdot \text{in.}$$

Figure 8-18c illustrates the procedures used to specify the true effort arm when the insertion angle is greater than 90 deg. Note that a new effort arm (EA') , identical to EA in length, is projected along the lever. The true effort arm is then applied perpendicular to the action line of $\mathbf{F}_T$ to Δ', the projected fulcrum. It can be seen that the true effort arm is of a lesser magnitude than EA, indicating a reduced tendency for the muscle to apply

TABLE 8–2

Tension Angle (deg)	True EA (in.)
10	
25	
60	
90	2
Insertion Angle	
110	

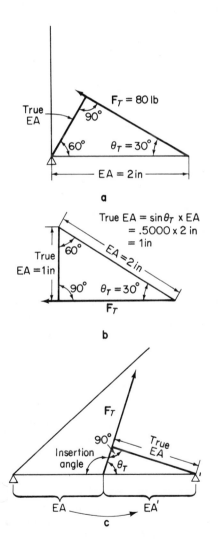

Figure 8–18. Determination of the true effort arm.

rotatory action to the lever. As would be expected, similar procedures would be followed to determine the true resistance arm.

→ *Perform the computations necessary to complete Table 8-2.*

Compensatory Mechanisms

Most but not all skeletal muscles are situated so that they operate in conjunction with poor effort-to-resistance arm ratios. This ratio may be interpreted to be an indication of the efficiency of muscle action through the lever system. As such, it represents one means of determining a lever system's *mechanical advantage, MA.* For perpendicular forces, this is the simple ratio EA/RA. The poor mechanical advantages demonstrated throughout the musculoskeletal system dictate a destiny of limited muscular forcefulness. However, certain compensatory mechanisms are available to improve the situation somewhat.

One means of compensation is to improve the angle at which the muscle approaches the bone. Effective tension angles are increased somewhat by changing the course of the muscle tendon where it joins with the bone. This turning action, although relatively limited in most situations, is accomplished by having muscle tendons pass over bony protuberances or to have *sesamoid* bones embedded in the tendons. The resulting pulley-like action improves the mechanical advantage of the system by lengthening the true effort arm. Specific coverage of these and other assistive mechanisms will be reserved for Part III of the text which details those specific anatomical functions. In doing so, the discussions will obtain the benefit of being applied within the context of the structural locations where they operate.

Another self-compensating mechanism is considered in greater detail here because it represents a natural extension and application of the content of this chapter. This mechanism is physiologically based and its compensation is automatically in operation when the musculoskeletal system is mechanically disadvantaged. Conversely, there is also a compensatory interplay in the opposite direction: a mechanical gain during physiological distress. Attending to the former first, it is a well-established physiological principle that muscles possess their greatest tension-producing abilities when near their greatest length within their structural environment. For a flexor muscle, this condition would occur when the joint which it crosses is fully extended. For an extensor muscle, the opposite would be the case. Generally, the relationship is as follows: When a muscle's tension angle is almost nonexistent, the muscle is in its prime physiological position to exert force.

The other clearly defined physiological principle is that as a muscle shortens during contraction, it rapidly loses its original ability to develop tension along its length. As a flexor muscle moves a segment through a flexion movement, its tension angle increases, as does its mechanical advantage. This is most certainly a useful compensatory action. However, these phenomena do not follow a one-to-one inverse relationship where the mechanical gains effectively rule out the physiological losses. It is particularly disproportionate as the muscle nears its point of greatest mechanical advantage. Certain muscles may, as noted before, shorten in their skeletal sites to a degree which allows the insertion angle to exceed 90 deg. When this occurs, both the physiological and mechanical advantages are compromised simultaneously to result in positions which are quite unstable muscularly. Fortunately, ranges of joint mobility as well as common experience tend to limit our use of such positions and save us much embarrassment.

A commonly cited physical task which illustrates the operation of these principles is the simple "chin-up" under conditions of muscular fatigue. After a series of chin-ups, fatigue develops rapidly in the elbow flexor musculature. Usually, the first evidences of distress show when the elbows are fully extended with the body at its lowest point directly below the bar. The distress manifests itself as an inability to begin the flexion movement. The combination of poor mechanical advantage and the weakened muscle, even though it is in its lengthened position, makes some "bouncing" or "cheating" necessary merely to begin a flexion tendency. After it is begun, the continuation of the flexion is usually possible. Often the bouncing is employed to facilitate flexion in one limb, usually the stronger of the two, which allows a lateral, swaying-climbing action to alternate the demands of the effort between the two limbs.

As the flexion movement progresses, the disproportionate loss of contractile force allows gravity to slow the movement. Finally, the body's own weight wins the battle and halts the motion completely. At this point, the chin has not reached the level of the chinning bar and no amount of continued effort will complete the task. The best that is possible under these terminal conditions is simply to balance out the force of gravity. Nevertheless, it is common to see youngsters kick their legs and flail their suspended bodies in search of those last few inches of movement that would lead to success.

Man appears to have always understood his basic limitations with respect to force application. This is implicit in his initiation of training programs which are designed to increase the physiological abilities of his muscles to exert force through the skeletal levers. This approach is based upon the realization that there is no viable way to change his basic musculoskeletal leverage arrangements. Consequently, training programs are instituted to condition the musculature to grow larger and stronger progressively. Even with remarkable changes in one's strength through training, man is still a relatively nonforceful being in the mechanical sense.

All is not lost, however, because man is an ingenious being. He has learned to employ many and varied means for overcoming his basic difficulties. Chief among these means is his design and development of machines which can be manipulated within his own force applying capabilities to provide the additional motive forces he lacks. Man's machines may well become his most successful hedge against his basic lack of forcefulness.

REFERENCES

Alexander, R. S. "Immediate Effects of Stretch on Muscle Contractility." *American Journal of Physiology* 196 (1959): 807.

Amar, Jules. *The Human Motor.* New York: E. P. Dutton & Co. Inc., 1920.

Anderson, T. McClurg. *Human Kinetics and Analysing Body Movements.* London: William Heinemann Medical Books, Ltd., 1951.

Bernstein, Nikolai A. *The Coordination and Regulation of Movements.* New York: Pergamon Press, 1969.

Bowne, M. E. "Relationship of Selected Measures of Acting Body Levers to Ball Throwing Velocities." *Research Quarterly* 31 (1960): 392.

Darcus, H. D. "The Range and Strength of Joint Movement." In *Human Factors in Equipment Design*, edited by W. F. Floyd and A. T. Welford. London: H. K. Lewis & Co., Ltd., 1954.

Della, D. G. "Individual Differences in Foot Leverage in Relation to Jumping Performance." *Research Quarterly* 21 (1950): 11.

Dempster, W. T. "Free-Body Diagrams as an Approach to the Mechanics of Human Posture and Motion." In *Biomechanical Studies of the Musculo-Skeletal System*, edited by F. G. Evans. Springfield, Ill.: Charles C Thomas, Publisher, 1961.

———— "Space Requirements of the Seated Operator: Geometrical, Kinematic, and Mechanical Aspects of the Body With Special Reference to the Limbs." WADC Technical Report 55-159. Wright-Patterson Air Force Base, Ohio: Wright Air Development Center, July 1955.

Dyson, Geoffrey H. G. *The Mechanics of Athletics.* 4th ed. London: University of London Press Ltd., 1967.

Elftman, H. "The Action of the Muscles in the Body." *Biological Symposium* 3 (1941): 191.

Fenn, W. O. "The Mechanics of Muscular Contraction in Man." *Journal of Applied Physics* 9 (1938): 165.

———— "Work Against Gravity and Work Due to Velocity Changes in Running: Movements of the Center of Gravity Within the Body and Foot Pressure on the Ground." *American Journal of Physiology* 95 (1930): 433.

Fox, M. G., and Young, O. G. "Placement of the Gravity Line in Antero-posterior Posture." *Research Quarterly* 25 (1954): 277.

Ganslen, R. V. "Do Athletes Defy the Law of Gravity?" *Sports College News*, October 1955.

Gaughran, G. R. L., and Dempster, W. T. "Force Analyses of Horizontal Two-Handed Pushes and Pulls in the Sagittal Plane." *Human Biology* 26 (1956): 67.

Gersten, J. W. "Mechanics of Body Elevation by Gastrocnemius-Soleus Contraction." *American Journal of Physical Medicine* 35 (1956): 12.

Hellebrandt, F. A.; Riddle, K. S.; Larson, E. M.; and Fries, E. C. "Gravitational Influences on Postural Alignment." *Physiotherapy Review* 22 (1942): 143.

Hopper, B. "Units and Measurements in the Mechanics of Track." *Track Technique* 29 (1967): 908.

Katz, B. "The Relation Between Force and Speed in Muscular Contraction." *Journal of Physiology* 96 (1939): 45.

Little, A. D., and Lehmkuhl, D. "Elbow Extension Force." *Physical Therapy* 46 (1966): 7.

Lissner, H. R. "Introduction to Biomechanics." *Archives of Physical Medicine and Rehabilitation* 46 (1965): 2.

McMurrich, Kathleen I. *Applied Muscle Action and Coordination.* Toronto: University of Toronto Press, 1957.

Murray, M. P., and Sepic, S. B. "Maximum Isometric Torque of Hip Abductor and Adductor Muscles." *Physical Therapy* 48 (1968): 1327.

Perry, J. "Structural Insufficiency." *Physical Therapy* 47 (1967): 848.

Physical Science Study Committee. *Physics.* 2d ed. Boston: D. C. Heath and Company, 1965.

Provins, K. A. "Maximum Forces Exerted About the Elbow and Shoulder Joints on Each Side Separately and Simultaneously." *Journal of Appiedl Physiology* 7 (1955): 390.

Provins, K. A., and Salter, N. "Maximum Torque Exerted About the Elbow Joint." *Journal of Applied Physiology* 7 (1955): 393.

Ralston, H. J. "Mechanics of Voluntary Muscle." *American Journal of Physical Medicine* 32 (1953): 166.

Rasch, P. J. "Effect of the Position of Forearm on Strength of Elbow Flexion." *Research Quarterly* 27 (1956): 333.

——— "Relationship of Arm Strength, Weight, and Length to Speed of Arm Movement." *Research Quarterly* 25 (1954): 328.

Rogers, J. A. "The Leverage of the Foot." *Anatomical Record* 16 (1919): 317.

Salter, N., and Darcus, H. D. "The Effect of the Degree of Elbow Flexion on the Maximal Torque Developed in Pronation and Supination of the Right Hand." *Journal of Anatomy* 86 (1952): 197.

Santschi, W. R. "Moment of Inertia and Centers of Gravity of the Living Human Body." Technical Documentary Report No. AMRL-TDR-63-36. Wright Patterson Air Force Base, Ohio: May 1963.

Smith, J. W. "The Forces Operating at the Human Ankle Joint During Standing." *Journal of Anatomy* 91 (1957): 545.

Steindler, Arthur. *Kinesiology of the Human Body.* Springfield, Ill.: Charles C Thomas, Publisher, 1955.

Swearingen, J. J. "Determination of Centers of Gravity of Man," Federal Aviation Agency Report 62-14 (1962): 37.

Williams, M., and Stutzman, L. "Strength Variation Through the Range of Joint Motion." *Physical Therapy Review* 39 (1959): 145.

Williams, Marian, and Lissner, Herbert R. *Biomechanics of Human Motion.* Philadelphia: W. B. Saunders Company, 1962.

9

Kinetic Characteristics of Linear Motion

We have considered a number of situations in which forces act to produce, control, and stop motion. The laws of motion which have been introduced in the course of these considerations have provided us with the opportunity to think in terms of expected outcomes when important qualities and quantities are known. In each case, an understanding of these relationships has improved our ability to describe the motion accurately or to explain why motion did not occur. A concept which has been inherent in the previous discussions of forces but never specifically defined is the role that forces play in allowing interacting bodies to do *work* on each other. Although work is a term which is in common use in our language, and although we have an intuitive grasp of its meaning, special attention will be given to a definition of work which does not suffer from the variability of interpretation which is usually present in ordinary usage.

WORK

In order that work may be done, the force-producing interaction between two bodies must result in motion. Either one or both of the bodies may be displaced. This does not mean to imply that applied forces which displace nothing are valueless. It simply restricts the description of forces as "work-producing" to those which move along with their resultant displacements. Figure 9-1 illustrates two interactions in which forces are applied. In Fig. 9-1*a*, the weight-lifter's hands move with the lifted barbell while the lifting force is being applied. The lifter's hands which apply the lifting force will not move, nor will the barbell move until the applied force just begins to exceed the weight of the barbell. When this requirement is met, the barbell and the lifter's hands are displaced equally in the direction of the superior force. The barbell is displaced and the force which produced the displacement has acted through that distance. The work done on the barbell is then the product of the force and the distance over which it acts, $W = Fd$. If the barbell and the 50-lb effort force were both displaced 2 ft, the amount of work done would be exactly 100 ft lb. In Fig. 9-1*b*, the lifting body is unable to move the barbell because its resistance force cannot be overcome. Although a force of large magnitude may well be acting on the barbell, it is a stationary force and no work is accomplished.

The situation illustrated in Fig. 9-1*a* identifies a displacement which has the same direction as the force producing it. In Chapter 8, it was made clear that forces may act to move objects and not be applied in precisely the same direction as the resulting motion. Under these conditions, work is done to a degree consistent with the component of the force in the direction of the motion. Figure 9-2 illustrates the elements of such a situation in which the force of gravity acts on the moving ball at an angle to the motion path. The path of the motion at that instant is represented by the velocity vector, **v**. Component vectors of $\mathbf{F}_g$ are illustrated: one parallel to the velocity vector and one perpendicular to it. The perpendicular component acts only to change the direction of the motion, while the tangential force component, $\mathbf{F}_t$, acts to increase the velocity of the moving ball. It is the tangential force component which accomplishes the work for the force

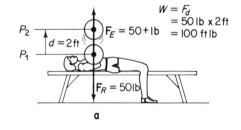

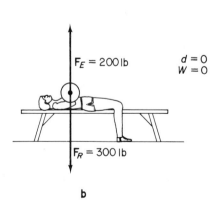

Figure 9–1. When displacement is the direct outcome of an applied force, work is done.

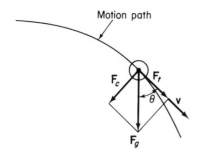

Figure 9–2. Forces, applied to objects in directions other than that of the resulting displacement or at right angles to it, are limited in magnitude to **F**cos θ with the displacement.

of gravity which continually acts across the motion path. Therefore it is necessary to compute the magnitude of the work-producing force from the force of gravity in terms of the angle θ. Consequently, work is derived from

$$W = (F \cos \theta)d$$

and is a scalar quantity.

The perpendicular force component in Fig. 9-2 acts at right angles to the ball's displacement and is not a work-producing force since cos 90 deg = 0. Figure 9-3 identifies the forces responsible for the horizontal displacement of the wrestler on the right who has momentarily lost his firm contact with the mat. Two constant forces are seen to be operating on this wrestler. One is produced by his opponent and the other is due to gravity. The force component, **F** cos θ, is responsible for the 1.5-ft horizontal displacement over the surface of the mat. The work done on the wrestler on the right is

$$W = (F \cos \theta)d$$
$$= (200 \text{ lb} \times .766) \times 1.5 \text{ ft}$$
$$= 153.2 \text{ lb} \times 1.5 \text{ ft}$$
$$= 229.8 \text{ ft lb}$$

The force of gravity plays no part in this horizontal work development since it acts perpendicular to the direction of the displacement under consideration.

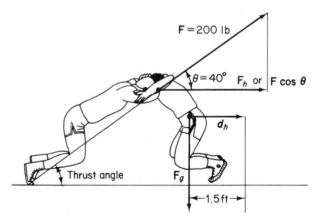

Figure 9–3. The horizontal displacement of the wrestler on the right is the result of the horizontal force component, **F**cos θ.

→ *Identify at least one effect of F_g on the motion even though it may be nearly imperceptible.*

POWER

In our everyday language, the word *power* is constantly in use. As might be expected, our intuitive understanding of the term leads to many differences in meaning. Power is related to work on the basis of time. When the time which is required for a quantity of work to be done is measured, the rate at which the work was performed may be determined. This rate of doing work is power, and like work, it is a scalar quantity. Power may be determined from

$$P = \frac{\Delta W}{\Delta t}$$

If the time which elapsed during the displacement illustrated in Fig. 9-3 had been measured to be exactly .8 sec, the power developed would be

$$P = \frac{229.8 \text{ ft lb}}{.8 \text{ sec}}$$

$$= 287.25 \text{ ft lb/sec}$$

When the power equation is written in the equivalent form,

$$P = \frac{F \, \Delta d}{\Delta t}$$

it can be seen that $\Delta d/\Delta t$ is average velocity to yield

$$\bar{P} = F\bar{v}$$

The velocity exhibited in the .8-sec time interval of Fig. 9-3 is 1.5 ft/.8 sec, or 1.875 ft/sec. Therefore the rate at which power was developed is

$$\bar{P} = F\bar{v}$$

$$= 153.2 \text{ lb} \times 1.875 \text{ ft/sec}$$

$$= 287.25 \text{ ft lb/sec}$$

the same outcome as above.

If the instantaneous power expended by a force on a moving body is required, Δt is reduced to a vanishingly small interval over which the displacement is measured. The equation then reads

$$P = F \lim_{\Delta t \to 0} \frac{\Delta d}{\Delta t} \quad \text{or} \quad P = Fv$$

As power values increase, it is customary to substitute the *horsepower* (hp) unit, which equals 550 ft lb/sec or 33,000 ft lb/min.

→ *What horsepower was developed in the wrestling sequence of Fig. 9-3?*

Power development is a difficult quantity to obtain accurately in complex human movements because the work units from which it is derived generally elude accurate determination. The primary problem resides in our inability to observe many force applications and in the difficulty of determining the changes in force magnitudes which operate on flexible, segmented bodies such as our own, particularly when applied over very short time intervals. When horsepower values are calculated, they are usually derived from energy expenditures which have been gathered by physiological means. At present, physiological methods are capable of identifying human power development far more accurately than mechanical methods. Although human horsepower figures in the low teens have been reported for activities such as short sprint running, it is likely that values of less than half that figure are more reasonable. Recent studies of the golf drive suggest that between 3 and 4 hp may be developed by the golfer's body during the downswing phase and that the large muscles of the legs and hips are mainly responsible.

Over longer time intervals, man, on the average, is seen to have a markedly reduced power capacity. It is also clear that large individuals with proportionately large musculatures have important force-generating advantages when compared to smaller individuals. If these large forces are optimally coupled to move objects rapidly, such an individual may appropriately be described as being "powerful." Beyond the point of force production, the pivotal consideration is seen to be time. In general, man is really not a very powerful being over extended periods of time.

IMPULSE

The important consideration of the period of time a force acts upon an object must continue beyond the realm of its importance in determining working rates. Numerous combinations of different force magnitudes and time intervals can be envisioned. For example, a force of great magnitude may act upon an object for a very short time interval, such as is the case in driving a golf ball from the tee. The period of interaction between the club and ball is very short. The opposite extreme would include a relatively small force acting over an extended time period. In comparison to the former example, delivering a bowling ball to the surface of the alley could generally represent the opposite case. The period of time the hand actually pushes the ball forward is quite long. The results of the two situations are very different when the velocities achieved at the end of interaction are examined. The former, short-termed force is called the *impulsive* force.

When a force and the time over which it acts on an object are combined as a product, the result, $F \Delta t$, is known as the *impulse* of the force because it represents the measure of what is required to change the motion of the object. It may be presented in the form of a graph in which force is plotted over time, as in Fig. 9-4. In Fig. 9-4a, a constant force acts over a period of time, $\Delta t = t_2 - t_1$, and the area under the force line represents the total impulse applied to the object. In Fig. 9-4b, the impulse areas for very small time intervals are summed to determine the total impulse of a varying force applied to an object over a time period, $t_2 - t_1$. Impulsive forces are so prominent in sports activities it would be a mistake to undervalue their importance.

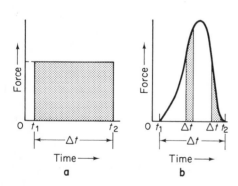

Figure 9–4. When force is plotted against time, the area under the force line represents the impulse.

→ *Identify additional examples of impulsive force interactions in games such as baseball, football, tennis, and boxing.*

At this juncture, it is once again necessary to return to the law of acceleration to continue the discussion of the results of force applications. When $F = ma$ is modified to include the velocities exhibited by objects under the motivations of impulsive forces, acceleration, a, is altered to read $\Delta v/\Delta t$. The equation then reads

$$F = m\frac{\Delta v}{\Delta t}$$

Clearing the right-hand side of the equation to leave the product of the object's mass and change of velocity, the equation becomes

$$F\,\Delta t = m\,\Delta v$$

The left-hand side of the equation is recognized as the impulse, which is a vector quantity whose direction is the same as the impulsive force. The right-hand side of the equation identifies the relationship between the object's change in velocity and its mass. As would be expected, massive objects are more reluctant to change their velocities than are smaller objects.

MOMENTUM

Investigating a simple situation, assume that an impulsive force is applied over a known interval of time to an object at rest, $v_o = 0$. After the time interval of application and the force are removed, the object's velocity is v_f. This is represented as

$$F\,\Delta t = m\,\Delta v = m(v_f - v_o) = mv_f - mv_o$$

Altering the equation once again, we get

$$F\,\Delta t = \Delta mv$$

with Δmv representing an equivalent measure of the total impulse over the time interval as demonstrated by the object. It is generally easier to determine Δmv from the observation of the object's movement behavior than it is to determine $F\,\Delta t$ directly. This is particularly true in athletic situations because of the difficulty of measuring force magnitudes directly.

From the foregoing, it is clear that Δmv, the right-hand side of the equation, $F\,\Delta t = \Delta mv$, is a most important concept in motion study and description. The product of an object's mass and velocity, mv, is known as its *momentum*, p. Therefore, Δmv represents the object's change of momentum as the result of the application of an impulsive force over a short time interval. Momentum is a vector quantity whose direction is the same as that of the applied force and resulting velocity. Since forces are the results of object interactions, they too may be determined from a knowledge of momentum changes as follows:

$$F = \frac{\Delta p}{\Delta t}$$

where the rate of change of momentum specifies the impulsive force applied over a very small time interval.

Suppose a hockey player applies an impulsive force to a stationary puck with his stick. Further, with $v_o = 0$, let $v_f = 100$ ft/sec at the instant the puck and stick separate. If the puck weighs 2 lb ($m = .0625$ slug), momentum at the moment of release is

$$p = mv$$
$$= .0625 \text{ slug} \times 100 \text{ ft/sec}$$
$$= 6.25 \text{ slug} \cdot \text{ft/sec}$$

its *impetus* or its tendency to resist any retardation of its motion.

Since a body's momentum is proportional to both its mass and velocity, it is logical that an object larger than the puck with the same velocity would be more difficult to resist or bring to a stop.

→ *Have you ever tried to stop a 16-lb shot as it rolled rapidly along the ground?*

The task is not so difficult when the rolling object is a tennis ball. In athletics, momentum was one of the earliest concerns of the football coach. It was understood that the small player must make up in velocity what he lacks in mass to compete with larger players. Looking back over football's history, it is clear that one of the most startling differences between early and present-day football play is that the players have continued to become larger as well as faster. Consequently, the small player finds it more and more difficult to compensate for his small mass with greater speed. Football has become a game for big men, that is, big, fast men. For that matter, the same may be said for other athletic activities, particularly basketball.

→ *Can you identify others?*

To return to the numerical example cited above, by determining the period of time the stick and puck were in contact (the time over which the force was applied), it is possible to calculate the impulsive force itself. Let us assume that .05 sec elapsed between the moment of first contact, t_1, and the moment of release, t_2. Momentum at t_1 is $p = 0$, while momentum at t_2 is 6.25 slug·ft/sec. Solving for F,

$$F = \frac{\Delta p}{\Delta t} = \frac{p_2 - p_1}{t_2 - t_1} = \frac{6.25 \text{ slug} \cdot \text{ft/sec}}{.05 \text{ sec}} = 125 \text{ lb}$$

If the impulsive force were graphed, it would appear as in Fig. 9-4b, rising sharply to a peak and then dropping off sharply over time. Since .05 sec is quite a small Δt in most human movement situations, we may accept the 125-lb force as being of an instantaneous nature.

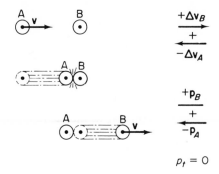

$p_t = 0$

Figure 9–5. Neglecting friction, the collision of the two pucks results in the total transfer of momentum from puck A to puck B without gain or loss.

TRANSFER AND CONSERVATION OF MOMENTUM

When two objects interact, as was the case for the hockey stick and puck, momentum changes are usually experienced by both of the objects. Our attention has been limited to only one of the objects, the puck, to simplify the discussion. Now, we must also investigate the momentum changes experienced by the objects which do the striking. To introduce this, a special situation is formulated. Another puck of identical mass with the first is used as the striking object rather than the stick. If the new puck, A, is accelerated toward the motionless puck, B, in rectilinear translation so that it will strike B on center, a very interesting thing will occur. The motionless puck, B, will move away in a continuation of the path of the striking puck A with the same velocity exhibited by the striking puck before the collision. In addition, the striking puck will stop immediately upon the collision, as illustrated in Fig. 9-5.

In this situation, the changes in momentum, Δp, were of equal magnitude but in opposite directions. Puck A lost exactly the same amount of momentum as was gained by B. Since their masses were identical, the changes in momentum were dependent on changes in velocity. For A, Δv was negative because the change occurred as the result of a decelerating force applied by B. Puck B demonstrated a positive Δv of equal magnitude because A applied an equal accelerating force upon B. Under these frictionless conditions, this account of the interaction satisfies the law of reaction in that equal and opposite forces were applied during the brief collision. Thus we may state that the total momentum, p_t, of the pair of pucks does not change as a result of the collision. That is, the total momentum before and after the collision is constant, $p_t = 0$, and momentum is thus *conserved*.

The masses of the two pucks need not be equal to satisfy the relationships cited above. Let puck B retain the same mass as in the original problem, .0625 slug. For the next collision, double the mass of puck A. In accordance with the law of reaction, the two pucks again interact with equal and opposite impulsive forces. However, the resulting, oppositely directed changes of velocity are not equal in magnitude owing to the unequal masses. The changes of momentum for the two pucks must be of equal magnitude but oppositely directed, $+\Delta p = -\Delta p$. If the instantaneous velocity of puck A just before contact was 20 ft/sec, its momentum was

$$p_{A_1} = m_{A_1} v_{A_1}$$
$$= .125 \text{ slug} \times 20 \text{ ft/sec}$$
$$= 2.5 \text{ slug} \cdot \text{ft/sec}$$

Puck B, just before contact, was at rest, $p_B = 0$. Upon examining the velocity of A after collision, it is noted to be exactly 15 ft/sec in the same direction. Therefore, after the collision, A had a momentum of

$$p_{A_2} = m_{A_2} v_{A_2}$$
$$= .125 \text{ slug} \times 15 \text{ ft/sec}$$
$$= 1.875 \text{ slug} \cdot \text{ft/sec}$$

The change of momentum for puck A is

$$\Delta p_A = p_{A_2} - p_{A_1} = 1.875 - 2.5 = -.625 \text{ slug} \cdot \text{ft/sec}$$

Although A lost momentum during the collision, its direction of motion remained unchanged, consistent with the direction of its momentum, 1.875 slug·ft/sec, after the collision. Because of the principle of momentum conservation, puck B must have gained the same amount of momentum that puck A lost. Knowing that $\Delta p_B = .625$ slug·ft/sec, we may solve for v_B immediately after the collision:

$$\Delta p_B = m_{B_2} v_{B_2}$$

$$.625 \text{ slug} \cdot \text{ft/sec} = .0625 \text{ slug} \times v_{B_2}$$

or

$$v_{B_2} = \frac{.625 \text{ slug} \cdot \text{ft/sec}}{.0625 \text{ slug}}$$

$$= 10 \text{ ft/sec}$$

Thus a gain in velocity of 10 ft/sec by a .0625-slug mass resulted from the loss of 5 ft/sec by a .125-slug mass during the collision to yield

$$+\Delta p_B = -\Delta p_A$$

$$m_B \Delta v_B = m_A \Delta v_A$$

$$.0625 \text{ slug} \times 10 \text{ ft/sec} = .125 \text{ slug} \times -5 \text{ ft/sec}$$

$$.625 \text{ slug} \cdot \text{ft/sec} = -.625 \text{ slug} \cdot \text{ft/sec}$$

The total momentum of the two-puck system, p_t, must be the same after the collision as before the collision. The p_t before the collision is

$$p_t = p_{A_1} + p_{B_1}$$

$$= 2.5 \text{ slug} \cdot \text{ft/sec} + 0 = 2.5 \text{ slug} \cdot \text{ft/sec}$$

After the collision, the total momentum is

$$p_t = p_{A_2} + p_{B_2}$$

$$= 1.875 \text{ slug} \cdot \text{ft/sec} + .625 \text{ slug} \cdot \text{ft/sec}$$

$$= 2.5 \text{ slug} \cdot \text{ft/sec}$$

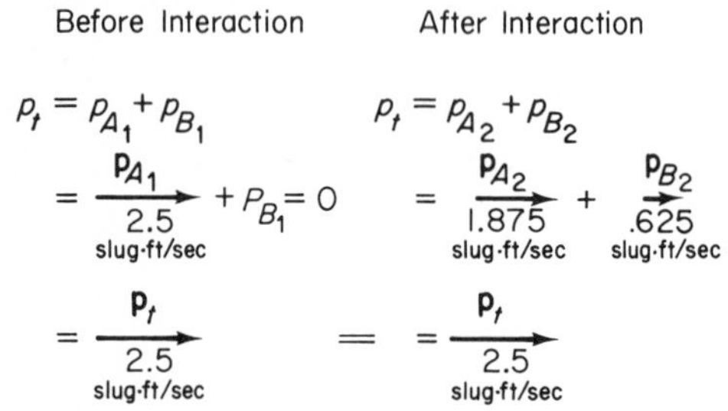

Before Interaction   After Interaction

$$p_t = p_{A_1} + p_{B_1} \qquad p_t = p_{A_2} + p_{B_2}$$

$$= \underset{\substack{2.5 \\ \text{slug·ft/sec}}}{\xrightarrow{p_{A_1}}} + p_{B_1} = 0 \qquad = \underset{\substack{1.875 \\ \text{slug·ft/sec}}}{\xrightarrow{p_{A_2}}} + \underset{\substack{.625 \\ \text{slug·ft/sec}}}{\xrightarrow{p_{B_2}}}$$

$$= \underset{\substack{2.5 \\ \text{slug·ft/sec}}}{\xrightarrow{p_t}} \qquad = \quad = \underset{\substack{2.5 \\ \text{slug·ft/sec}}}{\xrightarrow{p_t}}$$

Figure 9–6

Figure 9-6 illustrates the conservation principles in vector form.

The preceding examples have included only one direction of movement. When objects interact in such a manner that the direction of motion of one is changed, the momentum changes may be described in vector form also. Figure 9-7 illustrates an example where a stationary puck is struck off center. Thus the two pucks move away from each other at an angle with different momenta. Let the momentum before the collision for puck A be $\mathbf{p}_A = 5$ slug·ft/sec. Puck A leaves the collision along a path which deviates from its original path by approximately 64 deg with a momentum of about

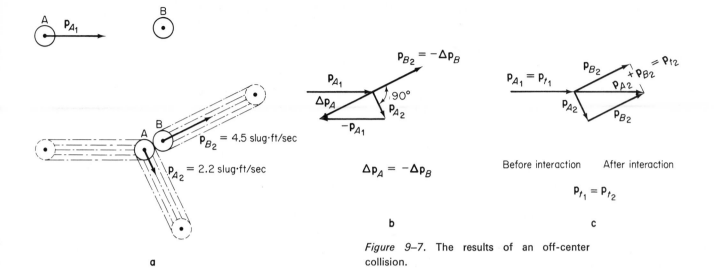

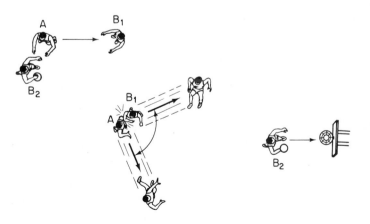

$$p_{A_1}$$

$$p_{B_2} = 4.5 \text{ slug·ft/sec}$$

$$p_{A_2} = 2.2 \text{ slug·ft/sec}$$

a

$$p_{A_1}$$

$$\Delta p_A$$

$$p_{B_2} = -\Delta p_B$$

$$90°$$

$$p_{A_2}$$

$$-p_{A_1}$$

$$\Delta p_A = -\Delta p_B$$

b

$$p_{A_1} = p_{t_1}$$

$$p_{B_2}$$

$$p_{A_2}$$

$$p_{A_2} + p_{B_2} = p_{t2}$$

$$p_{B_2}$$

Before interaction   After interaction

$$p_{t_1} = p_{t_2}$$

c

Figure 9–7. The results of an off-center collision.

2.2 slug·ft/sec. Puck B is seen to move away from the collision along a path which forms a 90-deg angle with the final path of A. Figure 9-7*b* shows the change in momentum for each puck to be equal in magnitude but opposite in direction. The change of momentum for B has been classified arbitrarily as negative in direction. In addition (Fig. 9-7*c*), conservation of momentum is illustrated in that the total momenta for the two pucks, before and after collision, are equal.

→ *Calculate the magnitude of p_{B_2} and the angle formed between it and p_{t_2}. Assuming that contact between the pucks lasted .005 sec, what was the approximate impulsive force applied during the interaction?*

Momentum-transferring collisions similar to those discussed above are common in sporting activities, with the exception that the interacting bodies are seldom inelastic as assumed above. In basketball, it is customary for an offensive player without the ball to set a stationary "pick" to block the path of his dribbling teammate's opponent. Figure 9-8 illustrates such a situation where much of the moving player's momentum is transferred to the stationary opponent.

Figure 9–8. A collision in basketball play.

Another interesting example of momentum transfer is demonstrated by the short, rapid "jab" in boxing. Because of the relatively small mass of the boxer's upper limb, the effectiveness of the jab, in part, depends on the object it strikes. If such a blow interacts with the massive trunk segment of an opponent, the mass ratio works to limit effective outcomes. However, if the aim is true and contact is made with the smaller head-neck segment of the opponent, the resulting momentum is capable of accelerating that segment to a point where equilibrium and timing can be badly upset, which can lead to openings for additional punches.

It should be evident that a useful way to limit the damaging effects of momentum transfer in collisions is to anticipate the moment of contact as well as the direction of the impulse. By moving with the striking object as contact is made, the momentum transfer is accomplished over a longer period of time. Moving the gloved hand backward when catching a rapidly moving baseball, moving with the punch in boxing, and riding a lunge in wrestling are examples of dissipating the forces of momentum by lengthening the time intervals over which they are applied. Since it is ultimately the average force of the impulse that does the damage, if the time (Δt) of momentum transfer is increased, the magnitude of the average force applied is decreased in accordance with $\bar{F} = \Delta p / \Delta t$.

KINETIC ENERGY

The technical definition of energy includes work. When defined in this manner it is commonly stated: Energy is the capacity to do work. We have seen that the product of moving forces and the displacements which result specifies the work done. This work may be used to represent the energy involved, and since it includes motion, a moving object's work-producing capacity is termed its *kinetic energy*, E_k. Kinetic energy is expressed in work units and is a scalar quantity. For our purposes, it is important to describe kinetic energy in terms of the object's motion characteristics covered previously, particularly in terms of its change of velocity.

If an object is set into motion by an applied force of constant magnitude, it is accelerated in accordance with $F = ma$. Suppose the object is a falling ball where a and F are constants. The displacement which results over time may be included in the left-hand side of the equation to represent the work done, Fd. The displacement then must be included in the same way in the right-hand side of the equation to result in $Fd = mad$. It will be remembered from Chapter 3 that a ball's instantaneous velocity may be obtained from the knowledge of its displacement and acceleration, $v^2 = 2ad$. Since the motion characteristic of interest is the change of velocity, $v_f - v_o$, rearrangement of this equation results in

$$a = \frac{(v_f - v_o)^2}{2d} = \frac{(v_f^2 - v_o^2)}{2d} = \frac{\Delta v^2}{2d}$$

With the ball at rest, its original velocity is $v_o = 0$. Therefore, the change of velocity, Δv, also represents the ball's instantaneous velocity, and $\Delta v^2/2d$

may be given as $v^2/2d$. When this term is substituted for a in $Fd = mad$, the outcome is

$$Fd = mad = m\frac{v^2}{2d}d = \frac{mv^2}{2} \quad \text{or} \quad \tfrac{1}{2}mv^2$$

The energy involved in the downward displacement of the ball as the result of gravitational attraction is its kinetic energy, $E_k = \tfrac{1}{2}mv^2$. Because the ball accelerated from rest, v_o, to some final velocity, v_f, the kinetic energy of the ball at these two moments in time may be given as $\tfrac{1}{2}mv_o^2$ or E_{k_o} and $\tfrac{1}{2}mv_f^2$ or E_{k_f}, respectively. The change of kinetic energy, $E_{k_f} - E_{k_o}$ or ΔE_k, represents the work done on the ball by the force of gravity.

For example, assume that a 16-lb shot has been elevated an appreciable distance and allowed to fall to the earth. After falling 1 sec, its velocity is 32 ft/sec. At that instant, its kinetic energy is

$$E_k = \tfrac{1}{2}mv^2 = \frac{1}{2} \times \frac{16\ \text{lb}}{32\ \text{ft/sec}} \times (32\ \text{ft/sec})^2$$

$$= 256\ \text{ft lb}$$

→ *What is the kinetic energy of the same object after it has fallen for 2 sec?*

It should be clear that a doubling of the object's velocity results in a fourfold increase in its kinetic energy. This explains the high degree of risk associated with collisions between rapidly moving bodies in athletic contests.

POTENTIAL ENERGY

The work done on the shot to elevate it above the ground is said to give it the potential to do work. When it is released, it increases its velocity throughout the period of fall until it strikes the ground. In striking the ground, the shot does work on the ground equal to $W = mgh$, or the product of its weight and height above the ground. A 16-lb shot elevated to a height of 16 ft has a *potential energy* of

$$E_p = mgh = wh$$

$$= 16\ \text{lb} \times 16\ \text{ft}$$

$$= 256\ \text{ft lb}$$

equal to the work required to raise it to that height. At the moment before contact with the ground, its velocity is 32 ft/sec ($v = \sqrt{2gd}$) and its kinetic energy equals its original potential energy, 256 ft lb, before release.

→ *Assume that you are going to jump into a swimming pool from an olympic tower, h = 33 ft approximately. What is your potential energy relative to the water's surface while in this elevated position? Calculate your velocity and kinetic energy at the moment your feet touch the water.*

CONSERVATION OF ENERGY

It is interesting to note that kinetic energy and momentum equations employ the same elements, namely, the object's mass and velocity. While momentum is a vector quantity, kinetic energy is a scalar quantity. The velocity terms used in the kinetic energy equations were scalars which were squared. Therefore, the direction of the motion is an item of concern when dealing with momentum but not when dealing with energy. Thus it can be seen that although these motion characteristics contain the same elements, they are independent phenomena and are employed independently in motion descriptions.

Additional similarities between kinetic energy and momentum may be noted. One of the most important is that kinetic energy transfer in collisions follows the same rule as does momentum transfer. That is, the energy lost by the striking object is exactly equal to the energy gained by the struck object. Second, the total energy of the two-object system before and after an interaction is the same. This is analogous to the principle of momentum conservation and is known as the *law of conservation of energy*. In the example of jumping from the olympic tower given above, the kinetic energy of your body at the moment of contact with the water is exactly equal to the potential energy it possessed atop the tower. What has occurred is the conversion of potential energy to kinetic energy with no loss or gain to indicate that

$$E_p = E_k$$
$$mgh = \tfrac{1}{2}mv^2$$

REFERENCES

Anderson, T. McClurg. *Human Kinetics and Analysing Body Movements*. London: William Heinemann Medical Books, Ltd., 1951.

Arkin, A. M. "Absolute Muscle Power: The Internal Kinesiology of Muscle." *Archives of Surgery* 42 (1941): 395.

Astrand, P. O. "New Records in Human Power." *Nature*, 12 November 1955.

Benedict, F. G., and Murschhauser, H. *Energy Transformations During Horizontal Walking*. Publication No. 231, Carnegie Institute of Washington: 1915.

Blader, F. B. "The Analysis of Movements and Forces in the Sprint Start." In *Medicine and Sport*, vol. 2. Basel, Switzerland: S. Karger AG, 1968.

Cochran, Alastair, and Stobbs, John. *The Search for the Perfect Swing*. Philadelphia: J. B. Lippincott Company, 1968.

Cotes, J. E., and Meade, F. "The Energy Expenditure and Mechanical Energy Demand in Walking," *Ergonomics* 3 (1960): 97.

Dempster, W. T., "Analysis of Two-Handed Pulls Using Free Body Diagrams." *Journal of Applied Physiology* 13 (1958): 469.

Dyson, Geoffrey H. G. *The Mechanics of Athletics*. 4th ed. London: University of London Press Ltd., 1967.

Eckert, H. M. "A Concert of Force-Energy in Human Movement." *Physical Therapy* 45 (1965): 213.

——— "The Effect of Added Weights on Joint Actions in the Vertical Jump." *Research Quarterly* 39 (1968): 943.

Elftman, H. "Forces and Energy Changes in the Leg During Walking." *American Journal of Physiology* 125 (1959): 339.

———— "The Work Done by Muscles in Running." *American Journal of Physiology* 129 (1940): 672.

Elmendorf, A. "Muscular Power and Endurance." *Science* (American Supplement) Aug. 11, 1917: 84.

Fenn, W. O. "Frictional and Kinetic Factors in the Work of Sprint Runners." *American Journal of Physiology* 92 (1930): 583.

———— "Mechanical Energy Expenditure in Sprint Running as Measured by Moving Pictures." *American Journal of Physiology* 90 (1929): 343.

———— "Work Against Gravity and Work Due to Velocity Changes in Running: Movements of the Center of Gravity Within the Body and Foot Pressure on the Ground." *American Journal of Physiology* 95 (1930): 433.

Fletcher, J. G.; Lewis, H. E.; and Wilkie, D. R. "Human Power Output: The Mechanics of Pole Vaulting." *Ergonomics* 3 (1960): 30, 89.

Gaughran, G. R. L., and Dempster, W. T. "Force Analyses of Horizontal Two-Handed Pushes and Pulls in the Sagittal Plane." *Human Biology* 26 (1956): 67.

Hay, J. G. "An Investigation of Take-Off Impulses in Two Styles of High Jumping." *Research Quarterly* 39 (1968): 983.

———— "Mechanical Energy in Pole Vaulting." *Track Technique* 33 (1968): 1047.

Henry, F. M. "Force-Time Characteristics of the Sprint Start." *Research Quarterly* 23 (1952): 301.

Henry, F. M., and Whitley, J. D. "Relationships Between Individual Differences in Strength, Speed, and Mass in Arm Movement." *Research Quarterly* 31 (1960): 24.

Hill, A. V. "The Maximum Work and Mechanical Efficiency of Human Muscles and Their Most Economical Speed." *Journal of Physiology* 56 (1922): 19.

Inman, V. T. "Conservation of Energy in Ambulation." *Archives of Physical Medicine and Rehabilitation* 48 (1967): 484.

Jammer, Max. *Concepts of Force: A Study in the Foundations of Dynamics*. New York: Harper & Row, Publishers, 1957.

———— *Concepts of Mass in Classical and Modern Physics*. New York: Harper & Row, Publishers, 1961.

Koepki, C. A., and Whitson, L. A. "Power and Velocity Developed in Manual Work." *Mechanical Engineering* 62 (1940): 383.

Lloyd, B. B. "The Energetics of Running: An Analysis of World Records." *Advancement of Science* 22 (1966): 515.

MacLachlan, James H.; McNeill, K. G.; and Bell, John M. *Matter and Energy*. New York: Noble and Noble, Publishers, Inc., 1964.

Margaria, R., and Cavagna, G. A. "Human Locomotion in Subgravity." *Aerospace Medicine* 35 (1964): 1140.

Massey, Benjamin H.; Manson, Frank R.; Freeman, Harold W.; and Wessel, Janet A. *The Kinesiology of Weight Lifting*. Dubuque, Iowa: Wm. C. Brown Company, Publishers, 1959.

Menely, R., and Rosemier, R. A. "Effectiveness of Four Track Starting Positions on Acceleration." *Research Quarterly* 39 (1968): 161.

Natsoulas, T. "Principles of Momentum and Kinetic Energy in Perception of Causality." *American Journal of Psychology* 74 (1961): 394.

Physical Science Study Committee. *Physics*. 2d ed. Boston: D. C. Heath and Company, 1965.

Shortley, George, and Williams, Dudley. *Elements of Physics*. 4th ed. Englewood Cliffs, N.J.: Prentice-Hall, Inc., 1965.

Starr, I. "Units for the Expression of Both Static and Dynamic Work in Similar Terms, and Their Application to Weight Lifting Experiments." *Journal of Applied Physiology* 4 (1951): 26.

Tricker, R. A. R., and Tricker, B. J. K. *The Science of Movement*. New York: American Elsevier Publishing Company, Inc., 1967.

Wilkie, D. R. "Man as a Source of Mechanical Power." *Ergonomics* 3 (1960): 1.

Zajaczkowska, A. "Constant Velocity in Lifting as a Criterion of Muscular Skills." *Ergonomics* 5 (1962): 337.

10

Kinetic Characteristics of Curved Motion

In Chapter 9, the concepts of work, power, impulse, momentum, and energy in linear situations were introduced. Those discussions were based upon understandings of straight-line displacement, velocity, and acceleration. The present discussions follow the same pattern of concept presentation, with rotatory motion being the center of attention, based upon understandings of angular displacement, velocity, and acceleration, respectively. While the discussions in Chapter 9 assisted in our ability to describe whole-body motion, this chapter's discussions should provide the same benefit for body segment motions, which are primarily rotational in nature.

ANGULAR WORK AND POWER

In Chapter 8, we developed the concept of torque, τ, which is obtained by multiplying the magnitude of the rotation-producing force by the length of the lever arm to which it is applied. In a rotational sense, the lever arm length acts as the radius of rotation about the fixed axis. Thus the torque of an applied, rotation-producing force is dependent on the perpendicular distance from the action line of the force to the axis of rotation.

The *angular work* done on a rotating object by an applied force depends on the angular displacement produced by its action, as in Fig. 10-1. Suppose a bicycle chain is wrapped around a sprocket wheel so that an effective force may be applied perpendicular to a radius of the sprocket wheel for more than just an instant. The sprocket wheel rotates through the angle $\Delta\theta$ in response to the off-center force, **F**. The straight-line distance traversed by the force is equal to the arc traversed by the sprocket wheel's rim and is related to the angle θ as $S = \theta R$. Because linear work is given by $W = Fd$, by substitution, angular work is given by the equation $W = \tau\theta$. If a 20-lb force is applied over a radius (actually the lever arm) of .5 ft and the rotation which results is .785 rad, the work done in rotation is

$$W = \tau\theta$$
$$= FR\theta$$
$$= 20 \text{ lb} \times .5 \text{ ft} \times .785 \text{ rad}$$
$$= 10 \text{ lb} \cdot \text{ft} \times .785 \text{ rad}$$
$$= 7.85 \text{ ft lb}$$

This is said to be the work done by the torque, τ.

If the angular work done is referred to the time over which it was accomplished, *angular power* is the result. In terms of the previous discussion of power, $P = (\tau \Delta\theta)/\Delta t$. It will be remembered that $\Delta\theta/\Delta t = \omega$ is angular velocity. Therefore, angular power is obtained from the product of the applied torque and the object's angular velocity, $P = \tau\omega$.

Figure 10-2 illustrates an application involving a body segment movement as the result of a muscular contraction. The leg-foot segment combination is rotated through $\Delta\theta = 90$ deg or 1.571 rad as the result of the

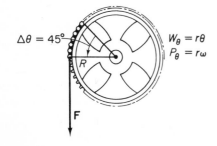

$\Delta\theta = 45°$

$W_\theta = r\theta$
$P_\theta = r\omega$

R

F

Figure 10–1. Angular work depends on the torque of the applied force and the resulting angular displacement. Angular power depends upon these same features relative to time.

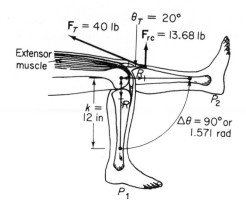

$F_T = 40$ lb

$\theta_T = 20°$

$F_{rc} = 13.68$ lb

Extensor muscle

R

$k = 12$ in

R

P_2

$\Delta\theta = 90°$ or 1.571 rad

P_1

Figure 10–2

tension force, $\mathbf{F}_T$, of the knee extensor muscle group. Note the similarity between the force application through the muscle tendon in this figure and that applied through the bicycle chain. However, the similarity ends when it is seen that the force in Fig. 10-1 always remains perpendicular to the radius of rotation. In the case of knee extension, the force is applied to the leg segment at an angle, $\theta_T = 20$ deg, which is far from being perpendicular to the radius of rotation at its point of insertion.

Following the procedures discussed in Chapter 8, the torque of the force is obtained by determining the rotatory force component and multiplying it by its perpendicular distance from the axis of rotation. If $\mathbf{F}_T = 40$ lb and the effort arm (radius) for the force application is 3 in. (.25 ft), the rotatory component is

$$F_{rc} = \sin 20° \times F_T = .3420 \times 40 \text{ lb} = 13.68 \text{ lb}$$

Assuming that $\mathbf{F}_{rc}$ remains constant throughout the rotation,

$$\tau = F_{rc}R = 13.68 \text{ lb} \times .25 \text{ ft} = 3.42 \text{ lb·ft}$$

Then the angular work done is

$$W = \tau\theta = 3.42 \text{ lb·ft} \times 1.571 \text{ rad}$$
$$= 5.37 \text{ ft lb}$$

If the extension movement, $\theta = 90$ deg, occurred over a time increment of 2 sec, the angular power developed was

$$P = \tau\omega$$
$$= 3.42 \text{ lb·ft} \times \frac{1.571 \text{ rad}}{2 \text{ sec}}$$
$$= 3.42 \text{ lb·ft} \times .786 \text{ rad/sec}$$
$$= 2.69 \text{ ft lb/sec}$$

→ *Calculate angular work and power for a similar situation where the force applied by the muscle group is 60 lb over an interval of 3 sec.*

MOMENT OF INERTIA

It was stated earlier that the resistance to a change in an object's motion is called its inertia and that its inertia is proportional to its mass. In fact, the usual measure of an object's inertia is its mass. When an object rotates around a fixed axis, its rotational inertia is also dependent on its mass. However, when an object is considered to be composed of a nearly endless quantity of individual particles, the distribution of each particle and its mass relative to the axis of rotation must be considered. In this case, each particle resides at a different location with respect to the axis of rotation. Each rotating particle's mass then acts through its own perpendicular distance from the axis to exhibit its individual inertia. The *moment of*

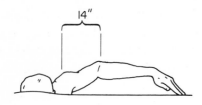

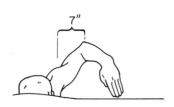

Figure 10–3. After J. E. Counsilman, *The Science of Swimming* (Englewood Cliffs, N. J: Prentice-Hall, Inc., 1968), p. 15.

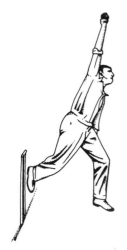

a cricket bowler

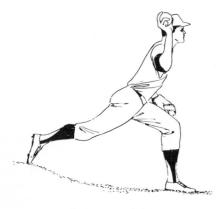

b baseball pitcher

Figure 10–4. Throwing with the elbow flexed (*a*) and extended (*b*).

inertia of each particle in rotation is obtained as the product of its mass and the square of its perpendicular distance from the axis of rotation, mR^2. All of these individual moments of inertia are then summed to provide the moment of inertia for the whole object:

$$I = \Sigma \, mR^2$$

The procedure described above is obviously a most difficult one and requires specific information about the object's density and shape. Moments of inertia for regularly shaped, rigid, rotating objects such as the sphere, hoop, cone, or rod may be readily calculated. However, irregularly shaped objects, such as the segments of the human body which also demonstrate inconsistent densities, require calculation procedures which are too complex and detailed for this text. Even when the body segments are assumed to approximate the shapes of the regular objects cited above, rotational inertia outcomes are limited as to accuracy. In addition, moments of inertia for the rotating segments must be computed for each new position the body assumes during a motion since the distribution of the mass is continually changing. Consequently, it is easy to understand why this motion characteristic is calculated so rarely on a large scale. When it is attempted, the computation procedure depends on the identification of a quantity known as the *radius of gyration*, k, relative to the axis of rotation.

If all the particle masses of a rotating object were assumed to be situated at a single point in the object, and this idealized location did not alter the object's moment of inertia obtained from normally distributed particle masses, the point's perpendicular distance from the axis of rotation is the radius of gyration, $k = \sqrt{I/m_t}$. This construct is **rather** like a special average of the perpendicular distances from the axis **of rotation** of all the object's particles and may be identified for objects of **any shape** and from any axis of rotation. If the object's total mass, m_t, were actually located at distance k from the axis of rotation, its moment of inertia is obtained from

$$I = m_t k^2$$

Note that the radial distance is again squared in keeping with $I = mR^2$.

In Fig. 10-2, the radius of gyration has been arbitrarily placed at a distance of 12 in. from the axis of rotation. Since all the mass of the 12.8-lb leg-foot segment combination is then considered to be concentrated at this point, the moment of inertia is

$$
\begin{aligned}
I &= m_t k^2 \\
  &= .4 \, \text{slug} \times (1 \, \text{ft})^2 \\
  &= .4 \, \text{slug} \cdot \text{ft}^2
\end{aligned}
$$

When a force is applied to a pivoted object, its tendency to resist angular acceleration depends on its moment of inertia. The smaller the moment of inertia of an object, the easier it is to accelerate in rotation.

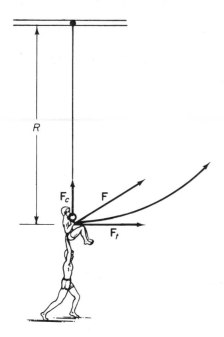

Figure 10–5. The hanging body is accelerated in the direction of F_t to begin its circular swing.

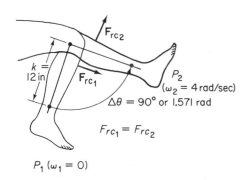

Figure 10–6

Thus in swimming, recovery movements of the arms are often accomplished with the limbs in shortened positions (Fig. 10-3). The elbow joint of the swimmer's left arm is flexed in recovery. The flexion distributes the limb's mass closer to the axis of rotation (reducing the average radius from the axis) so that the limb may be recovered as rapidly as possible. Similarly, it is easier to accelerate the throwing arm if the limb is shortened (Fig. 10-4) by flexing the elbow.

→ *Discuss the effects of the differing moments of inertia for the bowling motion in cricket shown in Fig. 10-4b with the pitching motion in Fig. 10-4a. Describe similar relationships in competitive diving, punting a football, figure skating, and ballet.*

Try the following to demonstrate different oscillatory rates of limb swing. First, flex the elbow joint completely and tie the arm and forearm segments together so that they may be moved as one. Swing the limb forward and backward as fast as possible for a 5-sec period through at least 45 deg. Count the number of complete oscillations. Next, repeat the procedure with the elbow fully extended. The speed of movement should be affected to the point where the totals differ. Sitting on the edge of a tall table, repeat the procedure with the more massive lower limb and compare your results.

Newton's law of acceleration may be applied to rotatory motion in a form which includes the rotating object's moment of inertia. When an applied force causes a rotation to occur as in Fig. 10-5, the tangential force component, F_t, is responsible for the resulting acceleration, a_t. Therefore the equation may be written as

$$F_t = ma_t$$

It will be remembered from Chapter 4 that a_t may be obtained by multiplying the radius of rotation by the magnitude of the angular acceleration, $a_t = R\alpha$. By substitution, the tangential force may be obtained from the equation $F_t = mR\alpha$, where α is proportional to the magnitude of F_t. Since the torque of F_t is F_tR, and the moment of inertia is mR^2, the result is

$$F_tR = mR^2\alpha \qquad \text{or} \qquad \tau = I\alpha$$

The gymnast's body, hanging from the rings, is then accelerated along the circular path to a degree which is directly proportional to the torque of the tangential force and inversely proportional to the moment of inertia of the body. This is seen to be the case by the rearrangement of the equation where $\alpha = \tau/I$.

→ *Identify three ways in which the body may have its angular acceleration increased by manipulating the elements involved in Fig. 10-5.*

Figure 10-6 illustrates an extension movement of the knee joint similar to that in Fig. 10-2. In this case, however, the knee joint is not completely extended after 90 deg of rotation because at P_1 the knee angle is seen to be less than 90 deg. Again, the focus of attention is upon the 12.8-lb leg-foot segment combination's radius of gyration which is located 12 in. from the axis of rotation. Using the rotational equivalent of the law of acceleration, $\tau = I\alpha$, we may solve for the moment of inertia by rearrangement to yield $I = \tau/\alpha$. Assuming that the force applied (rotatory component of the muscular force) to the segment combination is constant throughout the .5-sec movement, angular acceleration is seen to be exactly 8 rad/sec². With a torque of 3.2 lb·ft, the moment of inertia is

$$I = \frac{\tau}{\alpha}$$

$$= \frac{3.2 \text{ lb·ft}}{8 \text{ rad/sec}^2}$$

$$= .4 \text{ slug·ft}^2$$

The rotatory component force which produced the acceleration is obtained from

$$F_{rc} = \frac{\tau}{R} = \frac{3.2 \text{ lb·ft}}{.25 \text{ ft}} = 12.8 \text{ lb}$$

Last, the muscular tension, F_T, may be determined from the rotatory component assuming the tension angle to be $\theta_T = 20$ deg:

$$F_T = \frac{F_{rc}}{\sin \theta_T} = \frac{12.8 \text{ lb}}{.3420} = 34.5 \text{ lb} \qquad \text{(approximately)}$$

As will be seen later, muscular forces may be applied during a motion to decelerate rather than accelerate segments. In this way, muscles may act to control the precision of a segment's movement which is being positively affected by an outside force such as gravity or by an entirely different muscle group. As an example, in walking, the lower limb is shortened by flexing the knee and accelerated by hip flexor muscles. The flexed limb then demonstrates a reduced moment of inertia and is easily accelerated. However, when the limb nears its most forward position, it must prepare to plant the heel of the foot to begin a supporting phase. The leg-foot combination is decelerated in preparation for heel plant by the knee flexors to allow proper control to take place.

ANGULAR IMPULSE AND MOMENTUM

As would be expected, impulse and momentum have their analogous counterparts in rotatory motion. The product of the torque of a force and the increment of time over which it acts on the object is the *angular impulse*, $\tau \Delta t$. In the case of *angular momentum*, moment of inertia, I, and angular velocity, ω, are combined in the same manner as m and v in linear situations, namely $L = I\omega$.

The application of an angular impulse to a body changes its angular velocity so that

$$\tau \Delta t = I \Delta\omega$$

When the equation is written as

$$\tau \, \Delta t = I(\omega_f - \omega_o)$$

an applied angular impulse is seen to result in a change in the object's angular momentum:

$$\tau \, \Delta t = I\omega_f - I\omega_o \qquad \text{or} \qquad \Delta I\omega = \Delta L$$

Again it is easier to work with angular momentum than angular impulse because of the difficulty in measuring force magnitudes.

When a muscle group contracts with great force over a short increment of time, the force, as we have seen, may be considered an impulsive force. The torque of the force, which is responsible for the rotation of the body segment, is then called an impulsive torque. If the muscle contraction is terminated after Δt, the segment's momentum will support continued rotation without additional muscle action. This type of movement is known as *ballistic movement* and it will persist until some counterforce is applied in opposition. Ballistic movements are not limited to rotatory situations, but it has been claimed that much of man's refined, rapid rotatory movement is of the ballistic type.

TRANSFER AND CONSERVATION OF ANGULAR MOMENTUM

As was the case for linear momentum, angular momentum may be transferred between interacting bodies. General principles hold true in both cases to establish that the total angular momentum before, L_t, and after, L_t', interaction remains constant if other constraining influences are absent. Because the mechanisms of angular momentum transfer are so very complicated when applied to the human body, only simplified examples will be treated here in quantitative form.

Angular momentum may be transferred from a smaller body segment to the whole body—and in the opposite direction as well. Starting with the former, it is common to see an ice skater prepare for a long leap, within which pirouettes are performed, in recognizable patterns (Fig. 10-7). As the skater prepares for projection into the air, his upper extremities are vigorously rotated in the desired direction of the pirouette to build momentum. When he becomes airborne, momentum is transferred to the whole body, which is no longer restricted by contact with the rigid ice. The body is now free to rotate about its polar axis. The amount of preliminary upper extremity rotation is limited structurally. As this limit is approached, there is a marked deceleration of the segments, and their momentum is auto-

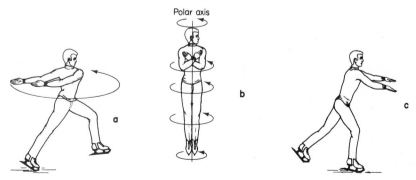

Figure 10–7. The transfer of angular momentum in an ice skater's leaping pirouette.

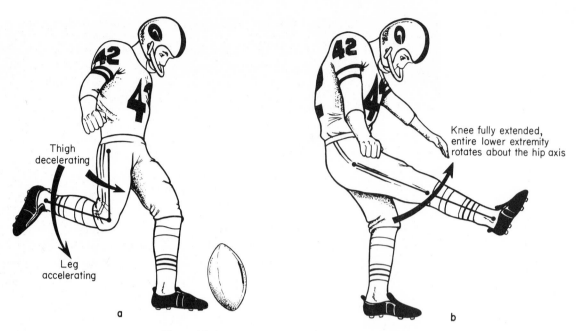

Figure 10–8. The transfer of angular momentum in place kicking a football.

matically transferred to the trunk, causing it to rotate. If this transfer coincides properly with the actual moment of loss of contact with the ice, the spinning effect on the whole body will be maximal. If the transfer occurs before the body is airborne, the trunk segment loses much of its acquired momentum to the supporting surface.

Figure 10-8 illustrates a place-kicking motion in which angular momentum is transferred from the whole body to the lower extremity. If a decelerating angular impulse, $-\tau \Delta t$, is applied during the motion to the thigh by the hip extensor muscles, some of the momentum of the thigh is transferred to the leg-foot segment combination. Both motions, hip as well as knee, are oriented in the same plane, so momentum transfer would not be unduly restricted. Limiting our attention to the lower limb, the momentum transfer from thigh to leg-foot is most easily recognized by changes in their angular velocities over Δt. Since the moments of inertia for the individual segments are structurally dependent, and therefore constant, the decelerating effect of the angular impulse on the thigh results in increasing the angular velocity of the adjacent, leg-foot segment combination. This is one of the most important principles in describing the motion of segmented structures such as the human body. Figure 10-9 illustrates that momentum transfer on the basis of velocity changes is very noticeable in stroboscopic photographs of the golf swing in which the segments of the upper limb are decelerated as the club is accelerated downward toward the ball. Plagenhoef has stated: "In whole body motions where a peak velocity is desired in the hands, the properly-timed stopping action of each segment in sequence from foot to hand produces the best results."[1] Figure 10-10 illustrates a baseball pitcher delivering a pitch.

[1]S. C. Plagenhoef, "Methods for Obtaining Kinetic Data to Analyze Human Motions," *Research Quarterly* **37** (March 1966), 110.

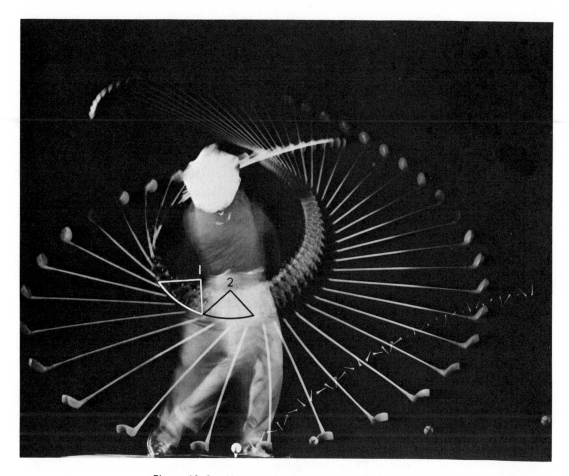

Figure 10–9. Although the club movement shown is not oriented in the plane of the photograph, it can be seen that the golfer's hands traverse a longer path in segment 1 than in segment 2 of the swing, demonstrating the deceleration required for momentum transfer. (Photo courtesy of Dr. Harold E. Edgerton, Massachusetts Institute of Technology, Cambridge.)

→ *Discuss the lead-up movements of the body segments in terms of proper timing of decelerating impulses and angular momentum transfers from massive to less massive segments.*

Because angular momentum is given as the product of an object's moment of inertia and angular velocity, a change in one of these elements must be accompanied by a compensatory change in the other if momentum is to be conserved. As I is increased, ω must decrease proportionately and vice versa. One of the most important outcomes of this phenomenon is that the angular velocity of a flexible, rotating object may be changed by altering the moment of inertia without the interaction of some external torque. Rigid bodies, of necessity, demonstrate constant moments of inertia because their masses are not deformable. Flexible bodies, such as our own, have variable moments of inertia depending on the positioning of their extremities owing to internal muscular forces. By careful manipulation of the positions of his body segments, man is capable of varying the velocity of his rotations through a rather wide range.

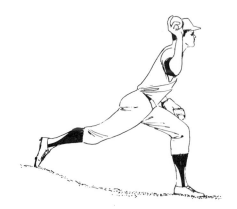

Figure 10–10. The folds in the fabric of the pitcher's uniform give excellent clues as to the movements of the body within it.

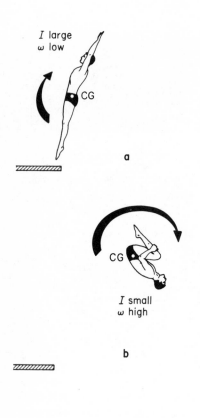

I large
ω low

CG

a

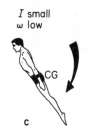

CG

I small
ω high

b

I small
ω low

CG

c

Figure 10–11. The interplay between the body's moment of inertia and angular velocity in a backward double somersault dive.

The backward double somersault shown in Fig. 10-11 illustrates both increases and decreases in angular velocity as the result of redistributing the body's mass. As the diver leaves the board in Fig. 10-11*a*, his body is extended to nearly its greatest length. Its reaction to the board is to rotate sagittally about its center of gravity. Because *I* is large in this position, rotational velocity is limited. By shortening the body into the "tuck" position (Fig. 10-11*b*), primarily by flexion movements, *I* is considerably reduced because the body's mass is now distributed as close to the axis of rotation as possible. Consequently, ω is commensurately increased. The maneuver allows the magnitude of rotation required by the dive to fit within the time available between the moment of leaving the board and contact with the water. Angular momentum is not altered because no significant external torque acts upon the diver's body to alter the magnitude of rotation beyond that resulting from the changes in *I*. At the proper moment, the diver will lengthen his body again, primarily by extension movements, to decelerate the rotation and allow a correct position for entry into the water (Fig. 10-11*c*). In this case, *I* is increased at the expense of ω to provide the proper control of the motion. Figure 10-12 illustrates additional examples of skillful rotation control about other axes. In addition, concurrent rotation about more than one axis is possible, as shown in Fig. 10-12*c*. Accelerations and decelerations about these multiple axes may occur simultaneously to provide the proper positions throughout a very complex movement.

When angular momentum is large, a large external torque is required to cause the rotating object's axis of rotation to change its orientation in space. That is, objects are afforded a great deal of stabilization when they are made to spin, particularly so when spinning about axes which are oriented along their paths of motion. Examples of thrown objects which require such stabilization are footballs and javelins as well as the discus. A spinning bicycle wheel provides an example of the resistance to change of axis orientation. If a bicycle wheel is held between the hands, as shown in Fig. 10-13, and is then set spinning with great velocity, large torques in the directions given by the arrows are required to alter its original position. The fact that some reorientation is possible is due to our being in contact with the ground, which resists our being turned by the spinning wheel.

If a pivoted platform which exhibited little friction were inserted between the feet and the ground (Fig. 10-13), the spinning wheel would resist the externally imposed torques and actually drive the body in rotation about its polar axis. Note that opposite torques applied to the wheel's axle result in opposite rotation reactions about the body's polar axis.

→ *Can you explain the reason for these opposite reactions?*

Pivoted platforms like that illustrated in Fig. 10-13 are available commercially for approximately $4.00.

From the foregoing, it is clear to see that the tendency of an isolated system (body, bicycle wheel, and turntable) is to conserve angular momentum. The use of a freely rotating platform to illustrate the rotational reactions of body parts relative to one another is a valuable adjunct to

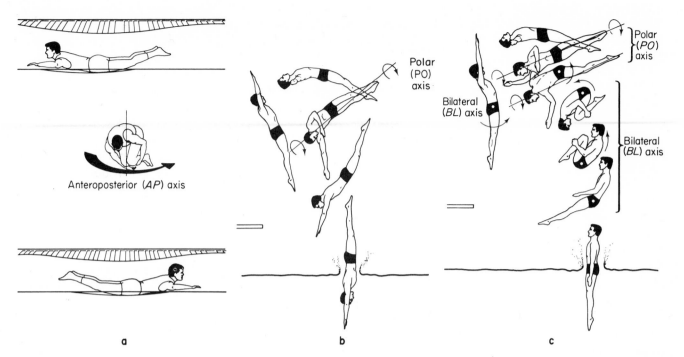

Figure 10–12. (a) The half-turntable on the trampoline. (b) The reverse dive, half twist. (c) The reverse dive, half twist, forward somersault tuck and its multiple rotations.

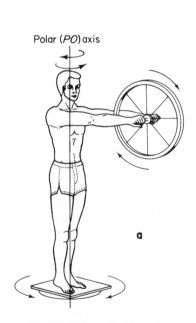

Figure 10–13. When the spinning bicycle wheel's axle is pivoted to the right, the platform and body rotate to the right, and vice versa. What would be the outcome if the same torques were applied to the wheel's axle while it was spinning in the opposite direction?

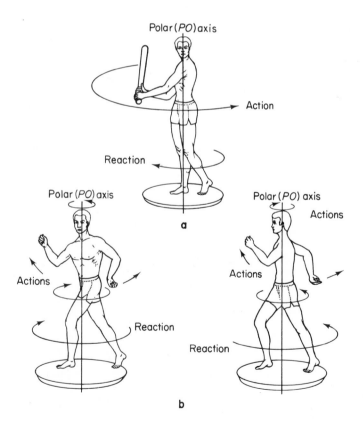

Figure 10–14

accurate motion description. Figure 10-14 illustrates additional action-reaction examples in athletic situations.

ROTATIONAL ENERGY

When an object at rest is set into rotation by a torque, the object's *rotational kinetic energy* exists in the particles of the object even though its axis of rotation is restricted to one location in space. Summing the individual particle energies is a process which identifies their individual moments of inertia as well. Consequently, it is reasonable that the equation from which rotational kinetic energy is derived is

$$E_{k_\theta} = \tfrac{1}{2} I \omega^2$$

which is seen to be analogous to the linear equation for a whole body. Like its linear counterpart, it is equivalent to the angular work done on the body, $\tau\theta$, and is a scalar quantity.

Suppose a torque of 4.8 lb·ft is applied to the upper limb by a shoulder abductor muscle to accelerate it uniformly from rest through 90 deg with a final angular velocity of 5.67 rad/sec, as in Fig. 10-15. With $I = .47$ slug·ft^2 for the limb ($m = .3$ slug, $k = 15$ in.), its kinetic energy at the horizontal position is

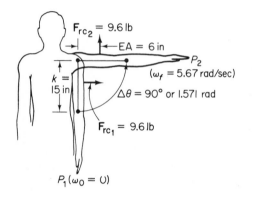

$$
\begin{aligned}
E_{k_\theta} &= \tfrac{1}{2} I \omega^2 \\
&= \frac{.47}{2}(5.67)^2 \\
&= .235 \times 32.08 \\
&= 7.54 \text{ ft lb}
\end{aligned}
$$

Checking to determine if $E_{k_\theta} = \tau\theta$, we see that

$$E_{k_\theta} = \tau\theta$$
$$7.54 \text{ ft lb} = 4.8 \text{ lb·ft} \times 1.571 \text{ rad}$$
$$= 7.54 \text{ ft lb}$$

→ *Knowing ω_o and ω_f, calculate the angular acceleration by applying $\alpha = \tau/I$. Next, compute the time increment required for the 90-deg abduction to take place by applying $\Delta t = \Delta\omega/\alpha$. If the muscle applying the force to the bone of the arm segment works through a tension angle, $\theta_T = 10$ deg, what was the approximate muscular force, F_T, applied?*

The total kinetic energy of an object demonstrating **both** translatory and rotatory motion is obtained by adding the translational kinetic energy of the object's center of gravity and its concurrent rotational kinetic energy about that point to give the total kinetic energy:

$$
\begin{aligned}
E_{k_t} &= E_k + E_{k_\theta} \\
&= \tfrac{1}{2}mv^2 + \tfrac{1}{2}I\omega^2
\end{aligned}
$$

In figure (left): $F_{rc_2} = 9.6$ lb; EA = 6 in; P_2 ($\omega_f = 5.67$ rad/sec); $k = 15$ in; $\Delta\theta = 90°$ or 1.571 rad; $F_{rc_1} = 9.6$ lb; $P_1(\omega_0 = 0)$

Figure 10–15

The energy to do work through rotation may be a function of an object's position. Elevated objects which become free to pivot about an axis demonstrate in the motion the stored potential energy given to them while reaching the elevated position. Gravity again represents the external force which is responsible for the stored capacity to do work. As before, when released, the rotating object transforms this stored energy into the kinetic energy of motion as the angular velocity increases. A common example illustrating this is that of "casting" the body forward and upward to begin a swinging motion on the horizontal bar in gymnastics. The elevating process is driven by muscular energy and forces against the resistance of gravity. Inevitably, gravity prevails to stop the elevation and at that moment begins to accelerate the gymnast's body about the bar in the opposite direction.

If a coiled spring is compressed, it, too, contains potential energy to do work. As it is being compressed, part of its total energy is kinetic and part is potential. Upon complete compression, the stored energy is poised to be recovered. The recovery depends on the reduction or release of the compressing force which generated the potential energy within the spring. Similarly, it is not difficult to see similar applications in man's musculoskeletal system where the muscles are the storehouses of potential energy.

When a muscle's pulling force on a body segment is resisted to an equal degree by an external force, the segment has the potential to move in response to the muscle force when released from the constraint. Figure 10-16 illustrates such a situation. It is a matter of common experience to have the potential energy released at an unexpected moment, causing the segment to be accelerated into another body part which must absorb its kinetic energy. Often, the result is a bruise. Athletic competition is replete with examples similar to the above, particularly in combative activities such as wrestling.

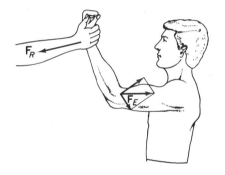

Figure 10–16. When the resistance force, **F**$_R$, is released, the original potential energy becomes the energy of motion and the forearm-hand segment combination is accelerated inward toward the body.

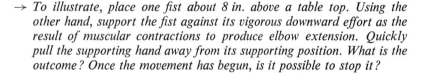

→ *To illustrate, place one fist about 8 in. above a table top. Using the other hand, support the fist against its vigorous downward effort as the result of muscular contractions to produce elbow extension. Quickly pull the supporting hand away from its supporting position. What is the outcome? Once the movement has begun, is it possible to stop it?*

The resisting force need not be applied by some object external to the body. Muscle forces applied to opposite sides of a joint which result in equal and opposite torques may be used to stabilize a body segment in a preparatory position. When one of the muscles is suddenly willed to relax, the segment responds in the direction of, and to a degree which is proportional to, the remaining torque.

REFERENCES

Anderson, T. McClurg. *Human Kinetics and Analysing Body Movements.* London: William Heinemann Medical Books, Ltd., 1951.

Benedict, F. G., and Murschhauser, H. "Energy Transformations During Horizontal Walking." Publication No. 231, Carnegie Institute of Washington: 1915.

Booyens, J., and Keatinge, W. R. "The Expenditure of Energy by Men and Women Walking." *Journal of Physiology* 138 (1957): 165.

Bouisset, S., and Pertuzon, E. "Experimental Determination of the Moment of Inertia of Limb Segments." In *Medicine and Sport*, vol. 2. Proceedings of the First International Seminar in Biomechanics, Zurich, August 1967. Basel, Switzerland: S. Karger AG, 1968.

Bouisset, S., and Goubel, F. "Influence of the Termination of Movement on the Relationship Between the Mechanical Work and the Integrated EMG of the Principal Agonist." *Electroencephalography and Clinical Neurophysiology* 25 (1968): 395.

Bowne, M. E. "Relationship of Selected Measures of Acting Body Levers to Ball Throwing Velocities." *Research Quarterly* 31 (1960): 392.

Carpenter, A. "A Study of Angles in the Measurement of Leg Lift." *Research Quarterly* 9 (1938): 70.

Clarke, H. H.; Irish, E. A.; Trzynka, G. A.; and Popowich, W. "Conditions for Optimum Work Output in Elbow Flexion, Shoulder Flexion, and Grip Ergography." *Archives of Physical Medicine & Rehabilitation* 39 (1958): 475.

Cochran, Alastair, and Stobbs, John. *The Search for the Perfect Swing.* Philadelphia: J. B. Lippincott Company, 1968.

Cotes, J. E., and Meade, F. "The Energy Expenditure and Mechanical Energy Demand in Walking." *Ergonomics* 3 (1960): 97.

David, H.; Hamley, E. J.; and Thomas, V. "Analysis of Leg Muscle Action in a Repetitive Locomotor Task." *Journal of Physiology* 197 (1968): 63P.

Dempster, W. T. "Space Requirements of the Seated Operator: Geometrical, Kinematic, and Mechanical Aspects of the Body with Special Reference to the Limbs." WADC Technical Report, 55-159. Wright-Patterson Air Force Base, Ohio: Wright Air Development Center, July 1955.

Dern, R. J.; Levene, J. M.; and Blair, H. A. "Forces Exerted at Different Velocities in Human Arm Movements." *American Journal of Physiology* 151 (1947): 415.

Dyson, Geoffrey H. G. *The Mechanics of Athletics.* 4th ed. London: University of London Press Ltd., 1967.

Eberhart, H. D.; Inman, V. T.; and Bresler, B. "The Principal Elements in Human Locomotion." In *Human Limbs and Their Substitutes*, edited by P. E. Klopsteg and P. D. Wilson. New York: McGraw-Hill Book Company, 1954.

Eckert, H. M. "Angular Velocity and Range of Motion in the Vertical and Standing Broad Jumps." *Research Quarterly* 39 (1968): 937.

——— "Linear Relationships of Isometric Strength to Propulsive Force, Angular Velocity and Angular Acceleration in the Standing Broad Jump." *Research Quarterly* 35 (1964): 298.

——— "The Effect of Added Weights on Joint Actions in the Vertical Jump." *Research Quarterly* 39 (1968): 943.

Elftman, H. "Forces and Energy Changes in the Leg During Walking." *American Journal of Physiology* 125 (1959): 339.

——— "The Work Done by Muscles in Running." *American Journal of Physiology* 129 (1940): 672.

Fenn, W. O. "Mechanical Energy Expenditure in Sprint Running as Measured by Moving Pictures." *American Journal of Physiology* 90 (1929): 343.

Ganslen, R. V. "Aerodynamic Factors Which Influence Discus Flight." *Discobolus* 5 (1958): 9.

Ganslen, Richard V., and Hall, Kenneth G. *The Aerodynamics of Javelin Flight.* Fayetteville, Ark.: University of Arkansas Press, 1960.

Hay, J. G. "Pole Vaulting: A Mechanical Analysis of Factors Influencing Pole-Bend." *Research Quarterly* 38 (1967): 34.

Henry, F. M., and Whitley, J. D. "Relationships Between Individual Differences in Strength, Speed, and Mass in Arm Movement." *Research Quarterly* 31 (1960): 24.

Hopper, B. "Rotation—A Vital Factor in Athletic Technique." *Track Technique* 15 (1964): 468.

Howell, A. Brazier. *Speed in Animals.* Chicago: University of Chicago Press, 1944.

Hubbard, A. W. "Homokinetics." In *Science and Medicine of Exercise and Sports*, edited by W. R. Johnson. New York: Harper & Row, Publishers, 1960.

———— "Muscular Force in Reciprocal Movements." *Journal of General Physiology* 20 (1939): 315.

Inman, V. T. "Conservation of Energy in Ambulation." *Archives of Physical Medicine and Rehabilitation* 48 (1967): 484.

Klopsteg, Paul E., and Wilson, Philip D., eds. *Human Limbs and Their Substitutes.* New York: McGraw-Hill Book Company, 1954.

Koepki, C. A., and Whitson, L. A. "Power and Velocity Developed in Manual Work." *Mechanical Engineering* 62 (1940): 383.

Lapp, V. W. "A Study of Hammer Velocity and the Physical Factors Involved in Hammer Throwing." *Research Quarterly* 6 (1935): 134.

Nubar, Y. "Energy of Contraction in Muscle." *Human Factors* 5 (1963): 531.

Passmore, R., and Durnin, J. V. G. A. "Human Energy Expenditure." *Physiological Review* 35 (1955): 801.

Plagenhoef, S. "Computer Programs for Obtaining Kinetic Data on Human Movement." *Journal of Biomechanics* 1 (1968): 221.

———— "Methods for Obtaining Kinetic Data to Analyze Human Motions." *Research Quarterly* 37 (1966): 103.

Provins, K. A. "Maximum Forces Exerted About the Elbow and Shoulder Joints on Each Side Separately and Simultaneously." *Journal of Applied Physiology* 7 (1955): 390.

Provins, K. A., and Salter, N. "Maximum Torque Exerted About the Elbow Joint." *Journal of Applied Physiology* 7 (1955): 393.

Ramsey, R. W.; Norris, A. H.; LeVore, N. W.; Shock, N. W.; Street, S.; Bower, J.; Miller, M. R.; Rosser, R.; and Szumski, A. "An Analysis of Alternating Movements of the Human Arm." *Federation Proceedings* 19 (1960): 254.

Rasch, P. J. "Relationship of Arm Strength, Weight, and Length to Speed of Arm Movement." *Research Quarterly* 25 (1954): 328.

Roberts, E. M., and Metcalfe, A. "Mechanical Analysis of Kicking." In *Medicine and Sport*, vol. 2. Basel, Switzerland: S. Karger AG, 1968.

Santschi, W. R., "Moment of Inertia and Centers of Gravity of the Living Human Body," Technical Documentary Report No. AMRL-TDR-63-36. Wright Patterson Air Force Base, Ohio: May 1963.

Schwartz, R. P.; Heath, A. L.; and Wright, J. W. "Kinetics of the Human Gait." *Journal of Bone and Joint Surgery* 16 (1934): 343.

Shames, Irving H. *Engineering Mechanics—Statistics and Dynamics.* 2nd ed. Englewood Cliffs, N.J.: Prentice-Hall, Inc., 1967.

Shortley, George, and Williams, Dudley. *Elements of Physics.* 4th ed. Englewood Cliffs, N.J.: Prentice-Hall, Inc., 1965.

Slocum, D. B., and Bowerman, W. "The Biomechanics of Running." *Clinical Orthopedics* 23 (1962): 39.

Spencer, R. R. "Ballistics in the Mat Kip." *Research Quarterly* 34 (1963): 213.

Stroup, F., and Bushell, D. L. "Rotation, Translation, and Trajectory in Diving." *Research Quarterly* 40 (1969): 812.

Tricker, R. A. R., and Tricker, B. J. K. *The Science of Movement.* New York: American Elsevier Publishing Company, Inc., 1967.

Whitley, J. D., and Smith, L. E. "Velocity Curves and Static Strength-Action Correlations in Relation to the Mass Moved by the Arm." *Research Quarterly* 34 (1963): 379.

Winter, F. W. "Mechanics of the Tuck Position in Executing the Forward Three and One-Half Somersault." *Athletic Journal* 45 (1965): 19.

11

Muscle Dynamics

Muscle is a specialized tissue which exhibits the ability to contract, and in so doing, it develops tension along its length. The study of the muscular systems of the body is known as *myology*. Although the human body contains three different types of muscle tissue, *smooth*, *cardiac*, and *skeletal*, we shall attend only to skeletal muscle in this chapter.

STRUCTURE OF SKELETAL MUSCLE

Skeletal muscles are found in varying shapes and sizes as befits their functions and locations within the body. Figure 11-1 illustrates a whole muscle in a generalized form so that its gross parts may be identified. Most of the muscles of the body attach at both ends to the skeleton. Often, the muscle narrows into strong *tendons*, which are dense, parallel bundles of white *connective* tissue. Tendons are continuations of connective tissue sheaths which bind together the muscle's central sections. The central portion of a whole muscle is often called the *belly*, which is encased in a connective tissue sheath known as the *epimysium*. These sheaths function mechanically to control and combine contractile action throughout the muscle. In addition, the whole muscle is held in its correct position within a body segment by extensive connective tissue layers of *fascia*.

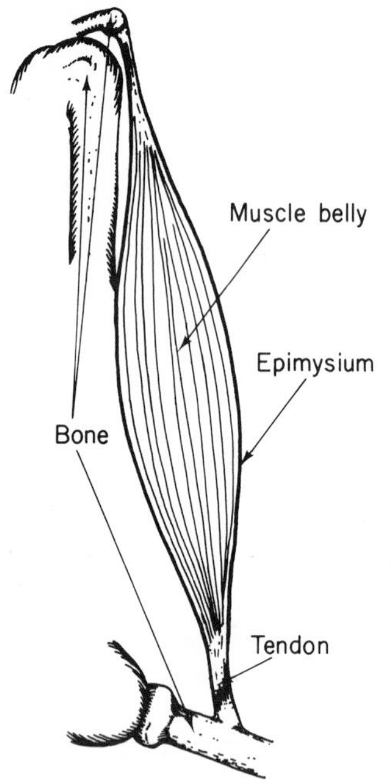

The epimysium penetrates into the muscle to divide it into separate, longitudinal compartments which house a group of muscle *fibers*. The bundle of fibers, consisting of as many as 150 individual fibers, is termed a *fasciculus* (Fig. 11-2). At this level of differentiation, the connective tissue sheath is called the *perimysium*. Fasciculi run parallel to one another in the muscle, as do the fibers housed within them. Surrounding each muscle fiber in a fasciculus is the *endomysium*. Note that in addition to the mechanical functions given above, these sheaths support capillaries and veins, lymph vessels, and nerve fibers which must course to and supply the contractile fibers.

Figure 11-3 illustrates a portion of a single skeletal muscle fiber which has its own cell membrane, the *sarcolemma*. Skeletal muscle cells (fibers) show many nuclei along their cylindrical lengths. They are located just

Figure 11–1. A whole muscle, illustrating its central belly and tendons.

Figure 11–2. Muscle cross section, showing fasciculi and associated structures. (Figures 11–2, 4, and 5 are reprinted with permission of the Macmillan Company from *The Human Body Its Structure and Physiology* by Sigmund Grollman. © Copyright Sigmund Grollman, 1969.)

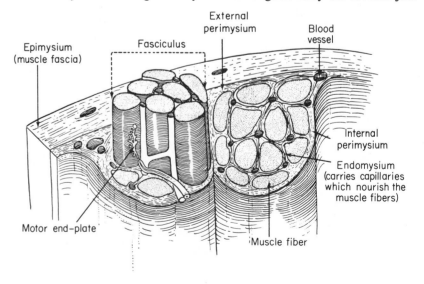

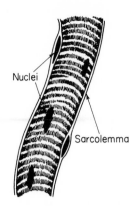

Figure 11–3. Section of a single muscle fiber, showing its nuclei and membrane (*sarcolemma*).

Figure 11–5. The step-wise organization of muscle to the level of the myofibril.

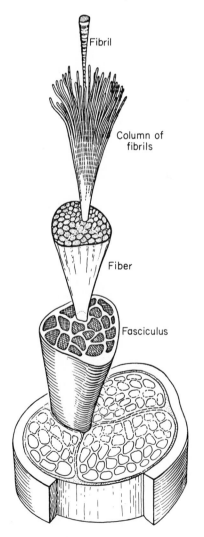

Fibril

Column of fibrils

Fiber

Fasciculus

Section of muscle

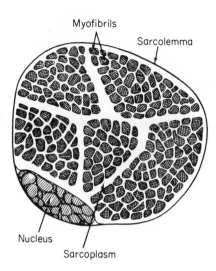

Figure 11–4. Cross section of a muscle fiber, illustrating the internal organization of myofibrils.

beneath the sarcolemma in a layer of cellular fluid known as the *sarcoplasm*. Figure 11-4 illustrates a cross-sectional view which identifies the internal structure of the muscle fiber.

Muscle fibers vary considerably in length, in some cases extending the entire length of a muscle and generally ranging from 10 to 100 μ (microns) in diameter.[1] These diameter dimensions indicate that muscle fibers are of microscopic size. Under special circumstances, skeletal muscle fibers exhibit transverse stripes or *striations*; this accounts for the common substitution of the term *striated* for skeletal when describing this class of muscle tissue. Figure 11-3 shows these stripes clearly. The striations are the result of even smaller units, *myofibrils*, located within the fiber which exhibit the same transverse stripes across their lengths. Myofibrils are located in clusters and run the length of the muscle fiber. Each myofibril is separated from its neighbor by the surrounding sarcoplasm. Figure 11-5 illustrates the stepwise differentiation of muscle structures to the level of the myofibril.

The myofibrils are the contractile elements below which we need not proceed, even though there are still smaller structures within them. These smaller structures, which are responsible for the myofibril's striations (Fig. 11-6), have been precisely identified, but the exact mechanism of the contractile process at that level is still in the theoretical stage of development. Myofibrils are composed of short, longitudinal sections called *sarcomeres* which contract upon suitable stimulation to reduce their lengths and develop tension. The result of this shortening is the shortening of the muscle fiber which houses them, with the development of considerable tension along the length of the fiber. The combined tensions of the many contracting fibers within the whole muscle's compartmentalized structure are transmitted to the body's bony levers through the network of connective tissue sheaths and the muscle tendons.

[1] One micron (μ) = 1/1000 mm (1.0×10^{-6} meter).

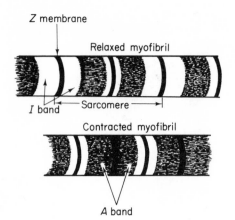

Z membrane

Relaxed myofibril

I band — Sarcomere

Contracted myofibril

A band

Figure 11–6. The myofibril in relaxed and contracted states. The sarcomeres shorten to draw their terminations (Z membranes) closer together.

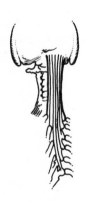
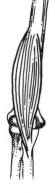

Figure 11–7. Two examples of longitudinal fiber arrangements.

VARIATIONS IN FIBER AND FASCICULUS ARRANGEMENTS

All muscles are composed of muscle fibers, but the positions of the fasciculi and the fibers within them, relative to the muscle's tendons, may vary. As a result, fiber arrangement figures prominently in an individual muscle's magnitude of shortening in contraction and its ability to exert force. In general, two groups of fiber arrangements exist, each with several variations, namely, *longitudinal* and *penniform*.

Fibers in longitudinal muscles run parallel or nearly parallel to each other along the length of the muscle. The fibers may be very long, such as those in the long, ribbon-like *sartorius*, or quite short, such as those of the *intercostals*. A variation which is rounded and increases in diameter from its ends to its belly is the *fusiform*, that is, spindle-shaped. It, too, is found in various sizes and shapes. A good example of fusiform arrangement is found in the *brachialis*, which crosses the anterior aspect of the elbow joint. Figure 11-7 illustrates examples of each.

The penniform (feather-like) group consists of several variations. *Unipennate*, the simplest form, exhibits fibers which approach a tendon obliquely from only one side. Examples of this sort of arrangement are the *tibialis posterior* and the *semimembranosus* of the lower limb. When fibers converge on a tendon from both sides, the muscle is called a *bipennate*. The *rectus femoris*, located on the front of the thigh, is a particularly good example. The middle portion of the *deltoid* muscle is an example of a *multipennate* fiber arrangement, which may be considered to be a combination of the two above. Figure 11-8 illustrates the penniform variations.

A comparison of longitudinal and penniform muscle shortening is illustrated in Fig. 11-9. It has been determined that skeletal muscle fibers may shorten approximately 50% during contraction. An uncontracted and relatively unstretched muscle in the body is said to be at its *resting length*. Thus in longitudinal muscles, with the fibers contracted to one half their resting length, $\mathscr{F}_{cl}$, the muscle is also of that length, where $\mathscr{F}_{cl} = \mathscr{M}_{cl}$. The same applies to the resting length, where $\mathscr{F}_{rl} = \mathscr{M}_{rl}$. Because the fibers of a penniform muscle are arranged so that they shorten at an angle to the direction the muscle shortens, the two are not equal in direction or magnitude. Assuming that the fibers shown in Fig. 11-9*b* are 5 in. long, contracting to .5 their resting length results in the whole muscle shortening:

$$\mathscr{M}_s = \mathscr{F}_s \cos \theta$$

$$= \frac{\mathscr{F}_{rl}}{2} \cos 30°$$

$$= 2.5 \text{ in.} \times .8660$$

$$= 2.165 \text{ in.}$$

→ *What is the muscle's contracted length, $\mathscr{M}_{cl}$, if its resting length, $\mathscr{M}_{rl} = 15$ in.?*

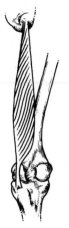

Unipennate

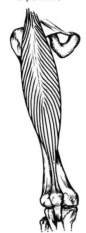

Bipennate

Multipennate

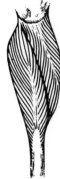

Figure 11–8. Penniform fiber arrangement variations.

This outcome is, of course, limited to penniform muscles whose fibers approach their tendons at 30-deg angles. As one would expect, the closer θ approaches 0 deg, the nearer the fiber and muscle lengths will be to being equal. It can be seen, therefore, that the penniform arrangement sacrifices magnitude of shortening when compared to longitudinal muscle of the same length.

→ *Satisfy your curiosity that this is the case by altering θ to 45 deg and 15 deg, respectively.*

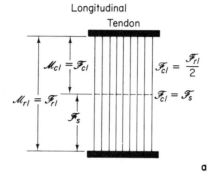

Longitudinal

$\mathcal{F}_{rl}$ = Resting fiber length
$\mathcal{M}_{rl}$ = Resting muscle length
$\mathcal{F}_{cl}$ = Contracted fiber length
$\mathcal{M}_{cl}$ = Contracted muscle length
$\mathcal{F}_s$ = Magnitude of fiber shortening
$\mathcal{M}_s$ = Magnitude of muscle shortening

a

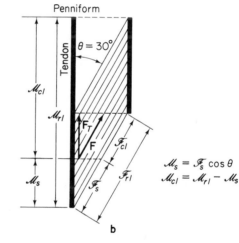

Penniform

$$\mathcal{M}_s = \mathcal{F}_s \cos \theta$$
$$\mathcal{M}_{cl} = \mathcal{M}_{rl} - \mathcal{M}_s$$

b

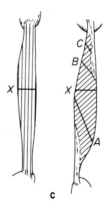

Figure 11–9. Comparison of longitudinal and pennate shortening. In (*c*), the cuts required to include all the fibers in the muscle to determine its physiological cross section.

c

The amount of tension a muscle may develop in a maximal contraction depends on many things. However, three structural factors are known to be directly related to a muscle's maximal tension-developing capabilities. They are (*1*) the number of muscle fibers, (*2*) the size or girth of the fibers, and (*3*) the internal fiber arrangement. The total force which a contracting muscle may exert on its bony lever has been found to be intimately related to the product of (*1*) and (*2*) above, that is, the total cross-sectional area of the muscle at its widest point. Studies over a span of years have yielded a rather wide range of force magnitudes. Recent sources have given figures ranging from about 42 to 71 lb/in.^{2} (3–5 kg/cm^2).

The determination of cross-sectional area requires the inclusion of all of the muscle's fibers, termed the *physiological cross section*. For longitudinal muscle, a cut at right angles to the muscle's length is sufficient generally to examine the whole, *x* in Fig. 11-9*c*. With the pennate arrangement, the number of fibers cut by such a section (*x*) depends on θ and the length of the muscle. It can be seen that only a few of the many fibers illustrated have been cut. Therefore, physiological cross section is determined by summing the areas of sufficient cuts at right angles to the fibers ($A + B + C$) to include them all. Obviously, such a procedure is limited to excised muscle of a laboratory preparation.

For a given muscle length, the penniform arrangement is said to allow for a greater number of fibers within a cross-sectional area. Assuming the force per fiber is constant, the greater number of fibers in the penniform arrangement per square inch of cross section yields a more forceful muscle. However, since the fibers approach the tendon at an angle, force along the muscle's action line is calculated on the basis of cos θ, where the usable tension of the fiber, $\mathbf{F}_T$, is

$$\mathbf{F}_T = \mathbf{F} \cos \theta$$

Refer once again to Fig. 11-9*b*. Even so, the penniform arrangement has advantages when compared to the longitudinal arrangement, as is evidenced by the fact that most of the strong muscles of the lower limbs are of this type, where maximal muscular forces are a premium. When extremely large forces are needed to motivate and control movement, the bipennate and multipennate arrangements are particularly advantageous in increasing the number of active fibers for a given muscle length. Beyond this, the number of fibers in a pennate muscle depends on its length; thus its ability to develop tension is also directly related to its length. This is not the case for longitudinal muscle, whose fibers are much longer and can extend over a large percentage of the muscle's length.

From the foregoing, it is clear that the penniform arrangement sacrifices the degree of shortening in favor of increased tension development. The longitudinal arrangement is reversed to facilitate wide ranges and greater speed of movement. Certainly both kinds of muscles are absolutely essential in human movement. In terms of the discussions of the work presented in Chapters 9 and 10, where both force and displacement are involved, muscle tissue clearly exhibits the characteristics necessary to be the source of potential energy, the capacity to do work.

Work Production

The determination of work capacity of longitudinal muscle is a relatively simple matter since fiber shortening is parallel to muscle shortening. It is the product of the tension and magnitude of shortening ($F\mathscr{F}_s$). Take, for example, a fusiform muscle whose body is 6 in. long. Assuming a circular cross section from the widest part of the belly to have a 1.5-in. diameter, cross-sectional area is

$$\pi R^2 = 3.142 \times (.75 \text{ in.})^2$$
$$= 3.142 \times .5625$$
$$= 1.8 \text{ in.}^2 \quad \text{(approximately)}$$

If we arbitrarily choose 70 lb/in.² as our tension figure, the muscle's total tension development capacity is

$$1.8 \text{ in.}^2 \times 70 \text{ lb/in.}^2 = 126 \text{ lb}$$

Assuming the fibers are capable of shortening one half their original length, 6 in./2 = 3 in., the work capacity is

$$W = F\mathscr{F}_s$$
$$= 126 \text{ lb} \times 3 \text{ in.}$$
$$= 378 \text{ in. lb} \quad \text{or} \quad 31.5 \text{ ft lb}$$

In penniform muscle, it was just shown that both tension development and magnitude of shortening are dependent on the cosine function of the angle the fibers make with the muscle's direction of shortening. Since work is $W = (F\cos\theta)d$, in the terms of Fig. 11-9,

$$W = F_T \mathscr{M}_s$$
$$= F\cos\theta\,\mathscr{F}_s\cos\theta$$
$$= F\mathscr{F}_s\cos^2\theta$$

With a hypothetical penniform muscle like that shown in Fig. 11-9b and the same cross section as above (1.8 in.²), a reduction in work capacity is quite evident:

$$W = F\mathscr{F}_s\cos^2\theta$$
$$= 126 \text{ lb} \times 2.5 \text{ in.} \times .8660^2$$
$$= 315 \text{ in. lb} \times .75$$
$$= 236 \text{ in. lb} \quad \text{or} \quad 19.7 \text{ ft lb}$$

a reduction of approximately 35%.

It is not likely that we would encounter a situation of this sort for the human body for two reasons: (*1*) We have not taken into account the increase in active fibers which would be present in a penniform muscle of

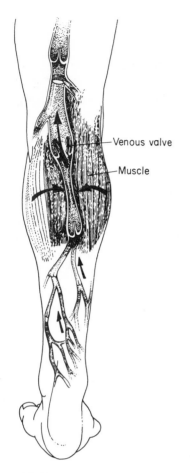

Figure 11–10. Internal compression forces upon veins impels blood toward the heart. (Reprinted by permission of Prentice-Hall, Inc. from *The Science of Health* by W. Guild, R. Fuisz, and S. Bojar, 1969.)

the same length, particularly those of the bipennate and multipennate arrangement, and (2) the angle θ is likely to be smaller for most pennate muscles. Under these circumstances, the work capacities of muscles of both types of equal size are nearly the same—the longitudinal muscle gaining the advantage of greater displacement and the penniform being more forceful.

NONAXIAL FORCES

The forces produced in muscular contractions are not directed entirely along the long axis of the muscle. As a muscle shortens, there is a very marked change in the shape of its belly in addition to its reduced length, namely, an increase in its diameter. This may be illustrated nicely by placing the thumb and fingers on opposite sides of the *biceps brachii* muscle on the front of the arm segment. As you forcibly contract the muscle through the range of elbow flexion, the change in shape is very noticeable. Even when the muscle is not allowed to shorten appreciably, these notably useful *internal compression* forces are developed—so much so, that when a maximal contraction is sustained over a period of time without shortening occurring, blood flow in the muscle is reduced drastically in magnitude.

One very beneficial outcome of these compression forces when they are applied intermittently is the work done in forcing blood in the veins back toward the heart. Figure 11-10 illustrates the phenomenon which may be voluntarily controlled to overcome the tendency for blood to pool in the lower limbs during prolonged standing. Contracting muscles in vigorous exercise play an important role in maintaining the required circulation to meet the demands of the active tissue.

In addition to compression forces within the contractile portion of the muscle, tendons crossing rounded bony protuberances enroute to their attachment points demonstrate another kind of forceful action. When tension is developed within the tendon, the underlying, curved bone surface acts to support a portion of the tension within the taut tendon. The action resembles, in part, the way a Fiberglas fishing rod supports a taut line. With the rod sharply curved, as in Fig. 11-11, it supports the line over parts of its smoothly curved upper surface, and the tendency for the line to break is reduced markedly. Consequently, lighter lines may be used with these rods than was the case with earlier, less flexible models.

Of course, bone ends do not bend under similar influences, but their curved surfaces do absorb large amounts of tension pressures which tend to increase the magnitude of stress that tendons may withstand without being inordinately thick. The quadriceps femoris tendon can serve as a particularly good example. In crouched positions, that is, weight bearing in flexed knee positions, the patella may apply forces more than five times a person's body weight to the distal surface of the femur.

→ *Can you describe any other practical outcome of these forces?*

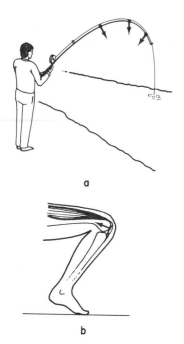

Figure 11–11. (*a*) The flexibility of the fishing pole along its length supports the line against breaking. In (*b*), a similar occurrence at the knee joint.

DISTENSIBILITY AND ELASTICITY

Our concerns to this point have centered around muscle important property, *contractility*. Now, two additional properties of muscle are to be discussed. They are (*1*) *distensibility* degree to which the muscle tissue will stretch in response to exter applied forces, and (*2*) *elasticity*, the propensity of muscle tissue to retur to its unstressed length after having been deformed. Putty is a material which may be deformed easily, but it will not return to its original. conformation. After deformation, a tennis ball quickly returns to its original shape. Thus it can be seen that materials may have one or both of these properties. Muscle tissue demonstrates both to a sizable degree.

Muscle distention is the usual case within the normally functioning musculoskeletal system. When a muscle is severed, its two ends retract from one another toward their opposing tendons. This is the reason for using the terms *relatively unstretched* when discussing the resting length of a muscle in its natural site. What was meant was that stretching was limited to a length which did not exceed the constraints of joint mobility. When an excised muscle is distended under laboratory conditions, tension within the muscle increases as the external load increases, but not linearly. That is, if muscle tension is plotted over muscle length, the plotted line is not straight, as in Fig. 11-12. Note that when the muscle is stretched (curve A), its resistance to further distension becomes greater. If the muscle is stimulated to contract after it has been distended, curve B shows the total tension exhibited by the muscle. It is seen that the maximal ability to develop tension during contraction occurs when the muscle is slightly longer than its normal length. Note also that the muscle can develop some tension after it has shortened beyond one half its normal length. Curve C represents the difference (B−A) between the tensions for the distended muscle under contractile and noncontractile conditions.

Because muscle is elastic, it exhibits a strong tendency to return to its normal length. This elasticity is claimed to reside within the network of connective tissues within and surrounding the muscle itself. Wilkie has likened this to the effect observed when a knitted stocking is stretched.[2] Since a part of this connective tissue lies alongside the muscle fibers, it has been called the *parallel elastic component* (*PEC*). The muscle's ability, when contracting, to increase the tension is called the *contractile component* (*CC*). There are additional elastic tendencies exhibited by the muscle fibers and tendons which are referred to as the *series elastic component* (*SEC*), because they are in line with the points between which the tension is developed. Upon examining Fig. 11-12, curve B, the maximal tension curve, is generally obtained by summing A (*PEC*) and C (*CC*). This would leave B as generally representing the muscle's total elastic tendency, between its points of attachment, to return to its normal length when released from the combination of external load and stimulation to contract.

[2]D. R. Wilkie, *Muscle* [London: Edward Arnold (Publishers) Ltd., 1968].

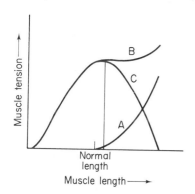

Figure 11–12. Muscle tension plotted against its length.

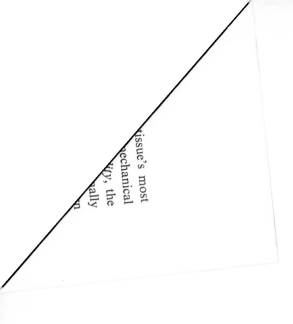

Like other elastic materials, muscle can be stretched to a point beyond which the ability to regain its original dimensions is lost. Within the normal ranges of joint mobility, the muscles are seldom in danger of stretching too far for their own good. It is well known, however, that violent contractions against formidable loads can produce sufficient tension to tear tendons and rupture muscle fibers. Elasticity and distensibility are seen to be two of man's most important mechanisms for safeguarding the functional integrity of the musculoskeletal system.

TENSION AND VELOCITY OF CONTRACTION

The length-tension phenomena which were described above were obtained under conditions known as *isometric*. When a muscle contracts under circumstances where little or no shortening can occur, it is called an isometric (equal-length) contraction. Theoretically, no work is done because no displacement through shortening has taken place, and the tension developed is termed *isometric tension*. True isometric contractions are only approximated within the musculoskeletal system even if a body segment is not allowed to move by being fixed externally. The muscle will be able to shorten approximately 7% before shortening is terminated because of the series elastic component (*SEC*). Since it is in line with the contractile component, early tension development is accompanied by the stretching of the *SEC*. This, in turn, slows the rate at which tension is developed. In terms of kinesiological description, these circumstances denote *static contractions*. Holding an object in a stationary position against the force of gravity and the application of equal and opposite muscular torques across a joint to hold a segment fixed are examples of static contractions. The important feature is that very little muscle shortening takes place in addition to that involved with stretching the *SEC*.

Isotonic contractions (equal tension) are those where shortening is allowed to take place, thus producing work in the process. This implies that some resistance is overcome and that the *isotonic tension* developed does not change throughout the displacement. In view of the previous discussions of musculoskeletal mechanics, equal tension is hardly likely to be maintained throughout the range of motion by a contracting muscle working across a joint. As would be expected, the shortening characteristics of isotonic contractions depend heavily on the magnitude of the loads moved. As load increases, total shortening decreases. This trend is followed until the isometric condition is reached. The velocity of shortening follows the same inverse relationship. When velocity of shortening is graphed against the load against which the muscle works, the outcome appears as in Fig. 11-13, curve A. If the baseline of the graph represented the tension developed in the muscle, it would show that as the velocity of shortening increases, tension developed by the muscle decreases. If the curve were followed below 0 with negative velocities, that is, when the muscle is being stretched or lengthened as it tries to resist an irresistible torque, the tension continues to rise somewhat. Curve B plots power output, where $P = Fv$, which is seen to reach a maximum at approximately

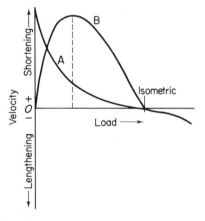

Figure 11–13. Curve A illustrates that as the load applied to a contracting muscle increases the velocity of shortening is reduced. Curve B plots power output of the contracting muscle.

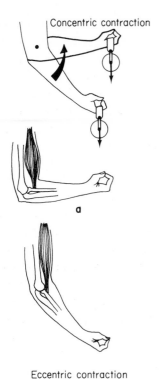

Concentric contraction

a

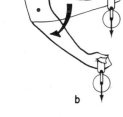

Eccentric contraction

b

Figure 11–14. Examples of (*a*) concentric and (*b*) eccentric contractions. Eccentric contractions are essential to dynamic stabilizations of body segments when control of displacement and velocity are crucial.

one third the maximal values of velocity and load. This suggests the possibility of adjusting the velocity of contraction to match fixed resistances to achieve the most favorable working conditions.

Two kinesiological terms are commonly employed to describe muscular contractions in terms of the direction of internal muscular displacements. When a muscle contracts and, in doing so shortens, the term *concentric contraction* is applied. Conversely, when a contracting muscle lengthens while still maintaining tension, it is known as an *eccentric contraction.* These terms avoid the issue of tension and velocity magnitudes. For instance, when the weight in Fig. 11-14*a* is carried upward as the result of elbow flexion, the elbow flexors are demonstrating concentric contractions. When the weight is lowered in Fig. 11-14*b*, its descent is controlled by the eccentric contractions of the same elbow flexors even though the movement illustrated is elbow extension. In either case, the tension developed and the velocity obtained may be large or small depending on the magnitude of the load. It is extremely important for the kinesiology student to recognize the immense importance of eccentric contractions in the description of the muscular control of body segment movements, particularly under the motivation of gravity. More will be said on this subject in Part III of the text, where the inclusion of more detailed anatomical descriptions may support the discussions.

MUSCULAR STRENGTH AND USE

It is a common observation that high levels of muscular *strength* are advantageous in tasks which include a high resistive component. The term *strength* is in common usage and is often incorrectly used as being interchangeable with other energetic terms. Consequently, we hear of feats of great potency, vigor, power, endurance, all used in evidence of the advantages of the proper applications of strength. From the standpoint of the following discussion, strength is defined as the maximum amount of *useful external force* which can be applied against some resistive medium. It goes beyond the muscle itself to include the skeletal levers through which the muscle operates and is measured externally. Although we speak of the strength of knee extension and shoulder flexion, this practice is not precisely correct because these movement terms do not entirely describe the functional conditions under which the measurements are made. In practice, such measurements are generally made isometrically at predetermined segment positions, with the aid of force registering instruments.

Elbow flexion strength is often measured with the joint in a flexed position: 90 or 115 deg. The useful external force measured in any one position within the range of joint mobility usually differs markedly from those of other positions for reasons already discussed. Therefore, it has been the practice to identify that position within a range of motion where the maximal isometric force may be applied and to use this position as a reference standard. The most recent evidence suggests that within the range of elbow flexion, the position is about 115 deg. In this way, there is some basis for comparison of muscular strengths of different individuals.

Training programs which continually work muscles near their maximal capacities with respect to load and intensity are effective in bringing about large increases in muscular strength. In addition to the measurable developments in strength, muscles usually grow in size, which is termed *hypertrophy*. The increased bulk of the muscle is the observable result of increases in the physiological cross section without a change in length or number of fibers present. Significant gains in connective tissue, fiber protein, sarcoplasm, nuclei, and capillaries yield the size changes.

Since strength is a measure of function, it would not be reasonable to attribute all of its development to structural changes. This is particularly true in view of evidence which charts threefold strength increases without commensurate increases in muscle size. One possible explanation for this phenomenon includes the changes in functional involvement of *motor units* during training regimens. A motor unit is made up of a motor neuron plus all of the muscle fibers which it supplies or innervates. The number of muscle fibers in a motor unit varies considerably, but it is clear that muscles which control fine movements contain fewer fibers per motor unit than those which control gross movements. Small muscles of the fingers have been reported to have approximately 100 fibers per motor unit, while the large muscles of the legs may have nearly 2000.

The muscle fibers of an individual motor unit are not limited to discrete fasciculi. They are found to be dispersed to intermingle with fibers of other motor units within the immediate vicinity. However, when the motor neuron is stimulated, all of the muscle fibers of that motor unit contract, although not simultaneously. Thus the tensions developed by individual fibers are mixed with those of others and fuse to develop a smooth wave of tension throughout the muscle. It is believed that as training progresses, motor unit activity becomes more efficient and more attuned to the specific modes of operation that the training demands. Consequently, it is not unreasonable to think of a *learning component* operating in the process of strength development which could function intramuscularly as well as intermuscularly.

MUSCULAR ACTIVITY MODES

Although there is much and proper attention paid to the group action of muscles, the fact remains that some muscles can and do act individually. In most cases, however, the movements which are the result of this individual muscle action are simple and not characterized as being highly resistive. An example is forearm pronation. When the opposite characteristics are in effect, either singly or combined, muscular action is communal. Of all of the factors contributing to the actions of muscle which have been identified, probably the most important factor is the muscle's position within the musculoskeletal system. Although there are many ways of describing the *functional position* of a muscle, the most common practice is to identify its attachment locations on the skeleton. In this way, an expected, thorough knowledge of skeletal anatomy would go far in

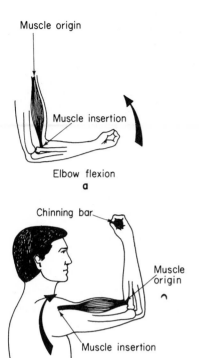

Muscle origin

Muscle insertion

Elbow flexion
a

Chinning bar

Muscle
origin

Muscle insertion

Elbow flexion in chinning
b

Figure 11–15. The reversal of muscle origin and insertion.

illuminating muscle action in terms of the joint structures crossed and muscle force action lines.

When a muscle contracts, tension is developed along its length so that the structures to which its ends are attached tend to perform all of the actions which are available to them under those circumstances. Historically, one of those circumstances has been identified as the stability of the structures to which the muscle ends attach. Thus the more stable or stationary attachment is referred to as the muscle's *origin.* The more easily moved attachment is called its *insertion.* In most cases, muscle origins are the more *proximally* (near center) located in the body, while insertions are more *distally* located. Hence, the terms *proximal* and *distal attachments* are commonly used as substitutes for origin and insertion, respectively.

The origin and insertion of a muscle may reverse when body segments are fixed in a manner that stabilizes the insertion end of the muscle. Figure 11-15 illustrates normal and reversed examples of elbow flexion. The muscle shown is the biceps brachii, and we shall be concerned only with its action at the elbow joint. In Fig. 11-15*a*, origin and insertion are in their conventional orientation, with the moving part being the forearm-hand segment combination. In Fig. 11-15*b*, the arm segment is the moving part because the hands are fixed to the stationary chinning bar, and origin and insertion are reversed. Thus a careful examination of the movement conditions coupled with a knowledge of the fiber course between attachment points can provide for quick identification of origin-insertion orientation as well as two of the most important muscle actions, namely, the approximation of origin and insertion and the drawing of origin and insertion fiber lines into the same plane.[3] Note that the proximal-distal orientation does not change under the circumstances of Fig. 11-15.

The purpose and outcome of muscular contraction need not always be limited to movement. In many cases the muscular force is applied to guide, resist, or stop movements from taking place. In analyzing human motion, muscles have been found to operate in the following activity modes.

Agonist

When a segment moves as the result of an applied muscular force, the muscle responsible for that movement is called the *agonist* or *mover.* Some muscles are named for their agonistic actions, such as the *pronator teres* and the *supinator.* A muscle may be an agonist for more than one movement, such as the *gastrocnemius,* which is involved with knee flexion and ankle plantar flexion. The gastrocnemius illustrates that agonistic activity may be major or minor. Its contribution to plantar flexion is major. However, its contribution to knee flexion is considered to be minor; then it is termed an *assistor.* When a given movement must be achieved against great resistance, several muscles may act as assistors to apply the required force effectively.

[3]M. A. MacConaill and J. V. Basmajian, *Muscles and Movements—A Basis for Human Kinesiology* (Baltimore, Md.: The Williams & Wilkins Company, 1969), pp. 86–88.

Antagonist

Most joints of the body are supplied with muscles which act to produce opposing movements. Thus the term *antagonist* is simply a convenient name for a muscle whose action could provide opposition for a designated agonist. If adduction is the movement in progress, abductor muscles are then potential antagonists and vice versa. Muscles may also be potential antagonists to movements motivated by gravity. In most cases of co-ordinated movement, antagonistic muscles do not contract, so that the desired agonistic action can take place. When they do act, they are usually employed to rule out an undesired movement or to check a high-velocity movement, which, if not decelerated, could lead to structural injury.

Stabilizer

A *stabilizer* muscle acts to secure or steady a bone or segment upon which an adjacent bone or segment moves. The stabilized part may then act as an anchor point so that a muscle attached to it may use that attachment as an origin. The other end of the muscle then functions as an insertion which is free to move the adjacent structure. Stabilization may also occur at some rather distant location in the body so that a rigid position may be maintained. An example can be found in a sit-up exercise. Of course, the lower limbs are stabilized so that the most important hip flexor muscles, normally originating above as well as below the hip joint, may both originate below the hip. If the sit-up required rigidly straight trunk and head-neck segments to increase the resistance torque, both of these segments would require some stabilizer action on the part of the posterior musculature of the vertebral column. Although it would appear that static contractions would be required, this is rarely the case with stabilization of the moving part's adjacent segment. These segments or bones nearly always require continuous position adjustments to provide optimal movement conditions for the moving parts. Arm movements at the shoulder joint are excellent examples. The *scapula* must move to adjust the position of the *glenoid fossa* with which the head of the *humerus* articulates. Therefore, the agonists for arm segment movement have a continuously adjusted anchor point from which to originate.

Synergist

Numerous attempts have been made in the past to develop a useful means of describing coordinated muscle teamwork. The term *synergist* comes from *synergy*, which means correlated or cooperative action. Although these words are appropriate for such descriptive purposes, usage and interpretation have varied greatly—so much so that some authors have avoided their use completely. This will not be the case in this text.

It can be seen that agonist and assistor teamwork is really an example of simple synergy in that they team up to accomplish a single objective. The *brachialis* and *biceps brachii* are agonists for elbow flexion and work together to arrive at that end. When added resistance to this movement is encountered, the *brachioradialis* may add its assistor function to the effort.

Of this group of muscles, only the brachialis is so situated to be limited to a single action.

Agonists and assistors frequently have secondary actions that tend to occur automatically as the result of tension development. Depending on the objective of the movement, some of these secondary actions may be inappropriate or undesired. It becomes necessary to rule out these secondary actions so that they do not impinge upon the desired outcome. This is accomplished through a process of antagonism where muscle action effectively neutralizes the undesired movements, leaving only those desired. When muscles cooperate to accomplish these two ends simultaneously, they are referred to as *synergists*. As an example, if the *rectus femoris* contracts, it has two agonistic functions, knee extension and hip flexion. If only knee extension is desired, a hip extensor muscle must be contracted to neutralize the hip flexion tendency. The hip extensor contributes to the desired outcome of knee extension through its antagonism or neutralizing action. Under these conditions, the hip extensor muscle is called a *pure synergist*. Assuming there were no other means available for ruling out the undesired secondary action, the pure synergist is as important to the desired outcome as is the agonist.

A second kind of synergic action occurs when two muscles operate agonistically to produce a desired movement and simultaneously neutralize each other's opposing secondary actions. When this happens, the cooperating muscles are termed *helping synergists* since both were involved in the neutralizing process. To help the reader gain a better understanding of how pure and helping synergy differ, refer to Table 11-1.

When it is remembered that muscle forces may be resolved into component forces, it is necessary to investigate their synergic contributions. In areas of the body such as the shoulder girdle and shoulder joint, force components are constantly at work to rule out one another to permit specialized actions to occur. When muscular involvements in movements are analyzed to the level of force component interactions, a muscle whose force component neutralizes an undesirable component of another may be classified further as a *component synergist*. Often a muscle's stabilizing

TABLE 11-1

	Pure Synergy			Helping Synergy		
Desired outcome	Forceful knee extension without concurrent hip flexion			Joint adduction without concurrent segment rotation		
Cooperating muscles	Muscle A	and	Muscle B*	Muscle A†	and	Muscle B†
	↓		↓	↓		↓
Actions	Knee extension and hip flexion	+	Hip extension	Adduction and inward rotation	+	Adduction and outward rotation
Outcome	Knee extension—hip flexion tendency neutralized			Joint adduction—segment inward and outward rotations mutually neutralized		

* Pure synergist.
† Helping synergist.

Shunt muscle

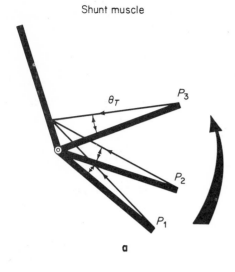

a

Spurt muscle

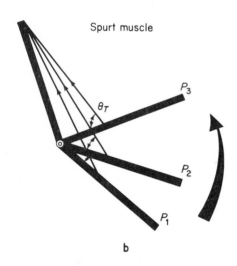

b

Figure 11–16. The positions of shunt and spurt muscles during joint flexion.

component acts to place a highly mobile bone in a position where further movement is badly restricted structurally. The dislocating component of another muscle may neutralize that unwanted movement of the bone, which allows a desired motion to be completed.

Shunt and Spurt

The action lines of muscular forces offer important clues as to the functions which muscles may perform. If a muscle is situated, with respect to the segment it motivates at a given joint so that its contractile action line remains very nearly parallel to the moving segment throughout its movement range, it is called a *shunt* muscle. Muscles of this type find their origins situated near the joint crossed, with their insertions a notably greater distance from the joint. The *brachioradialis* of the elbow joint and forearm is situated in this manner. It originates a short distance above the joint on the *humerus* and inserts near the end of the *radius* of the forearm. Upon contraction, its action line creates a small tension angle throughout its contractile range (Fig. 11-16*a*), which indicates its continually strong joint stabilization function.

→ *Examine the leg segment and the knee joint. What muscle crossing the back of the joint is so situated?*

If a muscle is situated to produce an obviously varying tension angle as the movement range is traversed, it is called a *spurt* muscle. At the elbow joint, the *biceps brachii* and *brachialis* are examples of spurt muscles. Their origins are farther removed from the joint crossed than their insertions. Consequently, as elbow flexion progresses, their tension angles improve to facilitate their rotatory functions.

→ *Can you identify a spurt muscle crossing the back of the knee joint?*

It can be seen that fixing the distal end of the forearm segment, as in performing a chin-up, necessitates origin and insertion reversal, which, in turn, generally necessitates shunt and spurt function inversion.

→ *Of what prime value are the biceps brachii and brachialis shunt forces during a chin-up?*

REFERENCES

Alexander, J. F.; Drake, C. J.; Reichenbach, P. J.; and Haddow, J. B. "Effect of Strength Development on Speed of Shooting of Ice Hockey Players." *Research Quarterly* 35 (1964): 101.

Alexander, R. S. "Immediate Effects of Stretch on Muscle Contractility." *American Journal of Physiology* 196 (1959): 807.

Arkin, A. M. "Absolute Muscle Power: The Internal Kinesiology of Muscle." *Archives of Surgery* 42 (1941): 395.

Bach, L. M. N. "Conversion of Red Muscle to Pale Muscle." *Proceedings of the Society for Experimental Biology and Medicine* 67 (1957): 268.

Bannister, R. G. "Muscular Effort." *British Medical Bulletin* 12 (1956): 222.

Barnett, C. H., and Harding, D. "The Activity of Antagonist Muscles During Voluntary Movement." *Annals of Physical Medicine* 2 (1955): 290.

Basmajian, J. V. "'Spurt' and 'Shunt' Muscles: An Electromyographic Confirmation." *Journal of Anatomy* 93 (1959): 551.

Beevor, Charles E. *The Croonian Lectures on Muscular Movements*. New York: The Macmillan Company, 1940.

Bender, J. A., and Kaplan, H. M. "The Multiple Angle Testing Method for the Evaluation of Muscle Strength." *Journal of Bone and Joint Surgery* 45-A (1963): 135.

Bennett, H. S. "The Structure of Striated Muscle as seen by the Electron Microscope." In *Structure and Function of Muscle*, edited by C. H. Bourne. New York: Academic Press, Inc., 1960.

Bernstein, Nikolai A. *The Coordination and Regulation of Movements*. New York: Pergamon Press, 1967.

Bourne, G. H., ed. *The Structure and Function of Muscle*. New York: Academic Press, Inc., 1960.

Brunnstrom, S. "Comparative Strengths of Muscles with Similar Functions." *Physical Therapy Review* 26 (1946): 59.

Buchthal, F. "Factors Determining Tension Development in Skeletal Muscle." *Acta Physiologica Scandinavica* 8 (1944): 38.

Clarke, H. Harrison. *Muscular Strength and Endurance in Man*. Englewood Cliffs, N.J.: Prentice-Hall, Inc., 1966.

Darcus, H. D., and Salter, N. "The Effect of Repeated Muscular Exertion on Muscular Strength." *Journal of Physiology* 129 (1955): 325.

DeLorme, T. L. "Restoration of Muscle Power by Heavy Resistance Exercises." *Journal of Bone and Joint Surgery* 27 (1945): 645.

deVries, H. A. "Muscle Tonus in Postural Muscles." *American Journal of Physical Medicine* 44 (1965): 275.

Doss, W. S., and Karpovich, P. V. "A Comparison of Concentric, Eccentric, and Isometric Strength of Elbow Flexors." *Journal of Applied Physiology* 20 (1965): 351.

Elftman, H. "The Action of the Muscles in the Body." *Biological Symposium* 3 (1941): 191.

———— "Biomechanics of Muscle: With Particular Application to Studies of Gait." *Journal of Bone and Joint Surgery* 48-A (1966): 363.

———— "The Function of Muscles in Locomotion." *American Journal of Physiology* 125 (1939): 357.

———— "The Work Done by Muscles in Running." *American Journal of Physiology* 129 (1940): 672.

Elmendorf, A. "Muscular Power and Endurance." *Science* (American Supplement), Aug. 11, 1917: 84.

Fenn, W. O. "The Mechanics of Muscular Contraction in Man." *Journal of Applied Physics* 9 (1938): 165.

Fenn, W. O.; Brody, H.; and Patrille, A. "The Tension Developed by Human Muscles at Different Velocities." *American Journal of Physiology* 97 (1931): 1.

Fick, R. *Handbuch der Anatomie und Mechanik der Gelenke*. Jena, Germany: G. Fischer, 1910.

Gratz, C. M. "Tensile Strength and Elasticity Tests on Human Fascia Lata." *Journal of Bone and Joint Surgery* 13 (1941): 334.

Haines, R. W. "The Laws of Muscle and Tendon Growth." *Journal of Anatomy* 66 (1932): 578.

Hellebrandt, F. A. "Special Review: Application of the Overload Principle to Muscle Training in Man." *American Journal of Physical Medicine* 37 (1958): 278.

Hellebrandt, F. A.; Cary, M. K.; Duvall, E. N.; Houtz, S. J.; Skowlund, H. V.; and Apperly, F. L. "Relative Importance of the Muscle Pump in the Prevention of Gravity Shock." *Physical Therapy Review* 29 (1949): 12.

Hettinger, Theodor. *Physiology of Strength.* Springfield, Ill.: Charles C. Thomas, Publisher, 1961.

Hill, A. V. "The Design of Muscles," *British Medical Bulletin* 12 (1956): 165.

——— "The Maximum Work and Mechanical Efficiency of Human Muscles and Their Most Economical Speed." *Journal of Physiology* 56 (1922): 19.

——— "The Mechanics of Voluntary Muscle." *Lancet* 261 (1951): 947.

——— *Muscular Movement in Man.* New York: McGraw-Hill Book Company, 1927.

Hoyle, Graham. *The Nervous Control of Muscular Contraction.* New York: The Cambridge University Press, 1958.

Huxley, H. E. "The Contraction of Muscle." *Scientific American,* November 1958.

——— "Mechanism of Muscular Contraction." *Scientific American,* December 1965.

Inman, V. T., and Ralston, H. J. "The Mechanics of Voluntary Muscle." In *Human Limbs and Their Substitutes,* edited by P. E. Klopsteg and P. D. Wilson. New York: McGraw-Hill Book Company, 1954.

Johnson, Warren R., ed. *Science and Medicine of Exercise and Sports.* New York: Harper & Row, Publishers, 1960.

Katz, B. "The Relation Between Force and Speed in Muscular Contraction." *Journal of Physiology* 96 (1939): 45.

Liberson, W. T.; Dondey, M.; and Asa, M. M. "Brief Repeated Isometric Maximal Exercises. An Evaluation by Integrated Electromyography." *American Journal of Physical Medicine* 44 (1962): 3.

Lockhart, R. D. "The Anatomy of Muscles and Their Relation to Movement and Posture." In *Structure and Function of Muscle,* edited by C. H. Bourne. New York: Academic Press, Inc., 1960.

Logan, G. A., and McKinney, W. C. "The Serape Effect." *Journal of Health, Physical Education, Recreation* 41 (1970): 79.

Lupton, H. "An Analysis of the Effects of Speed on the Mechanical Efficiency of Human Muscular Movement." *Journal of Physiology* 57 (1923): 337.

McCloy, C. H. "Some Notes on Differential Actions of Partite Muscles." *Research Quarterly* 17 (1946): 254.

MacConaill, M. A. "The Movements of Bones and Joints: II. Function of the Musculature." *Journal of Bone and Joint Surgery* 31-B (1949): 100.

——— "Some Anatomical Factors Affecting the Stabilizing Functions of Muscles." *Irish Journal of Medical Science* 6 (1946): 160.

MacConaill, M. A., and Basmajian, J. V. *Muscles and Movement: A Basis for Human Kinesiology.* Baltimore: The William & Wilkins Company, 1969.

McMorris, R. O., and Elkins, E. C. "A Study of Production and Evaluation of Muscular Hypertrophy." *Archives of Physical Medicine and Rehabilitation.* 35 (1954): 420.

Mommaerts, W. F. H. "Fundamental Aspects of Muscle Function." *Journal of Bone and Joint Surgery* 41-A (1959): 1315.

Monod, H. and J. Scherrer. "The Work Capacity of a Synergic Muscular Group." *Ergonomics* 8 (1965): 329.

Morris, C. B. "The Measurement of the Strength of Muscle Relative to the Cross Section." *Research Quarterly* 19 (1948): 295.

Paul, W. M.; Daniel, E. E.; Kay, C. M.; and Moncton, G. *Muscle.* New York: Pergamon Press, Inc., 1965.

Perry, J. "Structural Insufficiency." *Physical Therapy* 47 (1967): 848.

Ralston, H. J. "Mechanics of Voluntary Muscle." *American Journal of Physical Medicine* 32 (1953): 166.

Ralston, H. J., and Libet, B. "The Question of Tonus in Skeletal Muscle." *American Journal of Physical Medicine* 32 (1953): 85.

Rodahl, Kaare, and Horvath, Steven M., eds. *Muscle as a Tissue.* New York: McGraw-Hill Book Company, 1962.

Scott, J. H. "Muscle Growth and Function in Relation to Skeletal Morphology." *American Journal of Physical Anthropology* 15(*NS*) (1957): 197.

Steinhaus, A. H. "Strength from Morpugo to Muller. A Half Century of Research." *Journal Association for Physical and Mental Rehabilitation* 9 (1955): 147.

———— "Your Muscles See More Than Your Eyes." *Journal of Health, Physical Education, Recreation* 37 (1966): 38.

Tricker, R. A. R., and Tricker, B. J. K. *The Science of Movement*. New York: American Elsevier Publishing Company, Inc., 1967.

Walls, E. W. "The Micro-Anatomy of Muscle." In *Structure and Function of Muscles*, edited by C. H. Bourne. New York: Academic Press, Inc., 1960.

Waterland, J. C. "Integration of Movement." In *Medicine and Sport*, vol. 2. Proceedings of the First International Seminar on Biomechanics, Zurich, August 1967. Basel, Switzerland: S. Karger AG, 1968.

Whitney, R. J. "Mechanics of Normal Muscular Activity." *Nature* 181 (1958): 942.

Wilkie, D. R. "The Mechanical Properties of Muscle." *British Medical Bulletin* 12 (1956): 177.

———— *Muscle*. London: Edward Arnold (Publishers) Ltd., 1968.

———— "The Relation Between Force and Velocity in Human Muscle." *Journal of Physiology* 110 (1950): 249.

Wright, Wilhelmine G. *Muscle Function*. New York: Hafner Publishing Company, 1962.

Zorbas, W. S., and Karpovich, P. V. "The Effect of Weight Lifting Upon the Speed of Muscular Contraction." *Research Quarterly* 22 (1951): 145.

12

The Electromotive Characteristics of Muscle

The contraction of muscle is preceded by the passage of neural impulses across the myoneural junctions of the muscles involved. When these impulses reach the muscle fiber membrane, a wave of electrical activity passes the length of the muscle fiber. This is known as the *excitation wave.* Since the neural impulses and the excitation wave are electrical in nature, they may be recorded by specialized equipment. In the case of the excitation wave exhibited in muscle, the recording apparatus is known as the *electromyograph* and the recording is the *electromyogram.* While the knowledge of this electrical phenomenon has been in existence for many years, it was considered little more than a curiosity until the electronic developments of recent times. The availability of equipment sensitive enough to monitor the minute electrical currents typifying the excitation process has resulted in the collection of a unified body of knowledge and the emergence of the field of *electromyography.*

Much of the value of electromyography has been in the area of medical science, particularly as a diagnostic tool for neuromuscular pathology. For that purpose the work has been directed toward the study of the motor units, singularly or in small groups. While electromyography continues to be of great medical value, it has also attracted the interest of exercise physiologists and kinesiologists. These investigators have been more interested in the study of the actions of whole muscles or groups of muscles than in individual motor unit activity. The use of electromyography in the analysis of human motion has become of greater interest in recent years. While it is the purpose of this chapter to review the electrical characteristics of muscle and muscular contraction and explore its uses in motion analysis, it is, by no means, complete. Therefore, the interested reader is directed to the more detailed information afforded by the sources included at the end of the chapter.

THE ELECTRICAL ACTIVITY OF MUSCULAR CONTRACTION

Underlying the excitation wave phenomenon is the concept that the resting muscle fiber wall (sarcolemma) acts as a semipermeable membrane, with a high concentration of sodium ions on the outside and a high concentration of potassium ions on the inside of the membrane. This arrangement results in an electrical differential which is known as the *membrane potential,* with the outside of the membrane being charged positively and the inside charged negatively. When a nerve impulse travels along the axon to the motor unit and is transmitted by means of the myoneural junction to the muscle fiber, the permeability of the sarcolemma is changed. The change in membrane permeability results in sodium and potassium ions exchanging places. As the excitation wave passes along the muscle fiber, the membrane then reverts to its resting, polarized state, a situation which causes the sodium and potassium ions to return to their original positions. The electrical activity accompanying the exchange of ions is known as the *action potential,* and it is likely that it traverses the fiber's length before appreciable tension develops. In electromyography, it is these action potentials which are monitored and recorded.

The basic functional structure of muscular contraction is the motor unit. The motor unit consists of the axon, its branches, and the muscle fibers innervated by them (refer to Chapter 11). A stimulus to a motor unit causes excitation of all the muscle fibers of that unit almost simultaneously. When stimulated, individual fibers may undergo excitation phases of only 1 or 2 msec in duration. The staggering of these individual fiber phases may give an excitation phase for the entire motor unit lasting from 5 to 12 msec. The amplitude of the action potential has been found to be about $\frac{1}{2}$ mV, while the frequency has been found to range between 6 and 60/sec. Basmajian suggests that the limit of the frequency of the action potential is related to the physiological limit of about 50/sec found in the frequency of the axonal impulses.[1]

A voluntary muscular contraction involves numerous muscle fibers being innervated on the motor unit basis. Since each motor unit may undergo an excitation phase of 5 to 12 msec, it is likely that some of these phases will overlap, resulting in an "interference pattern" electromyogram (Fig. 12-1). As the intensity of muscular activity is increased, two changes have been found to occur: (1) The frequency of excitation of the muscle fibers of each active unit increases, and (2) more motor units will be called into action. Either of these changes will bring about an increase in the *total electrical activity* monitored from the muscle.

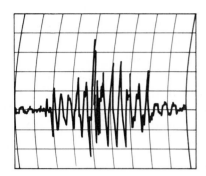

Figure 12–1. A typical interference pattern electromyogram from the biceps femoris muscle of a subject walking.

Relationship Between Excitation and Contraction

It has been established that the excitation wave may precede the contraction of the muscle by as much as 2 msec, indicating that the action potential may not be a direct trigger for contraction but possibly the initiator of some intermediate operation. It has been suggested that the intermediate operation may involve a change in the calcium concentration within the muscle fiber. It is possible that the role of the action potential is to initiate a sequence of reactions involving the calcium concentration which results in the contraction of the muscle fiber. A great deal of electromyographic research, particularly that in the area of fatigue, has indicated that action potentials may be present with no evidence of coincident contraction. If the biochemical environment of the muscle cell is such that the excitation wave cannot trigger the intermediate mechanisms which lead to contraction, then it can be seen that measurement of the excitation wave is not measurement of the contractile process.

The recording of action potentials without accompanying muscular contraction has occurred primarily in studies of muscular fatigue. It would appear that while laboratory situations may be set up in which the contractile response and the action potentials may appear to be unrelated, the voluntary innervation of a muscle in the living organism produces muscle action potentials and contractions which are essentially parallel.[2]

[1]J. V. Basmajian, *Muscles Alive—Their Functions Revealed by Electromyography* (Baltimore: The Williams & Wilkins Company, 1967), p. 8.

[2]G. N. Loofbourrow, "Neuromuscular Integration," in *Science and Medicine of Exercise and Sports* (W. R. Johnson, ed.) (New York: Harper & Row, Publishers, 1960).

RECORDING OF MUSCLE ACTION POTENTIALS

Electromyography is concerned with the measurement and analysis of muscle action potentials. Numerous techniques for recording and various methods of analyzing the data have been developed over the years. The person interested in using electromyography must determine exactly what his objectives are and then what instrumentation would best provide valid data. Whatever his choice, some type of electrodes must be attached to the subject to act as the first element between the bioelectric source and the recording device. The electrodes are then connected by wire or a telemetry device to a specialized piece of equipment (electromyograph) which receives and then records the action potentials as electromyograms.

The electrode type used depends very much on the objective of the measurement. When the objective is to examine and measure the electrical activity of motor units individually or in small groups, then the choice would suitably be an electrode which is inserted directly into the muscle, either the needle or wire type. When measurements of the whole muscle or groups of muscles are to be made, surface electrodes may often be of value. Since surface electrodes monitor the electrical activity of the muscle fibers underlying them, information concerning specific frequencies, single motor unit activity, and action potential shape cannot be obtained but should be monitored by intramuscular electrodes. It has been reported that electrical activity measured from surface electrodes and intramuscular electrodes tends to be highly correlated with respect to quantitative features.

The use of surface electrodes requires very careful preparation of the electrode site. The electrical energy must pass through the tissue located between the muscle and the electrode. These tissues offer a resistance to the flow of an alternating current known as *impedance*. The tissues lying below the skin have been shown to have relatively low impedance, while the skin itself has a high level of impedance. The preparation of the electrode site involves removing excessive hair from the surface, abrasion of the skin with a fine grade of sandpaper to remove some of the epidermal cells, and the application of an alcohol solution to the area to remove surface oils. When these steps have been completed, an electrolyte paste or jelly is rubbed into the prepared area. The electrolyte is then applied to the electrode, which is then secured to the prepared skin area. A measure of the impedance should then be taken. The maximal level of impedance considered acceptable depends in part on the objective of the study. Recordings of contractions of great magnitude will be influenced less by high impedance levels than will recordings of resting muscles. Levels ranging from 10,000 to 30,000 ohms (Ω) have been suggested. It is obvious that one should strive for low impedance conditions.

The electrode configuration is usually one of two types: (*1*) unipolar and (*2*) bipolar. The former configuration consists of one electrode positioned over the muscle to be monitored and a second electrode positioned over an area which will be electrically inactive, possibly over an area where bone resides just under the skin. The bipolar configuration, on the other hand, consists of two "active" electrodes positioned close together over the muscle and a third, "indifferent" electrode placed over an inactive site. The electrodes used to monitor the action potentials sample only the electrical activity in the muscle mass in close proximity to the point of electrode application. While the unipolar recording is felt to be more easily analyzed than the bipolar regarding the waveform produced, when the activity of the whole muscle is being monitored, waveform is usually of little importance.

A more important factor in the total electrical activity recorded is that of its tendency to spread from one muscle to another. The bipolar configuration samples only the area of the muscle lying under and between the two active electrodes. The size of the area sampled may be increased or decreased by altering the space between these electrodes. The bipolar configuration allows for more control over the possibility of electrical activity from adjacent muscles being monitored and recorded. On the other hand, the unipolar configuration monitors all of the electrical activity from the muscle mass around and under it, making it more susceptible to the electrical conditions of surrounding muscles.

The electrical activity monitored by the electrodes can be recorded by several different instruments. The most common methods are photographing the wave produced on an oscilloscope and adapting the action potentials to drive a pen-writer which then produces an ink or heat tracing on moving paper. Whatever method is used to record the action potentials, the mode of operation must be determined by the investigator. A common mode of recording when one is interested in the activity of individual motor units, small groups of motor units, or the pattern of excitation is known as *direct* recording (Fig. 12-2*a*). In this mode, the electrical activity of the muscle fibers is recorded as it is monitored. From the baseline, the recording pen may move both positively (upward) and negatively (downward). This type of recording can be valuable when studying the very small magnitudes of activity produced during relaxation. When the amount of activity increases, however, the individual waveforms of motor units are no longer visible. If one is interested in the concurrent actions of several muscles during a movement, the direct recording mode can be used to help determine the relationships of these muscles to each other.

The second mode of recording is that known as *integration* (Fig. 12-2*b*). The integrated recording is the result of electronic treatment of the electrical signals so that the frequency, duration, and amplitude of the current are averaged. The tracing thus produced is indicative of the amount of electrical activity produced during a particular activity or contraction. While the direct reading is more adaptable to subjective evaluations, the integrated recording is more useful in quantitative terms where statistical treatments are desired.

Another method of recording the muscle action potentials is similar to the integrated method just discussed. However, after the integration procedure has been accomplished, the signal is treated by a voltage-to-frequency converter, the pulsed frequency output of which is proportional to the quantity of electrical energy monitored. The frequency output is then directed into an electronic counter which produces a digital figure

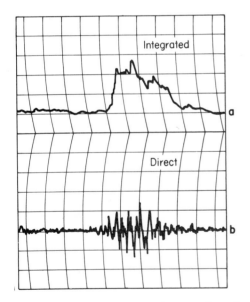

Figure 12–2. Simultaneous, integrated, and direct electromyograms from the rectus femoris muscle of a subject rising from a seated position.

representing the magnitude of the action potentials. These readings may be recorded over various time intervals and may be submitted to statistical treatment.

ANALYSIS OF THE ELECTROMYOGRAM

The recording of the muscle action potentials by any of the popular methods leaves the investigator faced with the problem of analyzing and interpreting the results. A review of the electromyographic literature indicates that there is no universally approved method of scoring and analysis. As would be expected, some investigators prefer to be rather subjective, while others lean toward a more objective approach. Regardless of the measurement approach taken, both qualitative and quantitative elements are available in the data for interpretation. Again, the choice of a measurement technique depends on the objectives of the investigation and it often boils down to a choice between methods of scoring.

One subjective method of scoring electromyographic data is in common use. It depends on subjective judgments which are based upon careful training and experience. It is a method of visual inspection of the electromyogram which employs a system of classification that establishes categories of electrical activity by assigning a series of symbols ($-$, 0, $+$, $++$) indicating relative magnitudes. Decisions regarding magnitudes involve amplitude and frequency primarily. An important value of this method is that it generally limits the investigator to the realm (a very productive realm to be sure) of relationships rather than strict quantification of numerical data. A second and more subjective method of analysis is performed by feeding the amplified action potentials into a loudspeaker. The result gives an audio impression of the quality and quantity of the excitation process which is quite dramatic. It has proved its value in clinical diagnostic practice as well as its use as a source of auditory feedback in studies involving muscle relaxation.

Many different scoring methods have been devised in attempting to make electromyogram analysis more objective. All rely on some form of quantitative appraisal which may be subjected to statistical treatment for interpretive assistance. Some investigators have counted the frequency of the spikes in interference patterns. Studies of muscles involved in high levels of tension development have often used some form of amplitude measurement. The amplitude has been averaged over a predetermined period of time in some cases, while in others the highest amplitude at a given time during a movement has been used. Others have employed combinations of frequency and amplitude appraisal from interference patterns. And, of course, the method of integration described earlier as averaging frequency, duration, and amplitude is in common use.

Attempts have been made to compare the results of spike counting with those of integration. For example, Bergström compared the number of spikes counted from a direct motor unit recording with the results of an integrated recording. He found a linear relationship up to a spike frequency

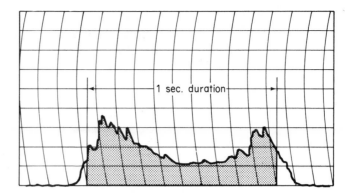

Figure 12–3

of about 500/sec.[3] He concluded that an estimation of the electrical activity of the whole muscle can be made by counting motor unit spikes. It should be pointed out that this study involved activity of small muscles of the hand and may not be entirely representative of the activity of larger muscles containing many more fibers under the control of fewer motor units per active fiber.

One basic problem involved in using the frequency or amplitude is that there are notable variations in the electromyogram during the period of contraction. Another lies in the nature of the direct reading taken from a maximal muscular contraction. The spike potentials usually represent the combination of the excitation phases from many motor units firing at their independent rates. The value of spike count and amplitude measurement probably lies in the study of small muscle activity.

The most common method of obtaining a measure utilizing both frequency and amplitude is by means of integration. This technique has been used by many investigators who have been interested in data which could be quantified with accuracy and submitted to statistical analysis. The typical procedure has been to measure the area under the curve drawn by the pen-writer, usually by means of a *planimeter*. Figure 12-3 illustrates an integrated electromyogram in which the area under the curve for a 1-sec duration has been shaded. The planimeter is made to trace the boldface line which acts as the perimeter of the shaded area. It then gives an indirect measure of the area, which is usually specified in *emg units*. Since the area measurement procedure remains the same, emg-unit values obtained from other electromyograms under similar conditions may be compared.

In summary, the best method of scoring is probably dependent on the objective of the study in question. If one is interested in the functioning of motor units, individual muscles, or the patterns of the action in a group of muscles, then the more subjective techniques are probably best. These types of studies are described later under "Qualitative Analyses." On the other hand, if one is interested in the relationships of force and electrical activity or joint angle and electrical activity, then the more objective, integrative techniques are probably more desirable. These will be discussed under "Quantitative Analyses" in subsequent pages.

[3]R. M. Bergström, "The Relation Between the Number of Impulses and the Integrated Electric Activity in Electromyograms," *Acta Physiologica Scandinavica* **45**, suppl. (1959), 97.

USES OF ELECTROMYOGRAPHY IN THE ANALYSIS OF MUSCULAR ACTIVITY

Electromyography (EMG) has been extremely important in the analysis of muscle action during movement. The analysis of the electrical activity during a skillful movement allows one to better understand how those muscles actually function. However, it is easy for the beginning student to assume that a particular movement occurs because of the action of the muscles which have been assigned that function in anatomy texts. The movement of elbow flexion, for example, is accompanied by action of the elbow flexors. To most, it should be obvious that forces other than muscular contraction can cause movement. Nevertheless, to some the assignment of elbow flexion to the biceps brachii indicates that whenever that movement occurs, the biceps brachii must be active. Actually, that muscle is often active during elbow extension. Because of space limitations, the Muscle Charts which accompany Chapters 14 through 20 do not include many actions such as the eccentric control of elbow extension by the elbow flexors. The mastery of these concomitant actions is left almost entirely to the student, whose inquiring nature will almost certainly impel him to accomplish the task.

Quantitative Analyses

The use of EMG to study muscle actions is not limited to determining when and if muscles act. When electromyograms are prepared for quantitative analysis, inferences may be drawn as to how and why muscles respond with varying magnitudes of activity.

Emg-Force Relationships

An assumption which seems to prevail in much of the literature is that there is a positive relationship between the force of muscular contraction and the electrical activity monitored from the contracting muscles. While this has been shown to be the case under many varied conditions, care should be taken in acceptance of this assumption under all conditions. The electrical activity monitored from active muscles is directly related to the number of muscle fibers being stimulated. Provided that the muscle fiber contracts when it is stimulated, then it would follow that a greater number of active muscle fibers would produce a greater amount of force.

Research into the change seen in the frequency and the amplitude of the action potentials during increased work loads indicates that these two factors do not respond identically. Frequency tends to increase linearly with force of contraction until some limiting point is reached, where it then tends to stabilize. On the other hand, amplitude seems to continue to increase throughout an increasingly heavy action. Integrated electromyograms include both of these elements and therefore show electrical activity to continue to increase when the contractions are isometric in nature. Figure 12-4 graphs the typical emg activity and force production of two elbow flexors during 2 min of maximal, isometric contraction at a flexion angle of 115 deg. As the muscles lose their ability to exert applicable

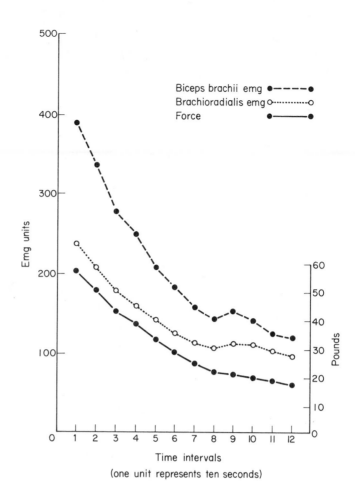

Figure 12–4. Mean emg and force (N = 31) for sustained, maximal isometric contractions. (Figures 12–4 and 5 from R. N. Aebersold, "An Electromyographic Study of Fatigue of the Biceps Brachii, Brachioradialis, and Triceps Brachii During Sustained Maximal Voluntary Contraction," unpublished Doctoral Dissertation, University of Maryland, 1969, by permission.)

force over the sustained contraction period, emg activity follows the same trend, with that of the biceps brachii being more accelerated.

While there is general agreement as to the relationship between emg activity and muscular force in isometric contractions, there is some disagreement regarding the relationship during isotonic contractions. Although the literature presents conflicting evidence, in studies where the rate of contractions and load intensity were controlled, the relationship was shown to be similar to that seen in isometric contractions.

Emg-Muscle Length Relationships

Muscles which function around a given joint can be seen to act more forcefully at one joint angle than another. The elbow flexors, for example, have been shown to produce their greatest amounts of force at an elbow angle approaching 120 deg. Physiologically, muscle fibers have been found to be most efficient during isometric contractions when operating at a length slightly longer than their resting length. It is evident, however, that muscle length is not the only factor influencing the force exerted by the limb in question. Variations in joint angles tend to influence the length of the muscles involved as well as their tension angles. The important factor would seem to be the composite, physiological-mechanical advantage resulting from a combination of these two factors, which are directly related to the joint angle.

169 The Electromotive Characteristics of Muscle

If the external force produced by a muscle were held constant while its physiological-mechanical advantage was varied, it would be seen that the number of active muscle fibers would also vary. More fibers would be required to perform the same task when the physiological-mechanical advantage was decreased, while less would be required when it was increased. As explained earlier, action potentials result from the excitation of muscle fibers. If a greater number of muscle fibers is stimulated or if the rate of stimulation is increased, a greater magnitude of electrical activity ensues. It follows then that a muscle operating from a favorable position would use fewer muscle fibers and therefore produce less electrical activity than under more unfavorable position conditions.

Although the graphs in Fig. 12-5 do not represent activity under constant external force application conditions, they were obtained under continuing conditions of maximal isometric exertion. It can be seen that emg activity was greatest for the biceps brachii in its shortest position (45-deg joint position) and remained that way throughout almost all of the contraction period. At 115 deg, the muscle is at its intermediate length and exhibits intermediate emg activity. At its greatest length (170-deg joint angle), emg activity was lowest throughout. Since these contractions were all maximal as to effort, we must assume that the rate of stimulation was similar under the three joint angle conditions. Therefore, it would appear that the differences were due to the number of active fibers involved. This

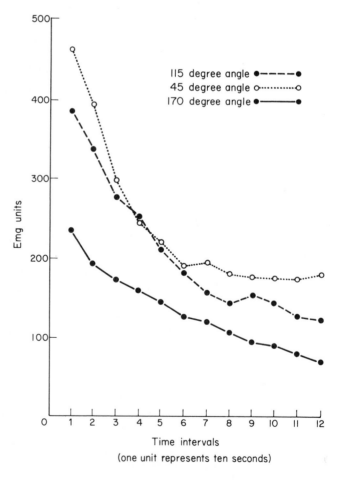

Figure 12–5. Mean emg (N = 31) for sustained, maximal isometric contractions for the biceps brachii at three different elbow joint angles.

suggests that of the two factors involved in the physiological-mechanical advantage, muscle length is the more important contributor to favorable conditions for efficient muscular action, as was pointed out in Chapter 8.

Numerous studies support the relationship given above concerning muscle length and electrical activity. Most of the data reported have been drawn from flexor muscles. A few authors who have examined extensor muscles have produced conflicting evidence. These studies show greater electrical activity in lengthened extensor muscles as opposed to their shortened states. Considering the conflicting nature of the data reported, it would appear advisable to consider the physiological-mechanical advantage of the muscles in question rather than simply their lengths.

→ *Is it likely that a shortened flexor muscle is disadvantaged to a greater degree than a shortened extensor muscle?*

More work needs to be undertaken in this area.

Worthy of careful attention is the approach taken by de Vries and others involving quantitative analysis.[4] The technique is that involving voltage measurement which was briefly described on p. 165. New insights into muscle tonus, muscular relaxation, and emg-force relationships, particularly with very low potential levels, have been among the notable outcomes of that effort. The reader should begin by referring to the text identified in footnote 4.

Emg-Muscular Fatigue Relationships

One of the factors which is known to influence the electrical activity of muscle is muscular fatigue. As used here, *fatigue* refers to the condition which develops within the neuromuscular system which prevents the maintenance of initial levels of contractive force. The discussion of fatigue in general is beyond the scope of this text, but the effects that fatigue may have upon the electromyogram are important.

Numerous investigators have used electromyography as a tool to study the problem of fatigue, with the results being somewhat at odds. Some results indicate that as fatigue develops, the recorded electrical activity increases. Others show that the decrease seen in the force exerted is accompanied by a similar decrease in the action potentials (refer again to Figs. 12-4 and 12-5). Under these maximal-effort, isometric conditions, it appears that those muscles which exhibit the greatest electrical activity early in the fatiguing bout show the most rapid reduction of that activity as fatigue sets in. The same sort of relationship seems to apply for the same muscle under varying length conditions (Fig. 12-5). If we compare different muscles or the same muscle under different conditions, fatigue acts as a great equalizer for electrical activity.

A closer investigation of the fatigue studies involving EMG suggests that changes in the electromyogram owing to fatigue may be dependent on the type of conditions employed to develop the fatigue. When submaximal

[4]Herbert A. de Vries, *Physiology of Exercise for Physical Education and Athletics* (Dubuque, Iowa: William C. Brown Company, Publishers, 1966).

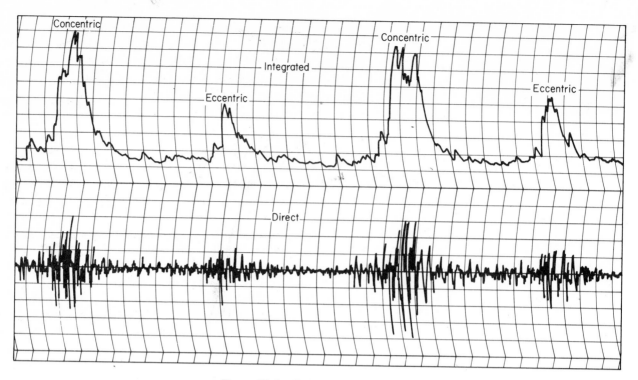

Figure 12–6. Concentric and eccentric contraction electromyograms from the rectus femoris muscle in integrated and direct modes, showing differences in magnitude.

contractions were used to bring about fatigue, the electrical activity was seen to increase. However, when maximal efforts were used, the resulting pattern of activity was one of decrease. It should be evident that care must be taken in comparing emg-force relationships of muscles undergoing fatiguing activity with these same relationships of rested muscles.

Concentric Versus Eccentric Contractions

A muscle can develop tension in conjunction with shortening its length as well as increasing its length. Evidence from a number of different approaches has shown that greater tension can be produced by muscles when contracting eccentrically than when contracting concentrically. Assmussen has indicated that only about one third as many muscle fibers are required to perform a task eccentrically than are needed to perform the reversed task concentrically.[5] In the latter, the contraction produces the movement, while in the former, the contraction controls the movement under extrinsic motivation. It is important to avoid any urge to refer to these two movement situations as constituting the same task.

It must be assumed that the eccentric operation, because of its considerably lower active-fiber demands, would result in a lower electrical activity output even though the force exerted might be the same. Figure 12-6 illustrates direct and integrated emg patterns for such a concentric-eccentric contraction cycle under conditions which were controlled with

[5]E. Assmussen, "Muscular Performance," in *Muscle As a Tissue* (K. Rodahl and S. M. Horvath, eds.) (New York: McGraw-Hill, Book Company, 1960), p. 173.

respect to contraction durations and movement ranges. It is apparent that the concentric operation elicits the greater magnitudes of electrical activity. Thus it can be seen that in relating the electrical activity to the force produced, care must be taken to consider the nature of the contraction involved.

Qualitative Analyses

The analysis of muscular activity in qualitative terms is extremely important in the discussion of skilled movement. Evaluation of the electromyogram qualitatively allows one to look at the pattern of the excitation of various muscles. The amount of electrical activity is important as an indication of the degree of activity rather than as an indication of the force produced by the muscle. By monitoring the electrical activity of a group of muscles, one can determine when each muscle was active, when it was most and least active, whether or not the muscles were active in cyclical sequences, and many other factors which may be of interest regarding a specific problem under investigation.

Testing Traditional and Theoretical Concepts

Logically inferred muscle actions, which for years have awaited confirmation as the result of careful research work, have been substantiated in some cases and refuted in others on the basis of electromyographic evidence. An example of confirmation can be found in the shunt and spurt theory of MacConaill, which was introduced in Chapter 11.[6] Mathematical analysis suggested that a muscle's position across its joint should indicate to some degree the conditions under which it will perform. Thus a shunt muscle should act in rapid movements to provide stabilizing support. The brachioradialis has been cited as an example of a shunt muscle. Muscles which act to produce the predominant rotatory forces because of their positions across the joint have been described as spurt muscles. At the elbow joint, the biceps brachii and brachialis fit this description. Electromyographic evidence shows the brachioradialis to be relatively inactive during slow elbow flexions and quite active during rapid flexions. The biceps brachii and brachialis tend to be active under most conditions of elbow flexion to offer their changing rotatory components to move the segment.

An example of refuting evidence is found in the very old function applied to the brachioradialis, namely, supination of the forearm. This supposed function was so firmly set in the anatomical literature that the muscle was named the supinator longus. Electromyographic study has shown that this muscle is not a true supinator and is active in supination only when it occurs with the elbow extended, under resistance. Even at that, its supinating assistance is suspect. Enough examples exist, such as

[6]M. A. MacConaill, "Some Anatomical Factors Affecting the Stabilizing Functions of Muscles," *Irish Journal of Medical Science* **6** (1946): 160; and "The Movements of Bones and Joints. II: Function of the Musculature," *Journal of Bone and Joint Surgery* **31-B** (1949): 100.

that just noted, to cause one to be cautious about assigning function to muscles without careful consideration of such factors as speed of contraction and resistance to the movement under question.

Ballistic and Sustained Movements

Electromyography has been employed by Hubbard in the study of muscular contractions to identify differences between the so-called ballistic and sustained types[7] (refer to Chapter 10 and its discussion of angular impulse and momentum). The ballistic contraction is said to produce a short impulse which sets the segment moving and continuing as a result of its momentum. A sustained contraction is one in which the muscle produces useful tension throughout the movement.

The electrical activity of the biceps brachii and triceps brachii was monitored during rapid elbow flexions and extensions in the transverse plane while the shoulder was abducted, 90 deg. It was shown that the elbow flexors were responsible for accelerating the forearm through the first few degrees of flexion, after which the segment tended to move at a uniform speed for a time until it was compelled to decelerate. The uniform speed period was called the momentum phase. During this phase, biceps brachii shortening was said to "take up slack" within itself rather than applying motivating force to the bone as was indicated by reduced electrical activity. It was concluded that during the momentum phase, the muscle was contracting but was not actually causing the continued motion. It was simply keeping up with the rapidly moving segment to which it was attached.

In a sustained movement, the electromyogram would indicate more uniform activity of the agonists throughout the action. It seems likely that sustained contractions occur in slow, refined activities where a momentum phase is never clearly evident. The literature tends to support the ballistic theory as the basis for rapid or violent movements but gives no clear answer for the action during slow movements. Consequently, care must be taken not to assume that monitored electrical activity from a muscle during a movement means that it is undergoing a sustained contraction. It may simply be keeping in step with the movement.

Emg Patterns of Muscle Groups

It was stated previously that the pattern of electrical activity of muscles during a specific movement is of interest to the kinesiologist because it gives him information about the way individual muscles function within a group. It is one thing to say that a muscle is merely involved in a particular activity, but quite another to specify precisely its correct function. Therefore, the kinesiologist finds not only general activities useful in electromyographic investigations but sports skills in particular because they reflect movement behavior which runs the gamut of abilities from the halting, beginning attempts of the novice to the beauty and precision of the professional athlete.

[7]A. W. Hubbard, "Homokinetics," in *Science and Medicine of Exercise and Sports* (W. R. Johnson, ed.) (New York: Harper & Row, Publishers, 1960).

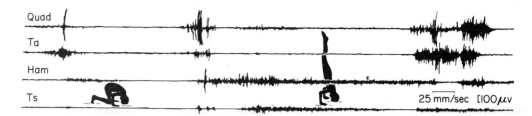

Quad

Ta

Ham

Ts

25 mm/sec [100μv

Figure 12–7. Electromyograms of a subject demonstrating a head stand. Starting from a standing position, the subject assumed the position on the left, pushed upward into the head stand which was held for about 10 sec, returned to the position on the left, and arose to a standing position again. Bursts along the quadriceps femoris record indicate the position changes. Quad, Quadriceps femoris group; Ta, Tibialis anterior; Ham, Hamstrings group; and Ts, Triceps surae (soleus and gastrocnemius). (Reproduced by permission of S. J. Houtz and the *Journal of Applied Physiology*, from "Influence of Gravitational Forces on Function of Lower Extremity Muscles," **19**: 999, 1964.)

Hermann studied the action potentials of the upper portion of the pectoralis major, the deltoid, the triceps brachii, and the teres major during shot-putting.[8] Six men were grouped according to their ability, with two being classed as "good," two as "average," and two as "poor." Motion pictures were taken and synchronized with the electromyograms. Specific points during the action were isolated (i.e., the body position as the shot was released from the hand) and compared on the basis of their action potentials. The degree of electrical activity for each muscle at each of the chosen body positions was determined.

The pattern of electrical activity tended to be different between good and poor subjects. In the case of the poor subjects, the greatest amount of electrical activity in most of the muscles monitored was found to occur after the shot had been released, a most wasteful circumstance. The muscles of the good shot-putters, however, were found to exhibit peak action potentials before the release of the shot. Thus maximal muscular contributions were applied where most needed, an excellent example of skill development. An interesting aspect of the study was the suggestion of a sequence of muscular actions which, according to the author's review of the electromyograms, should prove most efficient.

The activity of any particular muscle during contraction will be influenced by changes in body and joint positions during the movement. Figure 12-7 illustrates electromyograms obtained from several lower extremity muscles during the movements required to perform a head stand in which gravitational forces affect the performance. The total movement involved was really of four parts: (*1*) the assumption of the first position shown (preliminary position), (*2*) the attainment of the three-point head stand stance which was held for about 10 sec, (*3*) the return to the preliminary position, and (*4*) the return to the standing posture. The onset points of the movements coincide approximately with the notable bursts of activity from the quadriceps group, as shown in the upper electromyogram

[8]G. W. Hermann, "An Electromyographic Study of Selected Muscles Involved in the Shot Put," *Research Quarterly* **33** (1962): 1.

from left to right. It can be seen that the quadriceps group and the tibialis anterior were active during the movements required to assume the preliminary position.

→ *Have a friend perform these movements and examine them carefully. After doing so, analyze the electromyograms in the figure and describe the muscular actions which they depict.*

REFERENCES

Adrian, E. D. "Interpretation of the Electromyogram." *Lancet* 5311 (1925): 1229, 5312 (1925): 1283.

Adrian, E. D., and Bronk, D. W. "The Discharge of Impulses in Motor Nerve Fibers." *Journal of Physiology* 67 (1929): 119.

Allen, C. E. L. "Muscle action Potentials Used in the Study of Dynamic Anatomy." *British Journal of Physical Medicine* 11 (1948): 66.

Assmussen, E. "Muscular Performance." In *Muscle as a Tissue*, edited by K. Rodahl and S. M. Horvath. New York: McGraw-Hill Book Company, 1960.

Basmajian, J. V. "Control and Training of Individual Motor Units." *Science* 141 (1963): 440.

——— *Muscles Alive: Their Function Revealed by Electromyography.* 2d ed. Baltimore: The Williams & Wilkins Company, 1967.

——— "'Spurt' and 'Shunt' Muscles: an Electromyographic Confirmation." *Journal of Anatomy* 93 (1959): 551.

Battye, C. K., and Joseph, J. "An Investigation of Telemetering of the Activity of Some Muscles in Walking." *Medical and Biological Engineering* 4 (1966): 125.

Bergstrom, R. M. "The Relation Between the Number of Impulses and the Integrated Electric Activity in Electromyograms." *Acta Physiologica Scandinavica* 45 Suppl. (1959): 97.

Bierman, W., and Yashmon, L. J. "Electromyography in Kinesiologic Evaluations." *Archives of Physical Medicine* 29 (1948): 206.

Bigland, B., and Lippold, O. C. J. "The Relation Between Force, Velocity, and Integrated Electrical Activity in Human Muscles." *Journal of Physiology* 123 (1945a): 214.

Broer, Marion R., and Houtz, Sara Jane. *Patterns of Muscular Activity in Selected Sport Skills: An Electromyographic Study.* Springfield, Ill.: Charles C. Thomas, Publisher, 1967.

Close, J. Robert. *Motor Function in the Lower Extremity.* Springfield, Ill.: Charles C. Thomas, Publisher, 1964.

Close, J. R.; Nickel, E. D.; and Todd, F. N. "Motor-Unit Action-Potential Counts. Their Significance in Isometric and Isotonic Contractions." *Journal of Bone and Joint Surgery* 42-A (1960): 1207.

Csapo, A. "Studies on Excitation-Contraction Coupling." *Annals of the New York Academy of Sciences* 81 (1959): 453.

Davis, John F. "Manual of Surface Electromyography." WADC Technical Report 59-184. Wright-Patterson Air Force Base, Ohio: Wright Air Development Center, December 1959.

Denslow, J. S., and Graham-Service, D. "The Spread of Muscle Action Potentials from Active to Inactive Areas." *Federation Proceedings* 7 (1948): 27.

deVries, Herbert A. *Physiology of Exercise.* Dubuque, Iowa: Wm. C. Brown Company, Publishers, 1966.

——— "Quantitative Electromyographic Investigation of the Spasm Theory of Muscle Pain." *American Journal of Physical Medicine* 45 (1966): 119.

Eccles, J. C., and Sherrington, C. S. "Numbers and Contraction Values of Individual Motor-Units Examined in Some Muscles of the Limb." *Proceedings of the Royal Society of Medicine* 106 (1950): 326.

Edwards, R. G., and Lippold, O. C. J. "The Relation Between Force and Integrated Electrical Activity in Fatigued Muscle." *Journal of Physiology* 132 (1956): 677.

Flint, M. M., and Gudgell, J. "Electromyographic Study of Abdominal Muscular Activity During Exercise." *Research Quarterly* 36 (1965): 29.

Floyd, W. F., and Silver, P. H. S. "The Function of the Erectores Spinae Muscles in Certain Movements and Postures in Man." *Journal of Physiology* 129 (1955): 184.

Gray, E. C., and Basmajian, J. V. "Electromyography and Cinematography of Leg and Foot ('Normal' and Flat) During Walking." *Anatomical Record* 161 (1968): 1.

Hermann, G. W. "An Electromyographic Study of Selected Muscles Involved in the Shot Put." *Research Quarterly* 33 (1962): 1.

Houtz, S. J. "Influence of Gravitational Forces on Function of Lower Extremity Muscles." *Journal of Applied Physiology* 9 (1964): 999.

Houtz, S. J., and Fischer, F. J. "An Analysis of Muscle Action and Joint Excursion During Exercise on a Stationary Bicycle." *Journal of Bone and Joint Surgery* 41-A (1959): 123.

Hubbard, A. W. "Homokinetics." In *Science and Medicine of Exercise and Sports*, edited by W. R. Johnson. New York: Harper & Row, Publishers, 1960.

Inman, V. T.; Ralston, H. J.; Saunders, J. B. deC. M.; Feinstein, B.; and Wood, E. W. "Relation of Human Electromyogram to Muscular Tension." *Electroencephalography and Clinical Neurophysiology* 4 (1952): 187.

Joseph, J. *Man's Posture; Electromyographic Studies.* Springfield, Ill.: Charles C. Thomas, Publisher, 1960.

Kamon, E. "Electromyography of Static and Dynamic Postures of the Body Supported on the Arms." *Journal of Applied Physiology* 21 (1966): 1611.

Kaplan, E. B. trans. *Duchenne's Physiology of Motion.* Philadelphia: W. B. Saunders Company, 1959.

Kennedy, J. L., and Travis, R. C. "Prediction of Speed of Performance by Muscle Action Potentials." *Science* 105 (1947): 410.

Kitzman, E. W. "Baseball: Electromyographic Study of Batting Swing." *Research Quarterly* 35 (1964): 166.

Knowlton, G. C.; Bennett, R. L.; and McClure, R. "Electromyography of Fatigue." *Archives of Physical Medicine* 32 (1951): 648.

Licht, Sidney, ed. *Electrodiagnosis and Electromyography.* 2d ed. New Haven, Conn.: Elizabeth Licht, Publisher, 1961.

Lipetz, S., and Gutin, B. "An Electromyographic Study of Four Abdominal Exercises." *Medicine and Science in Sports* 2 (1970): 35.

Lippold, O. C. J. "The Relation Between Integrated Action Potentials in a Human Muscle and its Isometric Tension." *Journal of Physiology* 117 (1952): 492.

Loofbourrow, G. N. "Neuromuscular Integration." In *Science and Medicine of Exercise and Sports*, edited by W. R. Johnson. New York: Harper & Row, Publishers, 1960.

MacConaill, M. A. "The Movements of Bones and Joints: II. Function of the Musculature." *Journal of Bone and Joint Surgery* 31-B (1949): 100.

——— "Some Anatomical Factors Affecting the Stabilizing Functions of Muscles." *Irish Journal of Medical Science* 6 (1946): 160.

——— and Basmajian, J. V. *Muscles and Movement: A Basis for Human Kinesiology.* Baltimore: The Williams & Wilkins Company, 1969.

McFarland, G. B.; Krusen, V. L.; and Weatherby, H. T. "Kinesiology of Selected Muscles Acting on the Wrist: Electromyographic Study." *Archives of Physical Medicine and Rehabilitation* 43 (1962): 165.

Merton, P. V. "Problems of Muscular Fatigue." *British Medical Bulletin* 12 (1956): 219.

Miwa, N.; Tanaka, T.; and Matoba, M. "Electromyography in Kinesiologic Evaluations. Subjects on Two Joint Muscle and the Relation Between the Muscular Tension and Electromyogram." *Journal of the Japanese Orthopaedic Association* 36 (1963): 1025.

Norris, Forbes M., Jr. *The EMG: A Guide and Atlas for Practical Electromyography.* New York: Grune & Stratton, 1963.

O'Connell, A. L., and Gardner, E. B. "The Use of Electromyography in Kinesiological Research." *Research Quarterly* 34 (1963): 166.

Perry, J. "The Mechanics of Walking: A Clinical Interpretation." *Physical Therapy* 47 (1967): 778.

Ralston, H. J. "Uses and Limitations of Electromyography in the Quantitative Study of Skeletal Muscle Function." *American Journal of Orthodontics* 47 (1961): 521.

Rodahl, Kaare, and Horvath, Steven M., eds. *Muscle as a Tissue.* New York: McGraw-Hill Book Company, 1962.

Scheving, L. E., and Pauly, J. E. "An Electromyographic Study of Some Muscles Acting on the Upper Extremity of Man." *Anatomical Record* 135 (1959): 239.

Slater-Hammel, A. T. "Action Current Study of Contraction-Movement Relationships in the Golf Stroke." *Research Quarterly* 19 (1948): 164.

——— "An Action Current Study of Contraction-Movement Relationships in the Tennis Stroke." *Research Quarterly* 20 (1949): 424.

Suckling, E. E. *Bioelectricity.* New York: McGraw-Hill Book Company, 1961.

Travill, A. A. "Electromyographic Study of the Extensor Apparatus of the Forearm." *Anatomical Record* 144 (1962): 373.

Walters, C. E., and Partridge, M. J. "Electromyographic Study of the Differential Action of the Abdominal Muscles During Exercises." *American Journal of Physical Medicine* 36 (1957): 259.

Waterland, J. C., and Shambres, G. M. "Electromyography: One Link in the Experimental Chain of Kinesiological Research." *Physical Therapy* 49 (1969): 1351.

Wheatley, M. D., and Jahnke, W. D. "Electromyographic Study of the Superficial Thigh and Hip Muscles in Normal Individuals." *Archives of Physical Medicine* 32 (1951): 508.

Wiesendanger, M.; Schneider, P.; and Villoz, J. P. "Electromyographic Analysis of a Rapid Volitional Movement." *American Journal of Physical Medicine* 48 (1969): 17.

The
Anatomy
of
Motion

13

Skeletal and Articular Considerations

The fundamental concern of this book is human motion and its description. While a great deal of accurate motion description may be accomplished without a thorough knowledge of musculoskeletal anatomy, as is in evidence in Parts I and II, to proceed without it is similar to traveling in unfamiliar locales without a road map. An understanding of the structures of human motion is essential and is the subject of this part of the book. Our earlier discussions have been mechanically oriented. Those presented in this part have mechanical foundations also because the human structure is, indeed, a very complex machine.

In studying any component of a machine, one must relate the part to the whole. Similarly, in studying the components of the living human body, we must be aware of the importance of the integrated system of parts. In addition, it is of utmost importance to emphasize here that it is a *living* body which is being studied rather than some inanimate, lifeless object. Just as muscle is a living tissue, so is bone a living, functioning tissue. Thus the ways in which the bones of the skeleton function in movement depend on their structural organization.

BONE STRUCTURE

Living bone must not be considered to be a dry, inelastic material. It is made up of cells, *osteocytes*, which reside in interconnecting chambers within the bone matrix. The outer layer of bone is covered with a connective tissue sheath called the *periosteum* and is very dense in character. Because of its density, it is termed *compact* bone. Microscopically, compact bone is seen to be a complex network of canals and cavities within which the bone cells reside. Figure 13-1 illustrates a microscopic view of a small section of bone in which the *Haversian* network of canals is identified.

Compact bone blends into *spongy* or *cancellous* bone as the inner reaches of bones are examined. Spongy bone has the same cell organization as compact bone but its architecture shows an intricate and varying arrangement of bony bars or rails which provide great structural strength without

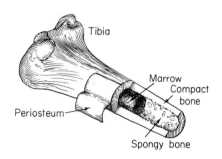

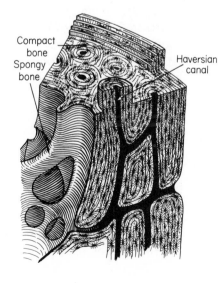

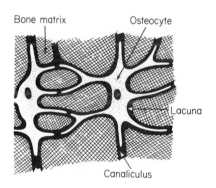

Figure 13–1. The structure of bone at three different levels. (Reprinted by permission of The Macmillan Company from *The Human Body Its Structure and Physiology* by Sigmund Grollman. © Copyright Sigmund Grollman, 1969.)

181

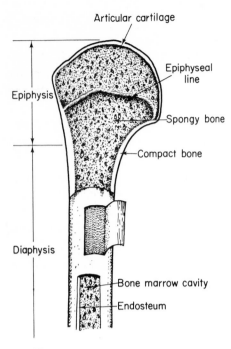

Articular cartilage

Epiphyseal line

Epiphysis

Spongy bone

Compact bone

Diaphysis

Bone marrow cavity

Endosteum

Figure 13–2

resulting in an inordinate increase in weight. These networks of spongy bone vary in organization from bone to bone. However, they generally follow patterns which provide maximal resistance to deformation under the stresses encountered in their skeletal locations. For example, the bones of the foot include spongy bone whose architectural patterns generally parallel the longitudinal curves of the foot. Hence, they provide internal rigidity against the stresses placed upon the arches in weight bearing.

Although bone exhibits some elasticity, in comparison to other body tissues, it is quite inelastic. Consequently, it depends on other means to resist the harmful effects of applied stresses. The ability to withstand compression and tension stresses appears to be shouldered predominantly by the compact bone, which in long bones is suitably oriented along the lines of weight-bearing force application. Spongy bone appears to act as a mechanism for energy absorption and internal stress distribution within the bones.

In a typical long bone, the *shaft* or *diaphasis* contains a tubular space called the *medullary* or *bone marrow* cavity. This cavity is lined with a delicate membrane, the *endosteum*, and is filled with bone marrow. The endosteum also covers the convoluted surfaces of spongy bone and lines the intricate networks of Haversian canals. At the rounded ends of long bones, the *epiphyses*, the periosteum gives way to *articular* cartilage. The epiphyses exhibit thin layers of compact bone within which is housed the spongy bone, as shown in Fig. 13-2.

Bone shapes vary considerably within the skeleton, as will be seen in later discussions. Their protuberances, depressions, perforations, etc., have been named to assist in the identification and clarification of location and function. Table 13-1 offers the most common of these *bony landmark* designations as well as examples of each.

THE SKELETON

For the purposes of classification, the skeleton has been subdivided into two sections: (*1*) the *axial skeleton*, consisting of the bones of the head, vertebral column, and rib cage, and (*2*) the *appendicular skeleton*, which includes the bones of the limbs. Figure 13-3 illustrates two views of the upright skeleton in which the appendicular bones are lightly shaded to differentiate them from the axial bones. Referring to the figure, it can be seen that the body segments, which were introduced in Chapter 6 for the purposes of kinematically classifying body movements, do not conform exactly to the axial and appendicular skeletal designations. The difference resides in the trunk segment, which, as used in this text, includes the shoulder and pelvic girdles. Skeletally, these bone groups are given as appendicular.

Bone classification may proceed further when shape becomes the identifying factor. This means of classification also brings to light many of the functions of the skeleton. For example, *flat bones* such as the scapula and ilium provide broad surface areas for the attachment of muscles and ligaments. The ilium offers shield-like protection for the soft tissues of

TABLE 13-1: Skeletal Landmarks

	Form	Description	Examples
I.	Surface	A broad bone area which is identified as to the direction it faces	Posterior surface of the sacrum or costal surface of the scapula
II.	Border	A narrow bone area which is identified as to the direction it faces; often serves as demarcation point between surfaces	Vertebral border of the scapula
III.	Depressions and perforations		
	A. Foramen	A clearly identified hole in a bone which may serve as a passageway	Obturator foramen of the hip bone
	B. Groove	A furrow which is used as a passageway for such structures as	
		1. Muscle tendons	1. Bicipital groove of the humerus
		2. Nerves	2. Groove for the radial nerve of the humerus
	C. Fossa	A rather large depression to	
		1. Receive a bone	1. Acetabular fossa of the hip bone
		2. Act as muscle attachment site	2. Supraspinatous fossa of the scapula
	D. Fovea	A small depression to	
		1. Receive a bone	1. Fovea atop the radial head
		2. Act as a ligament attachment site	2. Fovea capitis of the femoral head
	E. Notch	A large or small indentation on the edge or border of a bone; when closed by a ligament, can become a foramen	Greater sciatic notch of the hip bone; greater sciatic foramen
IV.	Prominences		
	A. Condyle	A bone end which is enlarged to better accommodate stress; may exhibit articular and nonarticular areas	Medial and lateral condyles of the femur
	B. Epicondyle	A projection upon a condyle	Medial and lateral epicondyles of the humerus
	C. Crest, ridge, lip, line	An elevated, elongated area of bone whose narrowness usually determines which term is used	Crest of the ilium; intertrochanteric ridge of the femur; internal and external lips on the iliac crest; gluteal lines of the ilium
	D. Facet	A flat area of bone which is often articular and often elevated	Superior and inferior articular facets of the vertebrae
	E. Head	A rounded end of a bone which is usually articular	Head of the humerus and femur
	F. Neck	A constricted area generally adjacent to the head of a bone	Neck of the femur
	G. Process	A projection of varying length and size depending on the bone of origin	Greater and lesser trochanters of the femur; malleoli of the fibula and tibia; spinous, transverse and articular processes of the vertebrae; styloid processes of the radius and ulna
	H. Tubercle, tuberosity	A rounded projection from any part of a bone; used interchangeably, but often tuberosity is used for a larger tubercle	Tuberosity of the calcaneus; dorsal radial tubercle of the radius
	I. Spine	A slender projection; it is often	
		1. Sharply pointed	1. Spine of the ischium
		2. Sharply bordered	2. Spine of the scapula

organs enclosed within the abdominal cavity. The skull performs the same service for the brain. *Long* bones, of which the femur and humerus are examples, serve the mechanical function of leverage in locomotion and act as weight-bearing columns in the extremities. The carpal and tarsal bones of the hands and feet, respectively, are classified as *short* bones. They are organized in closely associated groups by ligamentous binding. In groups, these bones perform supportive, shock absorption, and movement functions. The vertebrae of the vertebral column are examples of *irregular* bones which perform most of the functions given for the three other classes. Table 13-2 lists the bones of the human skeleton which will be of concern to the user of this book.

→ *With this list at hand, identify the bones illustrated in Fig. 13-3.*

TABLE 13–2: Bones of the Adult Skeleton

BODY SEGMENTS:

Foot (paired)		Leg (paired)		Thigh (paired)	Trunk (single)	
BONES:						
Phalanges	(28)	Tibia	(2)	Femur (2)	Hip bones:	(2)
Metatarsals	(10)	Fibula	(2)		Ilium	
Tarsals	(14)				Ischium }fused	
					Pubis	
					Coccyx	(1)
					4 coccygeal }fused vertebrae	
					Sacrum	(1)
					5 sacral }fused vertebrae	
					Lumbar vertebrae	(5)
					Thoracic vertebrae	(12)
					Ribs 12 pair	(24)
					Sternum	(1)
					Clavicle	(2)
					Scapula	(2)
Totals	52		4	2		50

BODY SEGMENTS:

Head-Neck (single)		Arm (paired)	Forearm (paired)		Hand (paired)	
BONES:						
Cervical vertebrae	(7)	Humerus (2)	Ulna	(2)	Phalanges	(28)
Skull			Radius	(2)	Metacarpals	(10)
Occipital	(1)				Carpals	(16)
Temporal	(2)					
Totals:	10	2	4			54
Grand total:	**178**					

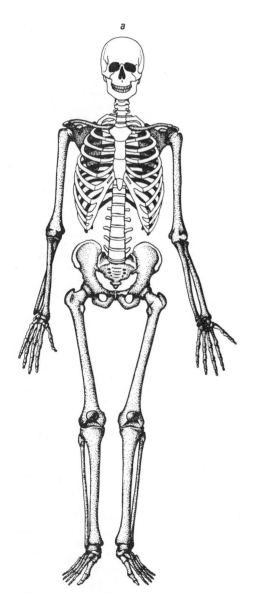

Figure 13–3. Anterior (*a*) and posterior (*b, opposite*) views of the human skeleton. Appendicular bones are shaded.

Skeletal Size

Animals of different species exhibit different sizes and shapes which allow them to be recognized as such. Each of the common animals has a skeletal framework which is of a size and shape which matches the circumstances of its livelihood. Man is a relatively large animal, and in accordance with his superior mentality, he is not just a larger replica of smaller animals. Furthermore, the examination of the skeletal structure of very large animals such as the hippopotamus makes it clear that large modifications in size are accompanied by marked changes in form. As would be expected, skeletal dimensions play a most significant role in the determination of form, and with larger skeletons come larger musculatures.

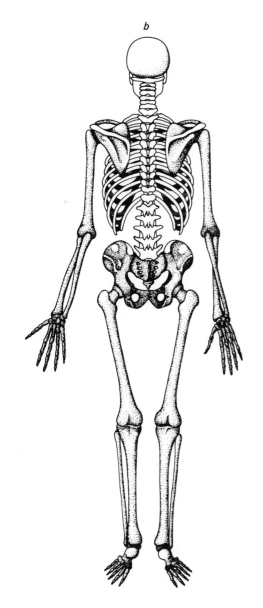

b

If the bones of the skeleton are to be capable of supporting their own weight and that of the rest of the body's parts in normal activities, they must demonstrate a thickness which is correct for their lengths. To cite a simplified example, the weight of the body's bulk depends on its three dimensions: height, breadth, and depth. Thus if these dimensions are increased 10 times, the body's weight increases $(10)^3$ or 1000 times. By imagining an individual who has the proportions of an average man but is 10 times his height, it is easy to see that gravity would pose real problems because he would weigh nearly as much as a large horse while preferring to stand on only two limbs.

The long bones of man's lower limbs demonstrate supporting strengths which are generally proportional to their cross-sectional areas. If their lengths were increased 10-fold, their strength would be increased only 100-fold, $(10)^2$. When the weight which must be supported by a structure is compared with its supporting strength, it is clear that there is a limit to how large a body can become and still maintain the same form or proportions. The skeletons of very large animals have bones which are, indeed, considerably thicker for their lengths than our own because they must support disproportionately greater masses.

Mythology is filled with human giants who possessed powers which were thought to be commensurate with their sizes. In addition, the Bible mentions many giants. Goliath is probably the most renowned of the biblical giants owing to his unfortunate encounter with David. Goliath was reputed to have measured six cubits and a span in height.

→ *How tall was he in feet and inches? Can you envision the movements of his battle with David?*

The heights of a number of authentic giants have been recorded since the time of ancient Rome. Both men and women are included with statures approaching and in some cases exceeding 9 ft in height. Certainly the great bulk of their bodies must have placed severe supportive demands on the bones and joints of their skeletons and, possibly, contributed to their generally short lives. Simple acts such as rising from a seated position or maintaining precarious balances must have required formidable muscular efforts to bring them about.

As it probably was with Goliath, we often find that there are advantages associated with a small stature. Certainly gravity is not the nuisance to very small animals that it is to man. However, some movements appear to be independent of body size. Haldane has pointed out that jumping height in animals is an example.[1] Because the energy expended in jumping is generally proportional to the weight of the jumper, and if it is assumed that the muscles used in jumping represent a constant percentage of the jumping animal's body, energy expenditure per ounce of muscle tissue is essentially independent of size. This reasoning depends on the speed with which the contractile force may be developed, especially in small animals.

SKELETAL ARTICULATIONS

The rigidity of bones limits their movements to those points where they join others. Although this is the case, the joining of two bones does not automatically mean that movement is possible. Whether movement can take place or not, these bone junctions are known as *articulations*. It is customary to substitute the word *joint* for articulation in ordinary usage.

Classification of Joints

The classification of joints has been a rather inexact process because of the complexity of the structures and movements which are available. The simplest form of classification is based on the amount of gross movement which is available at the joint as

1. *Synarthroses*—immovable
2. *Amphiarthroses*—slightly movable
3. *Diarthroses*—freely movable

An example of a synarthrodial joint is the skull *suture* whose bones are held together tightly by fibrous tissue. The slightly movable amphiarthrodial joints may be joined by fibrous or cartilaginous tissue. In the case of the *distal tibiofibular* joint, a fibrous interosseous ligament provides great stability while still allowing some "give" in weight bearing and movements at the ankle joint. The junctions between the vertebral bodies as well as that for the *symphysis pubis* employ cartilage in uniting the adjacent bone surfaces of the joint. It is easy to see that of the three classes of joints listed above, the diarthroses, because of the freedom of movement they allow, are of utmost interest to the study of kinesiology.

Diarthroses

In addition to the provision for greater freedom of movement, diarthrodial joints differ from those of the other classes by including a *joint cavity*. This category represents the highest level of development, and many variations in structure are found. Before proceeding with the classes of diarthrodial joints, we must first discuss their general structural characteristics. Generally, the joint cavity is bounded by two different structures, the

[1]J. B. S. Haldane, "On Being the Right Size," in *World of Mathematics*, vol. II (James R. Newman, ed.) (New York: Simon and Schuster, Inc., 1956), p. 956.

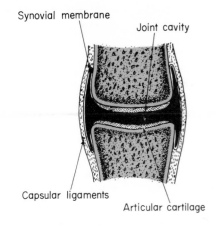

Synovial membrane

Joint cavity

Capsular ligaments

Articular cartilage

Figure 13–4. The diarthrodial joint and its parts.

articular cartilage of the bone ends and the *joint capsule* walls. Figure 13-4 illustrates these structures.

ARTICULAR CARTILAGE: Bone ends within joint cavities are covered with a molded jacket of articular cartilage, usually *hyaline* cartilage. The quantity of the cartilage usually depends on the amount of movement permitted in the joint. Cartilage thickness varies considerably, but with the more rounded bone ends, it is seen to be thickest at the borders of concave surfaces and at the center of convex surfaces. It is claimed that such articulating surfaces may more accurately fit one another and thus increase the joint's stability under stress.

Articular cartilage reacts to short-term deformation forces by compressing and quickly returning to its original shape. However, under conditions of prolonged stress, the cartilage acts much like a *damped* spring, which returns to its original shape slowly. Under intermittent stress conditions, these bone coverings show little sign of wear. Obviously, bone ends are suitably prepared to function in a wide variety of activity modes, offering their elastic cartilaginous support in conjunction with their very smooth surfaces.

JOINT CAPSULE: The capsule walls resemble elastic sleeves which encircle the joint. They vary in shape to match the joint borders and may be quite different in extent on opposite sides of the same joint, e.g., the elbow joint. The capsule wall is made up of two clearly defined structures: the innermost *synovial membrane,* which is covered externally by the ligamentous or fibrous capsule. The synovial membrane also covers intra-articular ligaments and tendons but not the articular cartilage. It is thought to secrete a *synovial fluid,* named because of its resemblance to egg white prior to heating, which performs extremely important lubrication functions within the joint.

Synovial fluid is found in small quantities in human joints and exhibits an interesting physical property associated with its viscosity. When two bone surfaces move across one another, a thin film of this viscous fluid acts as a boundary layer between them, reducing frictional effects and offering significant pressure support between the contacting surfaces. The fluid shows a much higher viscosity to slow action between articulating surfaces than it does to rapid action.[2] Under conditions of accelerated limb movement, the fact that synovial fluid viscosity is significantly reduced provides for an efficient mechanism where resistance is suitably low when high velocities are required.

The fibrous capsule may attach to ligaments as well as to bone. This is the case at the knee joint on its medial aspect. Capsule walls are often thickened in places where functional demands are greatest. These thickenings are referred to as *capsular ligaments* and provide binding and guiding functions in a manner similar to ligaments which are completely free of attachment to the capsule. The capsule may offer significant support

[2]C. H. Barnett, D. V. Davies, and M. A. MacConaill, *Joints, Their Structure and Mechanics* (Springfield, Ill.: Charles C Thomas, Publisher, 1949), p. 37.

against dislocation of bones which normally hang as the result of gravity. This is particularly so in the case of the humerus in the shoulder joint capsule.

JOINT LIGAMENTS: Aside from the capsular ligaments, freely movable joints are abundantly supplied with additional ligaments, both *extra-* and *intra-articular*. Extra-articular ligaments come in several forms which suit their functions and locations. Some are cord-like; others are flat. Some ligaments receive common names which reflect their shapes. For example, the *tibial collateral* ligament of the ankle joint is usually referred to as the *deltoid* ligament because of its triangular shape. The strongest ligament in the body, the *iliofemoral*, carries the name of the *Y* ligament because it resembles that letter somewhat if inverted.

When ligaments unite with each other to cross many joints, they can transmit their support and stabilization effects over a widespread area. This is particularly true in the foot where many small bones are combined to form a relatively small body segment. Some ligaments have been said to contain elastic fibers, which would add typical elastic properties to their otherwise inelastic nature. The *plantar calcaneonavicular* ligament is a noteworthy example which has borne the name *spring* ligament as a result. There is, however, strong objection to the claimed elastic constituents of this ligament.

Intra-articular ligaments appear to function in the same manner as other joint ligaments. They simply reside within the capsule. These ligaments are not widespread in the synovial joints of the body, being limited to the shoulder, hip, and knee joints. The *cruciate* ligaments of the knee are particularly important in limiting excessive movement of the tibia on the femoral condyles. When the knee is injured in athletic contests, the degree of tibial motion is often a valuable clue as to which cruciate ligament is damaged. When a joint contains an intra-articular structure such as a fibrocartilage, it may be bound to a bone end by ligaments within the capsule. The *coronary* ligaments perform that stabilizing function for the fibrocartilages of the knee joint.

OTHER JOINT STRUCTURES: Several freely movable joints contain intra-articular cartilage in addition to the knee. They are the hip, wrist, and the *sternoclavicular* and *acromioclavicular* joints of the shoulder girdle. In some cases, these disks separate a joint cavity into two discrete chambers, e.g., the sternoclavicular joint, while in others they may be incomplete, e.g., the knee joint. They perform numerous functions in their individual skeletal locations, which will be covered in detail in later chapters. General among these functions are the distribution of weight-bearing stresses, shock absorption, and the establishment of a better "fit" between articulating surfaces.

Occasionally, muscle tendons pass through joint capsules. This occurs at the shoulder and knee joints. The tendons of the long head of the *biceps brachii* and the *popliteus* pass through those joint capsules, respectively. Each is enclosed in a special sheath of synovial membrane. Intra-articular fat pads are also in evidence, functioning sometimes as padding in weight-bearing joints.

TABLE 13–3

Diarthrodial Class	Axial Designation	Degrees of Freedom (DF)*	Examples
1. Plane (gliding)	Nonaxial	2	Carpal and tarsal
2. Hinge	Uniaxial	1	Elbow
3. Pivot	Uniaxial	1	Proximal radioulnar
4. Ellipsoid	Biaxial	2	Wrist
5. Condylar	Biaxial	2	Knee
6. Saddle	Biaxial	2	First carpometacarpal
7. Ball and socket	Triaxial	3	Hip and shoulder

* DF are based upon active movements.

Diarthrodial Joint Classification

Returning again to the classification of diarthroses, the seven classes along with other pertinent data are compiled in Table 13-3. Refer to the table as discussions of them develop.

1. PLANE OR GLIDING JOINT: Small amounts of gliding movement are allowed between these joint surfaces even though they are not truly flat or plane as the name suggests. The gliding motion must then be classified as translation. Two degrees of freedom (DF) are available because the bone may move in two distinct planes, both of which are perpendicular to the plane of the articulating surfaces.[3] That is, if the plane of the articulating surfaces is thought to be frontally oriented, either bone of the pair may glide over that surface to trace sagitally or transversely oriented paths. A third translation, where the two adjacent articular surfaces are pulled directly away from each other, is not included. Because no rotation is encountered, these joints are classified as being nonaxial.

2. HINGE JOINT: Hinge joints are uniaxial and thus allow only 1 DF, in the plane of rotation at right angles to the axis of rotation. Because human hinge joints differ in architecture from standard door hinges, the swinging motions they allow are not as pure as those of a door on its hinges. The elbow joint and interphalangeal joints of the fingers provide excellent examples where large magnitudes of flexion and extension are allowed.

3. PIVOT JOINT: The single axis of rotation in pivot joints, allowing only 1 DF in rotation, is of polar orientation in the standing anatomical reference position. The rotations provided in the proximal radioulnar joint allow the radius to pivot about its mechanical axis to produce forearm segment rotations known as supination and pronation. In the anatomical position, the planes of these rotations are transversely oriented.

---

[3]When the bone movements which are allowed in diarthrodial joints are examined in terms of spatial orientation, the identification of the planes of movement is helpful. When a bone movement is restricted to tracing only a single plane in space, the joint is said to have 1 DF. Although this procedure may be applied to translatory as well as rotatory movements, DF designations have, more often than not, been applied only to rotation. Therefore, if a bone can rotate about two perpendicular axes in two perpendicular planes, the joint has 2 DF.

4. ELLIPSOID JOINT: The articulating surfaces of ellipsoid joints generally exhibit two radii of curvature, one longer than the other. If the convex surface of a football is examined, its curvature is seen to be greater around its center than from end to end. When such a shape articulates with a matching concave counterpart, an ellipsoid joint is the result. As such, 2 DF are available. The metacarpophalangeal joints of the hand allow flexion-extension and abduction-adduction. If these individual movements are sequentially performed, circumduction can result.

5. CONDYLAR JOINT: The knee joint is an excellent example of a condylar joint. The pair of femoral condyles (markedly convex) articulate with the pair of tibial condyles (slightly concave). Two degrees of rotation freedom are available in planes associated with bilateral and polar axes in the anatomical position. Flexion-extension and rotation are available, respectively, about these axes. The pair of condylar surfaces may be located in separate joint capsules but perform the same singular movement functionally.

6. SADDLE JOINT: Saddle joints exhibit *sellar* (saddle-like) surfaces which are both convex and concave at right angles to each other. If an English saddle were sectioned centrally from front to rear (pommel to cantle) and then viewed from the side, the section would be concave upward. If the same saddle were sectioned centrally from skirt to skirt and viewed from the direction of its pommel, the section would be convex upward. Saddle joints are junctions between two such surfaces which are reciprocally received by one another. They are formally classified as being biaxial, but some axial rotation is usually allowed. The carpometacarpal joint of the thumb is probably the best example in the entire skeleton.

7. BALL AND SOCKET JOINT: When a rounded head articulates with a bowl-shaped socket, it fits the general description of a ball and socket joint. Like the hinge joint, skeletal ball and socket joints such as the shoulder joint do not conform precisely to the specifications of their counterparts in engineering structures. They are classified as triaxial and possess 3 DF. Thus flexion-extension, abduction-adduction, rotations, and circumductions are allowed, usually in rather large magnitudes.

Control of Joint Movement

In Chapter 6, body segment movements were classified without concern for the articular actions being performed within and between those segments. That terminology is applicable to bone movements within articulations as well. Now that some background in musculoskeletal anatomy has been introduced, it is time to focus our attentions upon joint movement functions, particularly in terms of the ways in which structural organizations dictate and control movement.

The simplest way to limit a motion is to place an obstacle in the motion path. Two kinds of body structures are available for use as obstructions: soft and rigid tissue. Under most conditions, rigid skeletal obstructions are not met, even at the extremes of movement. Notable exceptions are the *facet* joints of the vertebral column. The reason for the lack of rigid-tissue obstruction is that soft tissues usually act as cushions between approaching segments. When the elbow is forcibly flexed, the soft contours of the two segments contact before the complete range of movement has been obtained, gradually resisting its continuance. The protruding abdomen of the very obese often make hip flexion so limited that "knee crossing" is most difficult to achieve and maintain.

The amount of resistance provided by soft tissues is, at first, small and increases as the tissues compress against each other. The quantity of soft tissue available for cushioning varies considerably from person to person but appears to be related primarily to muscular development and the sex of the individual. It has been shown, however, that despite remarkable muscular development, excessive movement limitation need not occur. If the developmental program undertaken is designed to carry the joints of the body through their complete ranges, no "muscle-boundness" need result. As muscle bulk is increased, so is the contractile force. The increased muscular strength may then be brought to bear upon compressing the more prevalent soft tissue. In fact, movement ranges often are increased as the result of properly executed programs for muscle development.

A second means of restricting movement ranges is to limit the range over which the motivating muscle is capable of applying its maximal force. It was noted earlier that as muscle shortening progresses during a concentric contraction, the muscle becomes more and more insufficient in terms of its force-generating capabilities. Consequently, as the point of soft-tissue contact and resistance is beginning to become prominent, the contracting muscle is often becoming progressively more ineffective. The two phenomena combine to serve a protective function.

The role of reflex muscular activity to resist and decelerate high-velocity movements is widespread throughout the body. In general, receptor bodies are situated in muscle, tendon, and joint tissues to signal the need for antagonistic muscle force applications near the ends of movement ranges or whenever there is an imminent danger of trauma. The signaling stimuli may be exhibited in such forms as mild or severe "stretch" tensions or pressure changes within articular cartilage. Unfortunately, the thorough discussion of these mechanisms is beyond the scope of this text. The pursual of this material is, however, encouraged strongly and will be assisted by referring to the bibliography at the end of this chapter.

Muscles may restrict movement ranges in another way. On occasion, a muscle which crosses a joint may not be able to lengthen sufficiently to allow the completion of a movement which would not be limited otherwise. Such a muscle is said to be "tight" and is a very common experience for athletes when beginning a training program which includes wide ranges of movement. The hamstrings muscle group is a notorious offender in such situations when prominent hip flexion and knee extension are concurrent.

→ *To demonstrate, sit on the floor with your knees completely extended in front of you. Now gradually flex at the hips to bring your trunk as close to your thighs as possible. Where do you experience the greatest discomfort?*

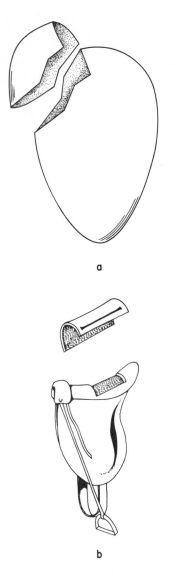

a

b

Figure 13–5. Ovoid and sellar joint surfaces.

Modern life, with its many comfortable conveyances, appears to have markedly reduced the demands for joint mobility. Consequently, sedentary individuals may find that their general mobility is bounded by the magnitudes of their habitual movement patterns.

Ligaments play an important role in joint movements. They function to mitigate the effects of violent movement and act as movement guides owing to their tautness and placement across the joint. Complex joint movements which include more than one rotation component as well as translation often owe their control to the guiding actions of ligaments. Some ligaments are essential in completing extension movements to the point of being *locked* in their terminal positions. The collateral and cruciate ligaments of the knee are good examples. Some ligaments prominently bring joint movements to a halt owing to their sinewiness. Indeed, some ligaments are referred to as *postural* ligaments because they bear chronic burdens in maintaining correct body alignments. The iliofemoral ligament of the hip joint is an able example. Among the most important of the ligamentous functions is that of working in concert with the articulating joint surface architecture to maintain the proper congruity between their generally dissimilar faces.

MacConaill has identified only two types of joint surface shape: the *ovoid* and the *sellar*.[4] The former may be either convex or concave and receives the name because of its similarity to eggshell surfaces. The latter has been described earlier in this chapter with respect to saddle joints. Figure 13-5 illustrates examples of each type of surface. It is important that the ovoid surface is not considered to be the same as a spherical surface. Unlike the spherical surface, the ovoid surface does not exhibit the same radius of curvature at all points.

Since articulating joint surfaces generally present differing curvatures to each other within the joint, only relatively small contact areas are the usual case. There are positions within joint ranges, however, which demonstrate maximal conformity between articulating surfaces. They generally occur at the terminal positions of joint ranges and are termed *close-packed* positions. In such positions, joints are afforded a high degree of stability by bony and ligamentous arrangements. In normally functioning joints, further movement in the directions required to reach the close-packed positions are negated.

Because of the varying degree of surface conformity, coupled with the rather lax ligamentous binding between the terminal joint positions, gliding (translatory) movements are made available in addition to those most often associated with the functional classification of diarthrodial joints. These gliding or sliding movements are not pure translations but accompany the rolling of one joint surface over another to become a combination of translation and rotation. A simple rule appears to generally characterize the elements of these joint surface movements, depending on which surface is regarded as moving over the other. For example, when a convex surface rolls over its concave mate, it tends to glide in a direction

[4]M. A. MacConaill, "Studies in the Mechanics of Synovial Joints," *Irish Journal of Medical Science,* **6** (1946): 223.

opposite that of its roll. With some risk of inaccuracy, think of trying to roll a rounded object out of a concave depression. As the object begins to climb the concave sides of the depression, it tends to slide back toward the center, particularly if the surfaces are lubricated and slick. When a concave surface rolls over its convex mate, it tends to glide in the same direction as its roll. Using the same slick surfaces as before, the rolling concave surface finds that the convex surface continually drops away from contact as the rolling progresses. Consequently, the concave surface tends to slide along in the direction approximating the borders of the convexity. Numerous referals are given to these movement characteristics in the chapters which follow.

REFERENCES

Adams, A. "Effect of Exercise Upon Ligament Strength." *Research Quarterly* 37 (1966): 163.

Barnett, C. H. "The Structure and Function of Fibrocartilages within Vertebral Joints." *Journal of Anatomy* 88 (1954): 363.

———— "Wear and Tear in Joints." *Journal of Bone and Joint Surgery* 38-B (1956): 567.

Barnett, C. H., and Cobbolo, A. F. "Lubrication Within Living Joints." *Journal of Bone and Joint Surgery* 44-B (1962): 662.

Basmajian, J. V. "Weight Bearing by Ligaments and Muscles." *Canadian Journal of Surgery* 4 (1961): 166.

Brantigan, O. C., and Voshell, A. F. "The Mechanics of the Ligament and Menisci of the Knee Joint." *Journal of Bone and Joint Surgery* 23 (1941): 44.

Brozek, Josef, ed. *Body Measurements and Human Physique.* Detroit: Wayne State University Press, 1956.

Camosso, M., and Marotti, G. "The Mechanical Behavior of Articular Cartilage Under Compressive Stress." *Journal of Bone and Joint Surgery* 44-A (1962): 699.

Darcus, H. D. "The Range and Strength of Joint Movement." In *Human Factors in Equipment Design*, edited by W. F. Floyd and A. T. Welford. London: H. K. Lewis & Co., Ltd., 1954.

Davies, D. V. "Aging Changes in Joints." In *Structural Aspects of Aging*, edited by G. H. Bourne. New York: Hafner Publishing Company, Inc., 1961.

———— "Synovial Membrane and Synovial Fluid of Joints." *Lancet* 2 (1946): 815.

Dempster, W. T. "The Anthropology of Body Action." *Annals of the New York Academy of Science* 63 (1955): 574.

Dintenfass, L. "Lubrication in Synovial Joints. A Theoretical Analysis." *Journal of Bone and Joint Surgery* 45-A (1963): 1241.

Elftman, H., and Manter, J. T. "The Evolution of the Human Foot, with Special Reference to the Joints." *Journal of Anatomy* 70 (1935): 56.

Evans, F. Gaynor. *Stress and Strain in Bones.* Springfield, Ill.: Charles C. Thomas, Publisher, 1957.

Fick, R. *Handbuch der Anatomie und Mechanik der Gelenke.* Jena, Germany: G. Fischer, 1910.

Frost, H. M. *An Introduction to Biomechanics.* Springfield, Ill.: Charles C. Thomas, Publisher, 1967.

Frost, Harold M., ed. *Bone Biodynamics.* Boston: Atlantic-Little, Brown and Company, 1964.

———— *The Laws of Bone Structure.* Springfield, Ill.: Charles C. Thomas, Publisher, 1964.

Gardner, Ernest; Gray, Donald J.; and O'Rahilly, Ronan. *Anatomy.* 3rd ed. Philadelphia: W. B. Saunders Company, 1969.

Goss, Charles Mayo, ed. *Gray's Anatomy of the Human Body.* 28th ed. Philadelphia: Lea & Febiger, 1966.

Haldane, J. B. S. "On Being the Right Size." In *The World of Mathematics*, vol. II, edited by J. R. Newman. New York: Simon and Schuster, Inc., 1956.

Hall, Michael C. *The Locomotor System, Functional Anatomy.* Springfield, Ill.: Charles C. Thomas, Publisher, 1965.

——— "The Trabecular Patterns of the Normal Foot." *Clinical Orthopedics* 16 (1960): 15.

Hardy, R. H. "Observations on the Structure and Properties of the Plantar Calcaneo-navicular Ligament in Man." *Journal of Anatomy* 85 (1951): 135.

Hertel, Heinrich. *Structure—Form—Movement*, translated and edited by M. S. Katz. New York: Reinhold Publishing Company, 1966.

Hill, A. V. "The Dimensions of Animals and Their Muscular Dynamics." *Proceedings of the Royal Institution of Great Britain* 34 (1950): 450.

Hirsch, C. "The Reaction of Intervertebral Discs to Compression Forces." *Journal of Bone and Joint Surgery* 37-A (1955): 1189.

Horton, W. G. "Further Observations on the Elastic Mechanism of the Intervertebral Disc." *Journal of Bone and Joint Surgery* 40-B (1958): 552.

Hoyle, Graham. *The Nervous Control of Muscular Contraction.* New York: The Cambridge University Press, 1958.

Hubay, C. A. "Sesamoid Bones of the Hands and Feet." *American Journal of Roentgenology, Radium Therapy, and Nuclear Medicine* 61 (1949) 493.

Koch, J. C. "The Laws of Bone Architecture." *American Journal of Anatomy* 21 (1917): 177.

Krogman, Wilton M. *The Human Skeleton.* Springfield, Ill.: Charles C. Thomas, Publisher, 1962.

Lamb, D. R. "Influence of Exercise on Bone Growth and Metabolism." *Kinesiology Review–1968.* Washington, D.C.: N.E.A., 1968, p. 43.

MacConaill, M. A. "Joint Movements." *Physiotherapy* (November 1964): 359.

——— "Mechanical Anatomy of Motion and Posture." In *Therapeutic Exercise*, edited by S. Licht. 2d ed. New Haven, Conn.: Elizabeth Licht, Publisher, 1961.

——— "The Movements of Bones and Joints: II. Function of the Musculature." *Journal of Bone and Joint Surgery* 31-B (1949): 100.

——— "The Movements of Bones and Joints: IV. The Mechanical Structure of Articulating Cartilage." *Journal of Bone and Joint Surgery* 33-B (1951): 251.

——— "Studies in the Mechanics of Synovial Joints." *Irish Journal of Medical Science* 6 (1946): 223.

MacConaill, M. A., and Basmajian, J. V. *Muscles and Movement: A Basis for Human Kinesiology.* Baltimore: The Williams & Wilkins Company, 1969.

McCormick, Ernest J. *Human Engineering.* New York: McGraw-Hill Book Company, 1957.

McMurrich, Kathleen I. *Applied Muscle Action and Coordination.* Toronto: University of Toronto Press, 1957.

Mathur, P. D.; McDonald, J. R.; and Ghormley, R. K. "A Study of the Tensile Strength of the Menisci of the Knee." *Journal of Bone and Joint Surgery* 31-A (1949): 650.

Morant, G. B. "Body Size and Work Space." In *Human Factors in Equipment Design*, edited by W. F. Floyd and A. T. Welford. London: H. K. Lewis & Co., Ltd., 1954.

Morton, Dudley J., and Fuller, Dudley D. *Human Locomotion and Body Form.* Baltimore: The Williams & Wilkins Company, 1952.

Rodahl, Kaare; Nicholson, Jesse T.; and Brown, Ernest M., Jr., eds. *Bone as a Tissue.* New York: McGraw-Hill Book Company, 1960.

Saaf, J. "Effects of Exercise on Adult Articular Cartilage." *Acta Orthopedica Scandinavica* 7 Suppl. (1950): 7.

Salter, R. B., and Field, P. "The Effects of Continuous Compression on Living Articular Cartilage." *Journal of Bone and Joint Surgery* 42-A (1960): 31.

Stein, Irvin; Stein, Raymond O.; and Beller, Martin L. *Living Bone in Health and Disease*. Philadelphia: J. B. Lippincott Company, 1955.

Steindler, Arthur. *Kinesiology of the Human Body*. Springfield, Ill.: Charles C. Thomas, Publisher, 1955.

Thompson, D. W. *On Growth and Form*, edited by J. T. Bonner. Abbreviated ed. Cambridge: Cambridge University Press, 1961.

Tobin, W. J. "The Internal Architecture of the Femur and its Clinical Significance." *Journal of Bone and Joint Surgery* 37-A (1955): 57.

Weinmann, Joseph P., and Sicher, Harry. *Bone and Bones*. 2d ed. St. Louis, Mo.: C. V. Mosby Company, 1955.

Williams, P. O. "The Assessment of Mobility in Joints." *Lancet* 2 (1952): 169.

14

Foot,

Ankle Joint,

Leg

THE FOOT SEGMENT

Man is a *plantigrade* animal in that he walks and stands on the soles of his feet. In its most inferior position within the erect body, the foot must withstand and transmit stresses associated with its contact with the ground in standing, walking, and vigorous running. These are formidable requirements which it can shoulder with little difficulty if cared for properly. If these functional demands are recognized by man, and it is obvious that this is the case, one of modern life's strangest problems is the degree to which man abuses his hard-working feet.

The Bones of the Foot

This distal segment of the lower extremity is composed of 26 separate bones. Figure 14-1 illustrates dorsal and plantar views of the foot with

Figure 14–1. The bones of the right foot from (*a*) dorsal and (*b*) plantar views.

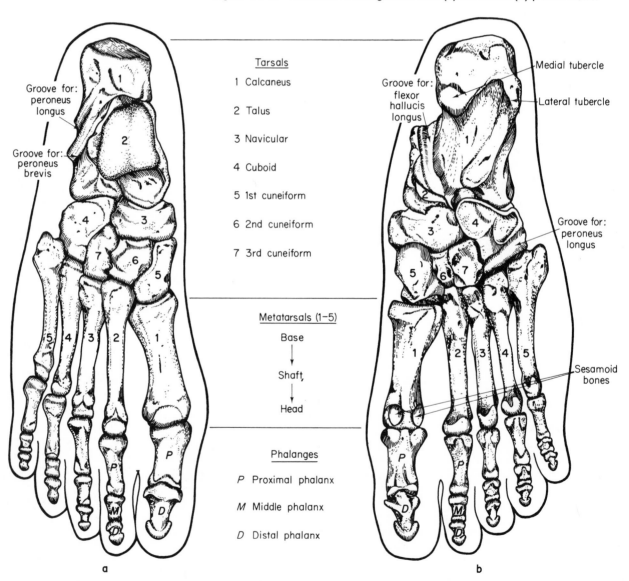

Tarsals

1 Calcaneus

2 Talus

3 Navicular

4 Cuboid

5 1st cuneiform

6 2nd cuneiform

7 3rd cuneiform

Metatarsals (1–5)

Base
↓
Shaft
↓
Head

Phalanges

P Proximal phalanx

M Middle phalanx

D Distal phalanx

Groove for: peroneus longus

Groove for: peroneus brevis

Groove for: flexor hallucis longus

Medial tubercle

Lateral tubercle

Groove for: peroneus longus

Sesamoid bones

a

b

each bone numbered and keyed. It is important that these views be studied carefully because they offer much information concerning the shape of the foot. For example, the second cuneiform (6) of the seven tarsal bones is more prominent from above than it is from below. This indicates a transversely oriented arch shape which is convex upward. Viewing the talus (2) and calcaneus (1) from below and then above indicates that the talus rides high upon the medial side of the calcaneus to act as the floor of the ankle joint. The calcaneus protrudes out behind the talus to act as a very useful lever as well as the posterior contact point of the foot. The forefoot serves the same purpose in front of the ankle.

Viewing the foot from the side (Fig. 14-2), it is possible to describe two longitudinal arches. They differ with respect to height, with the five metatarsal bones disposed to complete the arches in the anterior direction. The metatarsals are small long bones, each exhibiting a *base*, *shaft*, and *head*. Since the heads of the metatarsals are located where the forefoot contacts the ground in standing (ball of the foot), it may be said that we can stand on our metatarsal heads.

The junctions between the phalanges are known as the *interphalangeal* (IP) joints, a distinction which applies as well to those related joints of the hand. The toes of the foot vary in girth and length. Each of the four lesser toes includes three phalanges: a proximal (P), middle (M), and distal (D) phalanx. The great toe or *hallux* includes only a proximal and distal phalanx. Each of the phalanges exhibits long bone characteristics with a

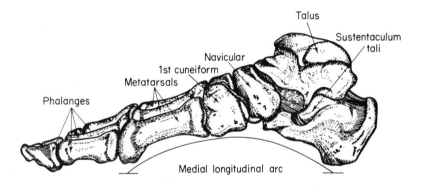

a

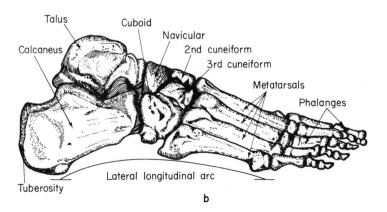

b

Figure 14–2. (*a*) Medial and (*b*) lateral views of the foot showing the difference between the longitudinal curvature of its two aspects.

base, shaft, and head, reading forward. Note the two elliptical *sesamoid* bones under the head of the first metatarsal. Since they reside at the ball of the foot, weight-bearing stresses must be transmitted through them in standing and pushing off in walking and running.

The junctions between the metatarsals and the phalanges are called the *metatarsophalangeal* (MP) joints. In balanced standing, they lie in the same plane as the base of the calcaneus. They reside at the ball of the foot and provide one of the most prominent sites where movement of the flexible forefoot may be observed.

The junctions between the forward tarsals and the metatarsal bases, the *tarsometatarsal* (TM) joints, show different elevations in the medial and lateral views of the foot. Note the differences in size among the metatarsals and that the fifth metatarsal has a very prominent projection at its base. Its position in the foot is easily seen and can be *palpated* (touched and felt with the fingers).

→ *Place your fingers on the foot's lateral border near the heel. Slide the fingers forward until they contact this bony landmark. Palpate as many other bony landmarks of the forefoot as possible.*

Weight Bearing and Shock Absorption Stabilization

The bones of the foot are tightly bound together by ligaments so that adequate movement is allowed in conjunction with the requirements of weight bearing and shock absorption. In the upright posture, the weight of the body is transmitted downward through the arched structures of the horizontal foot to the ground. Compared to lower primates, man's foot has gained strength at the expense of mobility, which may be considered a reasonable trade for continued use of upright postures.

Three weight-bearing mechanisms have been described for the foot by Hicks.[1] They are the beam, the arch or truss, and a muscular mechanism, each of which is capable of considerable individual support. However, they tend to function together to bear the body's weight. As a curved beam, the foot's primary resistance to the downward-directed body weight is provided by the tough plantar ligaments. Its upward curve is reduced somewhat in bearing the weight of the body to cause marked tension in those ligaments. When the body's weight is balanced over the ankle joint, surprisingly little intrinsic or extrinsic muscle action occurs. Even the metatarsals themselves may act as smaller beams in the forefoot.

As a longitudinal arch, the foot requires some means of fixing (a *tie*) the heel and ball piers so that they do not become further separated in weight bearing, thus reducing its curvature. The *plantar aponeurosis* (Fig. 14-3) is given credit for this binding function since it runs from heel to ball just under the skin of the foot's plantar surface. When the MP joints are hyperextended, tension in the aponeurosis is increased, tending to draw heel and ball closer together and increasing the foot's curvature.

[1]J. H. Hicks, "The Three Weight-Bearing Mechanisms of The Foot," in *Biomechanical Studies of The Musculo-Skeletal System* (F. G. Evans, ed.) (Springfield, Ill.: Charles C Thomas, Publisher, 1961), pp. 161–91.

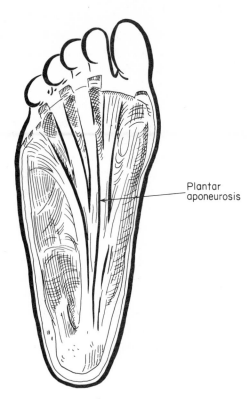

Plantar
aponeurosis

Figure 14–3. The plantar aponeurosis of the foot.

→ *Demonstrate this with your own foot and palpate the increased firmness of the plantar surface about midway between heel and ball. Notice that this phenomenon is far more pronounced on the medial side than on the lateral side.*

This would be expected since the lateral side demonstrates a far more limited mobility than the medial owing to its naturally lower contour. In the strictest of terms, only the medial longitudinal arch qualifies as being a true arch by architectural arrangement.

The *transverse tarsal* curvature, located at the TM joints, is not a true arch either in the engineering sense because there is no tie to bind together its two ends. The often mentioned *transverse metatarsal arch* at the ball of the foot suffers from the same limitations. Its transverse curvature is evident only when the toes are flexed.

→ *Palpate this curve on the ball of the foot while flexing the toes. Note how it disappears when the toes are extended.*

The muscles which control the position of the body's weight over the foot can have, indirectly, a marked effect in weight bearing. These effects are in addition to the usual direct actions compiled in this chapter's muscle chart (Muscle Chart 1). Those muscles which tend to pivot the leg backward above the standing foot, the plantar flexors, can control eccentrically a forward-leaning position, where the body's weight is balanced considerably in front of the ankle axis, nearly over the ball of the foot. In doing so, tension in the plantar aponeurosis is increased to nearly double that when the weight is balanced directly above the ankle. In this position, the tendency of the body weight to flatten the longitudinal curvature is greatest. The dorsiflexors, which can provide the opposite kind of eccentric balance so that the weight vector passes through the heel, tend to reduce the aponeurotic tension to near zero. In this position there is little or no tendency for the longitudinal curvature to flatten. For individual muscles, those which pass behind the ankle joint axis indirectly increase the body's tendency to flatten the foot, while those which pass in front of that axis function oppositely. Similar balancing mechanisms have been described as occurring in the frontal plane in which inversion and eversion of the leg on the fixed foot are employed to maintain equilibrium.

In walking, the heel and ball of the foot act as the striking points. Most of us have examined the footprint left on the deck of a swimming pool by a wet foot. The print generally is continuous along its lateral border from heel to ball but not so along the medial border. Thus it would be expected that the lateral and medial parts of the foot might serve somewhat different functions. Indeed, the responsibility for maintaining balance has been described as a function of the lateral side of the foot. The medial side acts to assist in propulsion. The path of weight bearing begins with the striking heel and passes forward, just off-center laterally, so that the forward pier of the lateral side makes contact slightly before its medial counterpart. The ball of the foot then is the site of a very rapid transfer of the weight from lateral to medial, a shift which places the burden of pushing off on the great toe at the first MP joint. The fact that deviations from the pattern of weight transfer cited above do occur is shown when footwear show accelerated deterioration predominantly along one border rather than being rather evenly distributed.

Whether or not the feet, with their twisted, half-domed shapes, actually contain true arches, their curvatures with their strong reinforcing ligaments act to absorb the shocks of weight bearing and locomotion. The natural elasticity of these structures allows them to be forced out of their natural form and then quickly return to their original shapes in a manner which resembles the action of prestressed concrete beams. Because of the many small bones and their numerous articulations, the energy of shock forces may be dissipated in many directions within the foot. As a result, the foot segment then acts as the first in a series of shock absorption mechanisms which are strategically placed in the lower limb.

Movements Within the Foot

The movements which can take place within the foot depend on the specific articulations involved, both individually and collectively. The locations within the foot which provide the primary mobility are now discussed.

INTERPHALANGEAL (IP) MOBILITY: These joints are hinge joints, allowing only flexion and extension. The proximal IP joints show the greater mobility. Each joint is reinforced by collateral and plantar ligaments. Placed as they are, active hyperextensions are all but ruled out.

→ *Examine and palpate the long extensor tendons coursing down the dorsal aspect of the foot to the four lateral toes and the great toe. Note that it is almost impossible to move these joints without hyperextending the next, more proximal row of joints.*

METATARSOPHALANGEAL (MP) MOBILITY: The greatest range of motion of the forefoot occurs at these ellipsoid joints. Flexion-extension and hyperextension are available about the shorter, bilateral axis of each joint, while slight abduction and adduction are allowed about the longer polar axis. It is possible to move these joints in such a manner that from a position of terminal hyperextension, each MP joint may be abducted and flexed in a sequence which first places the little toe in contact with the floor, followed in order by the fourth, third, second, and first toes. The reversed sequence may be performed, but usually with more difficulty.

→ *Attempt these actions and see if you concur.*

TARSOMETATARSAL (TM) MOBILITY: Dorsal, plantar, and interosseous ligaments tie these joints together. They are formed from the bases of the metatarsals and the anterior surfaces of the cuboid and the cuneiforms. Some gliding movements are allowed, but they are of limited magnitudes which favor the medial side of the foot. Even though they are slight, far medial and far lateral movements in opposing directions may occur simultaneously to cause the forefoot to twist slightly.

MIDTARSAL (MT) MOBILITY: This joint demonstrates 3 DF within its four-bone complex. The calcaneus articulates with the cuboid laterally while the talus and navicular articulate medially. Viewing the foot from above (Fig. 14-1), a flattened S shape is revealed which is convex forward on the medial side and convex backward on the lateral side. This compound joint is known technically as the *transverse tarsal* joint and often is used as the boundary line which separates the forefoot from the posterior pair of tarsals.

The forefoot may rotate about three axes at this joint. However, the movements are combined to result in a flexion plus adduction-extension plus abduction mode and a supination-pronation mode. Following the movement terminology set forth in Chapter 6, it is seen that the adduction-abduction components combine with inversion-eversion components, respectively, to result in supination-pronation. In other words, adduction-abduction contributes to both modes, with the supination-pronation mode being of greater consequence. Since the foot is placed within the body to interact with horizontal surfaces, MT joint adjustments are particularly important when the anterior and posterior parts of the foot must move in opposition when walking over irregular surfaces.

SUBTALAR MOBILITY: The talus and calcaneus are bound together by anterior, posterior, lateral, medial, and interosseous *talocalcaneal* ligaments (Fig. 14-6). Because of this binding arrangement, motion is limited. Although it is classified by some as a gliding joint, subtalar movements

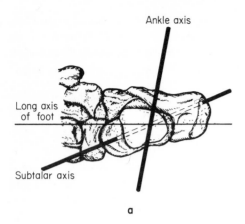

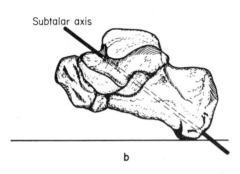

Figure 14–4. The subtalar and ankle axes. Note the oblique orientations with respect to the long axis of the foot in (*a*) and the horizontal in (*b*).

may be described as occurring about an oblique axis. Figure 14-4 illustrates the subtalar axis from dorsal and medial views. Note that it deviates from a true *AP* axis in two ways. Thus it is clear that subtalar movements are composites of other, simpler movements, as was the case for the midtarsal joint. When the foot is viewed from the rear, subtalar contributions to its movement are inversion-eversion, the former exceeding the latter in magnitude.

The talus and calcaneus are of particular interest because so few muscles find insertion attachments on their surfaces. In fact, the talus is free of muscle attachments entirely, while only the achilles tendon muscles have a significant motivating influence on the foot through the calcaneus. Because of the doubly oblique subtalar axis, muscles which are ideally placed to produce abduction (the *peroneus brevis*) are, at the same time, obligated to produce subtalar eversion. Occurring under similar circumstances are subtalar adductions and inversions. Because of these multiple muscular influences, the combined actions of the subtalar and ankle joints are often characterized by synergic activity.

THE ANKLE JOINT

The ankle or *talocrural* joint is formed by the joining of the tibia and fibula of the leg segment to the talus of the foot. Of the two leg bones, the tibia is the larger and is placed so that it articulates with the upper and medial surfaces of the talus. Figure 14-5 makes it clear that this junction is naturally situated to transmit vertical forces from the tibia to the talus. The lateral and medial surfaces of the talus articulate with the *fibular* and *tibial malleoli*, respectively. The malleolar surfaces form a partial *mortise*, into which the body of the talus fits.

The talus may be conceived generally as being partially analogous to the *tenon* of the carpenter's mortise and tenon joint except that its sides flare obliquely outward and downward, and it is wider anteriorly than posteriorly. Weight forces acting across the joint may be resolved into two components (Fig. 14-5b). Those forces (F_c) which are directed perpendicular to the talar surfaces act to clamp it in the *tibiofibular mortise*. The forces (F_s) which run parallel to the joint surfaces, if allowed, would tend to produce sliding of the tibia and fibula downward over the sides of the talus. This action is countered by the tight binding of the *distal anterior* and *posterior tibiofibular* ligaments (Fig. 14-6). Because they do not allow the tibia and fibula to be separated bilaterally, clamping is the result, and distal sliding is minimized.

Joint Stability

In terms of stability, the bony architecture results in a relatively stable joint. The fibular malleolus crosses the joint to a greater extent than does the tibial malleolus; hence the lateral side is said to be stronger than the medial side by bony arrangement. When dorsiflexed maximally, the broader anterior aspect of the talus tends to wedge mildly between the malleoli. This position, because of its compact bone arrangement, is said

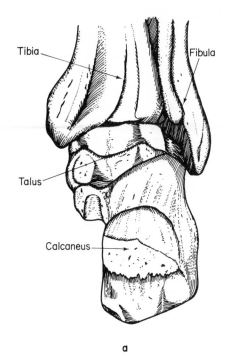

Tibia

Fibula

Talus

Calcaneus

a

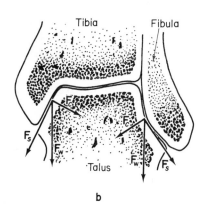

Tibia

Fibula

F_s

F_c

F_w

F_w

F_s

Talus

b

Figure 14–5. (a) The ankle joint from behind, and (b) in frontal section. Clamping forces, **F**$_c$, are generated due to the interaction of gravity and ligamentous bindings across the joint, adding to the joint's stability.

Figure 14–6. (a) Lateral and (b) medial views of the ligaments of the ankle joint and adjacent foot bones.

to be more stable than when the joint is plantar-flexed, where the narrower, posterior aspect is rotated upward between the malleoli. Brunnstrom has commented that the general increase in ankle joint instability as the result of wearing high-heeled shoes is due to the reduced congruity of the articular surfaces.[2]

When the primary ligaments of the ankle joint are considered, the joint is strengthened further. Figure 14-6 illustrates lateral and medial views of the joint, with the important ligaments included. The *fibular collateral* ligament includes three components. They are the *posterior* and

[2]Signe Brunnstrom, *Clinical Kinesiology*, 2d ed. (Philadelphia: F. A. Davis Company, 1966), p. 196.

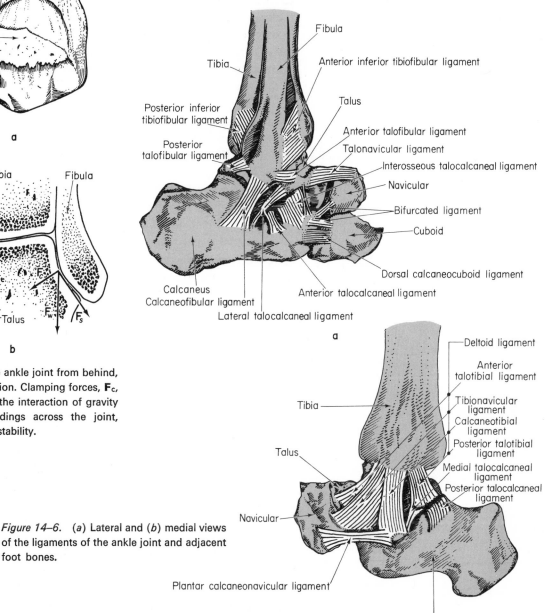

Fibula

Tibia

Anterior inferior tibiofibular ligament

Posterior inferior tibiofibular ligament

Posterior talofibular ligament

Talus

Anterior talofibular ligament

Talonavicular ligament

Interosseous talocalcaneal ligament

Navicular

Bifurcated ligament

Cuboid

Dorsal calcaneocuboid ligament

Calcaneus

Calcaneofibular ligament

Anterior talocalcaneal ligament

Lateral talocalcaneal ligament

a

Deltoid ligament

Anterior talotibial ligament

Tibionavicular ligament

Calcaneotibial ligament

Posterior talotibial ligament

Medial talocalcaneal ligament

Posterior talocalcaneal ligament

Tibia

Talus

Navicular

Plantar calcaneonavicular ligament

Calcaneus

b

anterior talofibular and *calcaneofibular* ligaments. Their positions across the joint give some indication of their roles in augmenting joint stability. They most notably resist excessive inversion of the foot on the leg as well as limit anterior and posterior displacement of the talus within the joint. These lateral ligaments are of particular interest because they are so often injured in athletic endeavors to result in the typical "inversion sprain."

The tibial collateral ligament is of triangular shape and as such is often called the *deltoid* ligament. It is composed of two parts: deep and superficial. Both parts arise from the medial malleolus. The tough deep fibers attach to the talus and are named collectively the *anterior talotibial* ligament. The superficial fibers fan downward to attach to the navicular, calcaneus, and talus. They are the *tibionavicular, calcaneotibial,* and *posterior talotibial* ligaments, respectively. As if to compensate for the lesser bony overlap on the medial side, the ankle joint is stronger medially than laterally by ligamentous arrangement. The deltoid ligament is in a position to resist excessive eversion of the foot and lateral displacements of the talus and calcaneus.

Muscles add significantly to the stabilization picture when their locations and actions are considered. For example, those which cross posterior to the joint (plantar flexors) act as posterior stabilizers to prohibit forward leg displacements on the talus. Those passing in front of the joint act as anterior stabilizers (dorsiflexors) to restrain any tendency for the leg to be displaced backward. Muscles which invert the foot offer some medial stabilization, while those which evert the foot offer some lateral stabilization. The muscular stabilization of the ankle joint just discussed must not be confused with muscular stabilization of the longitudinal arch of the foot. It has been shown that such stabilization of the foot contours is primarily shouldered by the ligaments of the foot, with the muscles playing secondary roles.

Joint Mobility

The usual designation of ankle movements is limited to dorsiflexion and plantar flexion. Actually, dorsiflexion is accompanied by a small amount of forward talar glide, while in plantar flexion, the situation is reversed. Upon examination, the axis of the joint is seen to deviate from a true bilateral axis (see Fig. 14-4). Since the axis courses essentially between the two malleoli, the medial end is somewhat anterior to the lateral end. Under experimental observation from the rear, the ankle joint axis is seen to pivot about its lateral end so that the medial end is elevated above the lateral in dorsiflexion and depressed below the lateral end in plantar flexion.

Referring to Muscle Chart 1, it will be seen that the muscles which move the foot are situated to produce combinations of movements. For example, contractions of the *peroneus tertius* generally elicit dorsiflexion of the ankle and eversion below. The same may be said for the *extensor digitorum longus* in addition to toe extension. On the other hand, the *tibialis anterior* and *extensor hallucis longus* act to dorsiflex the ankle joint and invert the foot below. When all four of these muscles act to dorsiflex the ankle, inversion and eversion are mutually excluded or ruled out, an example of helping synergy. Dorsiflexion mobility is limited to approximately 20 deg above the point where the foot is at right angles to the leg.

The muscles which pass behind the ankle joint are primarily plantar flexors. The *gastrocnemius* and *soleus* pass directly behind the ankle to the calcaneus. The *peroneus longus* and *brevis* tendons course behind the lateral malleolus, using it as a pulley to alter the pulling direction of their tendons. Because of the subtalar axis, they may evert the foot below the ankle. Coursing behind the medial malleolus are the *tibialis posterior*, the *flexor digitorum longus*, and the *flexor hallucis longus*. In addition to producing plantar flexion at the ankle, this group is situated to invert the foot below the ankle. Operating as a unified group, very forceful, balanced plantar flexion through approximately 50 deg is available, with the tendencies to invert and evert negating each other in helping synergy. According to Steindler, the working capacity of the combined plantar flexors is four to five times that for the combined dorsiflexors.[3] Given as a reason for this imbalance is the assistance given to dorsiflexion by gravity in upright standing. The gravital line passes in front of the ankle axis, which greatly augments the dorsiflexion tendency at the expense of plantar flexor stabilization.

→ *Place your foot and ankle, or that of a friend, in a well-illuminated position in which the superficial structures may be examined and palpated. Slowly combine sequential ankle and foot movements to produce a circumduction of the foot on the leg. Near the end of balanced dorsiflexion, produce forcible eversions and inversions. Have your friend stand on one foot so that you may examine the muscular actions which are called into play to maintain balance. Describe the movements and stabilizations of the foot and ankle which are required in football punting vs. place kicking or the differences between extreme positions of the frog and flutter kicks in swimming.*

---

[3]Arthur Steindler, *Kinesiology of the Human Body* (Springfield, Ill.: Charles C Thomas, Publisher, 1955), pp. 390–91.

Muscle Chart 1: Foot, Ankle Joint, Leg

Muscle	Attachments		Innervation
	Origin	Insertion	

I. The Intrinsic Foot Muscles

A. The Dorsal Group

Muscle	Origin	Insertion	Innervation
1. Extensor digitorum brevis	Upper and lateral surfaces of the calcaneus and the limbs of the extensor retinaculum	Three lateral tendons fuse with those of the extensor digitorum longus to the 2nd, 3rd, and 4th toes	Deep peroneal nerve (sometimes superficial peroneal nerve)
a. Medial part is called the extensor hallucis brevis		a. Dorsal surface of the base of the 1st phalanx of the great toe	

B. The Plantar Group—Layer I

Muscle	Origin	Insertion	Innervation
1. Abductor digiti minimi	Lateral tubercle and adjacent parts of the plantar surface of the calcaneus anterior to the tubercles	Lateral side of the proximal phalanx of the small toe	Lateral plantar nerve
2. Abductor hallucis	Medial tubercle of the calcaneus, the flexor retinaculum, and the plantar aponeurosis	Medial sesamoid and the base of proximal phalanx of the great toe	Medial plantar nerve
3. Flexor digitorum brevis	Medial tubercle of the calcaneus and the plantar aponeurosis	Sides of the middle phalanx of the four lateral toes	Medial plantar nerve

C. The Plantar Group—Layer II

Muscle	Origin	Insertion	Innervation
1. Lumbricales	Tendons of the flexor digitorum longus	Medial side of the base of the proximal phalanx of the four lateral toes	First lumbrical by the medial plantar nerve; 2nd, 3rd, and 4th by the lateral plantar nerve
2. Quadratus plantae	Medial side of the plantar surface of the calcaneus and the lateral side of the plantar surface of the calcaneus near the lateral tubercle	Deep surface of the tendon of the flexor digitorum longus	Lateral plantar nerve

Assists in extension and hyperextension of the MP joints
and extension of the IP
joints of the 2nd, 3rd, and
4th toes

a. Assists in extension and
   hyperextension of the MP
   joint of the great toe

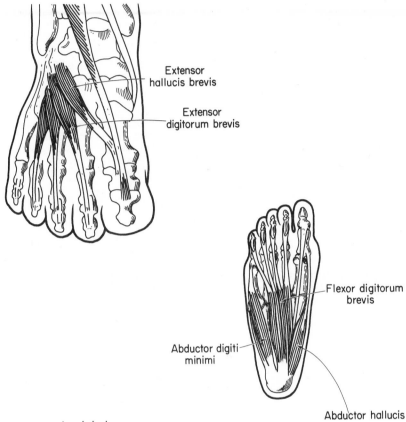

Extensor
hallucis brevis

Extensor
digitorum brevis

Flexion of the small toe

Abduction of the great toe;
assists in flexion of the MP
joint of the great toe

Flexion of the proximal IP
joints of the four lateral toes

Flexor digitorum
brevis

Abductor digiti
minimi

Abductor hallucis

Extension of the IP joints and
flexion of the MP joints of
the four lateral toes

Assists the flexor digitorum
longus tendons in flexion of
the IP joints of the four
lateral toes

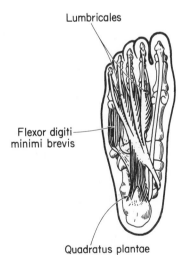

Lumbricales

Flexor digiti
minimi brevis

Quadratus plantae

(*continued*)

Muscle	Attachments		Innervation
	Origin	Insertion	

D. The Plantar Group—Layer III

1. Adductor hallucis

a. Oblique head	a. Anterior end of the long plantar ligament and the sheath of the peroneus longus	a. Sesamoid and proximal phalanx in common with the lateral part of the flexor hallucis brevis	a. Lateral plantar nerve
b. Transverse head	b. Plantar ligaments of the MP joints of the four lateral toes	b. Side of the fibrous sheath of the flexor hallucis longus	b. Lateral plantar nerve
2. Flexor digiti minimi brevis	Sheath of the peroneus longus	Proximal phalanx of the small toe	Lateral plantar nerve
3. Flexor hallucis brevis	Medial part of the plantar surface of the cuboid bone, contiguous portion of the lateral cuneiform and the prolongation of the tendon of the tibialis posterior	Medial and lateral sides of the base of the first phalanx of the great toe	Medial plantar nerve

E. The Plantar Group—Layer IV

1. Dorsal interossei	By two heads from adjacent sides of the metatarsals	Bases of the first phalanges of the 2nd, 3rd, and 4th toes, and the aponeurosis of the tendons of the extensor digitorum longus	Lateral plantar nerve
2. Plantar interossei	Base and medial sides of the shafts of the 3rd, 4th, and 5th metatarsals	Medial sides of the bases of the 1st phalanges and into the aponeuroses of the tendons of the extensor digitorum longus	Lateral plantar nerve

II. The Extrinsic Muscles of the Foot and Ankle Joint

A. The Anterior Crural Group

1. Extensor digitorum longus	Lateral condyle of the tibia, proximal three fourths of the anterior surface of the shaft of the fibula, and the proximal part of the interosseous membrane	Second and 3rd phalanges of the four lateral toes	Deep peroneal nerve
2. Extensor hallucis longus	Anterior, middle two thirds of the fibula, and same portion of the interosseous membrane	Base of the distal phalanx of the great toe	Deep peroneal nerve
3. Peroneus tertius	Distal third of the anterior surface of the fibula, distal part of the interosseous membrane	Dorsal surface of the base of the metatarsal of the small toe	Deep peroneal nerve
4. Tibialis anterior	Lateral condyle, proximal two thirds of the lateral surface of the tibia, and the adjoining part of interosseous membrane	Medial and plantar surfaces of the first cuneiform	Deep peroneal nerve

a. Adduction of the great toe; assists the flexor hallucis brevis in flexion of the MP joint of the great toe

b. Adduction of the great toe

Flexion of the MP joint of the small toe

Flexion of the MP joint of the great toe

Adductor hallucis (transverse head)

Adductor hallucis (oblique head)

Flexor hallucis brevis

Extension of the IP joints, and flexion of the MP joints of the 2nd, 3rd, and 4th toes; 2nd, 3rd, and 4th interossei draw the 2nd, 3rd, and 4th toes laterally; 1st interosseous draws the 2nd toe medially

Extension of the IP joints, and flexion of the MP joints of the three lateral toes; draw those toes toward the 2nd toe

Plantar interossei

Dorsal interossei

Extension of the MP joints of the four lateral toes; eversion and abduction of the foot; dorsiflexion of the ankle joint

Extension of the MP joint of the great toe; inversion and adduction of the foot; dorsiflexion of the ankle joint

Eversion and abduction of the foot; dorsiflexion of the ankle joint

Dorsiflexion of the ankle joint; inversion and adduction of the foot when accompanied by dorsiflexion of the ankle joint

Tibialis anterior

Extensor digitorum longus

Extensor hallucis longus

(continued)

| Muscle | Attachments | | Innervation |
	Origin	Insertion	
B. The Lateral Crural Group			
1. Peroneus brevis	Distal two thirds of the lateral surface of the shaft of the fibula	Tuberosity at the base of the 5th metatarsal on the lateral side	Superficial peroneal nerve
2. Peroneus longus	Head and proximal two thirds of the lateral surface of the shaft of the fibula	Lateral side of the base of the 1st metatarsal and lateral side of the 1st cuneiform	Superficial peroneal nerve
C. The Posterior Crural Group—Superficial Layer			
1. Gastrocnemius	By two heads to the popliteal surface of the femur above the medial and lateral condyles	Forms the achilles tendon with the soleus to end on the middle part of the posterior surface of the calcaneus	Tibial nerve
2. Soleus	Posterior surface of the head of the fibula, proximal one third to one half of the posterior surface of the shaft of the fibula, popliteal line, and middle one third of the medial border of the tibia	Forms the achilles tendon with the gastrocnemius to end on the middle part of the posterior surface of the calcaneus	Tibial nerve
D. The Posterior Crural Group—Deep Layer			
1. Flexor digitorum longus	Posterior surface of the shaft of the tibia below the popliteal line	Bases of the distal phalanges of the four lateral toes	Tibial nerve
2. Flexor hallucis longus	Distal two thirds of the posterior surface of the fibula	Base of the terminal phalanx of the great toe	Tibial nerve
3. Tibialis posterior	Posterior surface of the interosseous membrane, the lateral portion of the posterior surface of the shaft of the tibia, and from the proximal two thirds of the medial surface of the fibula	Tuberosity of the navicular, the plantar surface of the cuneiforms, cuboid, bases of the 2nd, 3rd, and 4th metatarsals, and the sustentaculum tali of the calcaneus	Tibial nerve

Eversion and abduction of the foot. Assists in plantar flexion of the ankle joint

Eversion and abduction of the foot; plantar flexion of the ankle joint

Plantar flexion of the ankle joint; assists in flexion of knee joint

Plantar flexion of the ankle joint

Flexion of the IP joints of the four lateral toes; inversion and adduction of the foot; assists in plantar flexion of the ankle joint

Flexion of the IP and MP joints of the great toe; assists in inversion and adduction of the foot, and plantar flexion of the ankle joint

Inversion and adduction of the foot; plantar flexion of the ankle joint

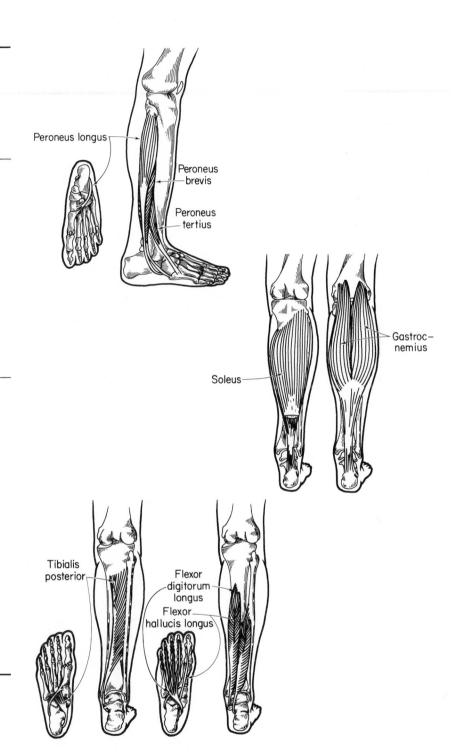

Peroneus longus

Peroneus brevis

Peroneus tertius

Gastroc-nemius

Soleus

Tibialis posterior

Flexor digitorum longus

Flexor hallucis longus

REFERENCES

Anderson, K. J.; LeCocq, J. F.; and Clayton, M. L. "Athletic Injuries to the Fibular Collateral Ligament of the Ankle." *Clinical Orthopedics* 23 (1962): 146.

Barnett, C. H. "Further Observations Upon the Axis of Rotation at the Human Ankle Joint." *Journal of Anatomy* 87 (1953): 449.

————— "The Normal Orientation of the Human Hallux and the Effect of Footwear." *Journal of Anatomy* 96 (1962): 489.

Barnett, C. H.; Davies, D. V.; and MacConaill, M. A. *Synovial Joints: Their Structure and Mechanics.* Springfield, Ill.: Charles C. Thomas, Publisher, 1961.

Barnett, C. H., and Napier, J. R. "The Axis of Rotation of the Ankle Joint in Man. Its Influence Upon the Form of the Talus and the Mobility of the Fibula." *Journal of Anatomy* 86 (1952): 1.

Basmajian, J. V. *Muscles Alive: Their Function Revealed by Electromyography.* 2d ed. Baltimore: The Williams & Wilkins Company, 1967.

————— "Weight Bearing by Ligaments and Muscles." *Canadian Journal of Surgery* 4 (1961): 166.

Basmajian, J. V., and Bentzon, J. W. "An Electromyographic Study of Certain Muscles of the Leg and the Foot in the Standing Position." *Surgery, Gynecology and Obstetrics* 98 (1959): 662.

Basmajian, J. V., and Stecko, G. "The Role of Muscles in Arch Support of the Foot." *Journal of Bone and Joint Surgery* 45-A (1963): 1184.

Bassett, David L. *A Stereoscopic Atlas of Human Anatomy.* Portland, Ore.: Sawyer's Inc., 1955.

Battye, C. K., and Joseph, J. "An Investigation of Telemetering of the Activity of Some Muscles in Walking." *Medical and Biological Engineering* 4 (1966): 125.

Bettmann, E. H. "The Human Foot." *Archives of Physical Therapy* 25 (1944): 13.

Brunnstrom, Signe. *Clinical Kinesiology.* 2d ed. Philadelphia: F. A. Davis Company, 1966.

Carlsoo, S. "Influence of Frontal and Dorsal Loads on Muscle Activity and on the Weight Distribution in the Feet." *Acta Orthopaedica Scandinavica* 34 (1964): 299.

Close, J. R. "Some Applications of the Functional Anatomy of the Ankle Joint." *Journal of Bone and Joint Surgery* 38-A (1956): 761.

Close, J. R.; Inman, V. T.; and Poor, P. M. "The Function of the Subtalar Joint." *Clinical Orthopedics* 50 (1967): 159.

Della, D. G. "Individual Differences in Foot Leverage in Relation to Jumping Performance." *Research Quarterly* 21 (1950): 11.

Eberhart, H. D.; Inman, V. T.; and Bresler, B. "The Principal Elements in Human Locomotion." In *Human Limbs and Their Substitutes*, edited by P. E. Klopsteg and P. D. Wilson. New York: McGraw-Hill Book Company, 1954.

Elftman, H. "A Cinematic Study of the Distribution of Pressure in the Human Foot." *Anatomical Record* 59 (1934): 481.

————— "The Functional Structure of the Lower Limbs." In *Human Limbs and Their Substitutes*, edited by P. E. Klopsteg and P. D. Wilson. New York: McGraw-Hill Book Company, 1954.

————— "The Transverse Tarsal Joint and its Control." *Clinical Orthopedics* 16 (1960): 41.

Elftman, H., and Manter, J. T. "The Axis of the Human Foot." *Science* 80 (1934): 484.

————— "The Evolution of the Human Foot, with Special Reference to the Joints." *Journal of Anatomy* 70 (1935): 56.

Evans, F. Gaynor, ed. *Biomechanical Studies of the Musculo-Skeletal System.* Springfield, Ill.: Charles C Thomas, Publisher, 1961.

———— *Stress and Strain in Bones.* Springfield, Ill.: Charles C. Thomas, Publisher, 1957.

Fenn, W. O. "The Mechanics of Standing on the Toes." *American Journal of Physical Medicine* 36 (1957): 153.

Fujikawa, K. "Functional Classification of Lower Limb Muscles." *Okajimas Folia Anatomica Japonica* 44 (1968): 383.

Gersten, J. W. "Mechanics of Body Elevation by Gastrocnemius-Soleus Contraction." *American Journal of Physical Medicine* 35 (1956): 12.

Gollnick, P. D. "Electrogoniometric Study of Walking on High Heels." *Research Quarterly* 35 (1964): 370.

Gollnick, P. D., and Karpovich, P. V. "Electrogoniometric Study of Locomotion and of Some Athletic Movements." *Research Quarterly* 35 (1964): 357.

Grant, C. Boileau. *An Atlas of Anatomy.* 5th ed. Baltimore: The Williams & Wilkins Company, 1962.

Gray, E. C., and Basmajian, J. V. "Electromyography and Cinematography of Leg and Foot ("Normal" and Flat) During Walking." *Anatomical Record* 161 (1968): 1.

Hall, Michael C. *The Locomotor System: Functional Anatomy.* Springfield, Ill.: Charles C. Thomas, Publisher, 1965.

———— "The Normal Movement at the Subtalar Joint." *Canadian Journal of Surgery* 2 (1959): 287.

———— "The Trabecular Patterns of the Normal Foot." *Clinical Orthopedics* 16 (1960): 15.

Harrison, T. J. "The Mechanics of the Ankle Joint." *Journal of Anatomy* 85 (1951): 432.

Haxton, H. A. "Absolute Muscle Force in the Ankle Flexors of Man." *Journal of Physiology* 103 (1944): 267.

Herman, R., and Bragin, S. J. "Function of the Gastrocnemius and Soleus Muscles." *Physical Therapy* 47 (1967): 105.

Hicks, J. H. "The Foot as a Support." *Acta Anatomica* 25 (1955): 34.

———— "The Function of the Plantar Aponeurosis." *Journal of Anatomy* 85 (1951): 414.

———— "The Mechanics of the Foot: I. The Joints." *Journal of Anatomy* 87 (1953): 345.

———— "The Mechanics of the Foot: II. The Plantar Aponeurosis and the Arch." *Journal of Anatomy* 88 (1954): 25.

———— "The Three Weight-Bearing Mechanisms of the Foot." In *Biomechanical Studies of the Musculo-Skeletal System,* edited by F. G. Evans. Springfield, Ill.: Charles C. Thomas, Publisher, 1961.

Houtz, S. J., and Fischer, F. J. "Function of Leg Muscles Acting on Foot as Modified by Body Movements." *Journal of Applied Physiology* 16 (1961): 597.

Houtz, S. J., and Walsh, F. P. "Electromyographic Analysis of the Function of the Muscles Acting on the Ankle During Weight Bearing with Special Reference to the Triceps Surae." *Journal of Bone and Joint Surgery* 41-A (1959): 1469.

Hubay, C. A. "Sesamoid Bones of the Hands and Feet." *American Journal of Roentgenology, Radium Therapy, and Nuclear Medicine* 61 (1949): 493.

Jones, F. W. *Structure and Function as Seen in the Foot.* 2d ed. London: Bailliere, Findall & Cox, Ltd., 1949.

Jones, R. L. "The Functional Significance of the Declination of the Axis of the Subtalar Joint." *Anatomical Record* 93 (1945): 151.

———— "The Human Foot. An Experimental Study of its Mechanics, and the Role of its Muscles and Ligaments in the Support of the Arch." *American Journal of Anatomy* 68 (1941): 1.

Joseph, J. *Man's Posture; Electromyographic Studies.* Springfield, Ill.: Charles C. Thomas, Publisher, 1960.

———— "Range of Movement of the Great Toe in Man." *Journal of Bone and Joint Surgery* 36-B (1954): 450.

Karpovich, P. V., and Wilklow, L. B. "Goniometric Study of the Human Foot in Standing and Walking." *Industrial Medicine and Surgery* 29 (1960): 338.

Klissouras, V., and Karpovich, P. V. "Electrogoniometric Study of Jumping Events." *Research Quarterly* 38 (1967): 41.

Lapidus, P. W. "Subtalar Joint, its Anatomy and Mechanics." *Bulletin, Hospital for Joint Diseases* 16 (1955): 179.

MacConaill, M. A. "The Postural Mechanism of the Human Foot." *Proceedings of the Royal Irish Academy* 50-B (1945): 159.

MacConaill, M. A., and Basmajian, J. V. *Muscles and Movement, A Basis for Human Kinesiology.* Baltimore: The Williams & Wilkins Company, 1969.

Mann, R., and Inman, V. T. "Phasic Activity of Intrinsic Muscles of the Foot." *Journal of Bone and Joint Surgery* 46-A (1964): 469.

Manter, J. T. "Distribution of Compression Forces in the Joints of the Human Foot." *Anatomical Record* 96 (1946): 313.

——— "Movements of the Subtalar and Transverse Tarsal Joints." *Anatomical Record* 80 (1941): 397.

Morton, Dudley J. *The Human Foot.* New York: Colombia University Press, 1935.

Quiring, Daniel P., and Warfel, John F. *The Extremities.* Philadelphia: Lea & Febiger, 1967.

Rarick, L., and Thompson, J. "Roentgenographic Measures of Leg Muscle Size and Ankle Extensor Strength." *Research Quarterly* 27 (1956): 321.

Ricci, B., and Karpovich, P. V. "Effect of Height of Heel Upon the Foot." *Research Quarterly* 35 (1964): 385.

Rogers, J. A. "The Leverage of the Foot." *Anatomical Record* 16 (1919): 317.

Royce, Joseph. *Surface Anatomy.* Philadelphia: F. A. Davis Company, 1965.

Rubin, G., and Witten, W. "The Talar-Tilt Angle and the Fibular Collateral Ligaments." *Journal of Bone and Joint Surgery* 42-A (1960): 311.

Sheffield, F. J.; Gersten, J. W.; and Mastellone, A. F. "Electromyographic Study of the Muscles of the Foot in Normal Walking." *American Journal of Physical Medicine* 35 (1956): 223.

Shepherd, E. "Tarsal Movements." *Journal of Bone and Joint Surgery* 33-B (1951): 258.

Smith, J. W. "Limitation of Movement at the Sub-talar and Calcaneo-cuboid Joints." *Journal of Anatomy* 84 (1950): 75.

——— "Muscular Control of the Arches of the Foot in Standing." *Journal of Anatomy* 88 (1954): 152.

——— "The Forces Operating at the Human Ankle Joint During Standing." *Journal of Anatomy* 91 (1957): 545.

Steindler, Arthur. *Kinesiology of the Human Body.* Springfield, Ill.: Charles C Thomas, Publisher, 1955.

Sutherland, D. H. "An Electromyographic Study of the Plantar Flexors of the Ankle in Normal Walking on the Level." *Journal of Bone and Joint Surgery* 48-A (1966): 66.

Viidik, A., and Magi, M. "The Motion Pattern of the Ankle Joint in Standing." In *Medicine and Sport*, vol. 2. Proceedings of the First International Seminar on Biomechanics, Zurich, August 1967. Basel, Switzerland: S. Karger AG, 1968.

Zitzlsperger, S. "The Mechanics of the Foot Based on the Concept of the Skeleton as a Statically Indetermined Space Framework." *Clinical Orthopedics* 16 (1961): 47.

15

Leg,
Knee Joint,
Thigh

THE LEG SEGMENT

The intermediate leg segment is between the foot and thigh segments. In the system of body segments, it is analogous to the smaller forearm segment of the upper limb in that it contains two bones. Unlike the forearm, the two bones of the leg differ markedly in size and must function in the weight-transmission line of the lower limb without appreciable movement occurring between them.

The Bones of the Leg

The two leg bones are situated parallel to each other—the tibia medially and the fibula laterally. Figure 15-1 illustrates anterior and posterior views of them in their natural positions, with the most important bony landmarks identified. The two bones differ greatly in size and shape, which would suggest differing functions. As would be expected, the tibia is a large, long bone since it is primarily responsible for transmitting body weight from the knee to the foot. Referring to Fig. 15-1, palpate the prominent tibial contours such as the *tuberosity*, *condyles*, *shaft*, *anterior crest*, and *malleolus*.

Figure 15–1. (*a*) Anterior and (*b*) posterior views of the leg segment bones.

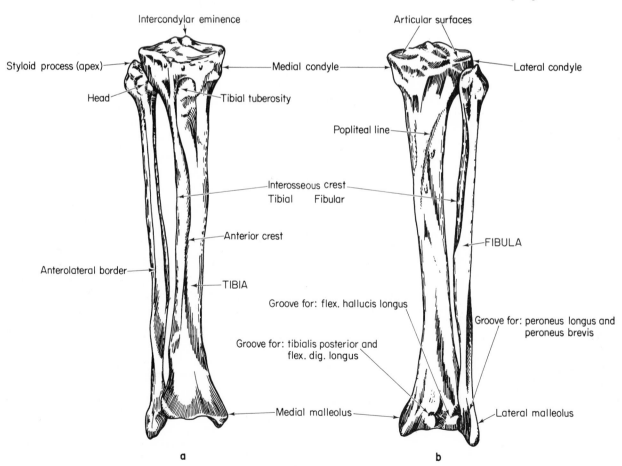

215

The fibula is very slender for its length, more so than any other long bone in the body. Situated as a lateral outrider to the tibia, it appears as though it might function as a splint or brace for the tibia. It has been accorded such a minor bracing function, but in conjunction with the *interosseous membrane*, it provides a major increase in suitable area for muscle attachments over that offered by the tibia alone. The fibula is not included in the structure of the knee joint and offers little aid to the tibia in direct weight bearing.

→ *Palpate the* head, styloid process, *lower* shaft, *and* malleolus *of the fibula.*

The Tibiofibular Joints of the Leg

It is obvious that the leg is not suitably constructed to be internally flexible. Its function in weight transmission generally sets the structural requirements for the junctions between its bones. The *distal tibiofibular* joint is of the amphiarthrodial type, containing neither hyaline cartilage nor a synovial membrane. As such, it exhibits tough ligamentous binding which is necessary for weight bearing (see Fig. 14-6). Little or no movement is allowed except for the resilient adjustments between malleolar ends of the tibia and fibula which are required to serve the ankle mortise. Close has identified some fibular rotation on the tibia as the leg moves on the stable foot.[1] The attainment of complete dorsiflexion of the ankle joint requires a small amount of inward rotation on the part of the tibia. In addition, the fibula makes small vertical adjustments on the lateral side of the talus during eversion and inversion.

The *middle tibiofibular* joint resides within the same class as its distal neighbor but is quite different in form. The shafts of the two bones do not articulate with each other in the usual joint sense but are linked structurally through an extensive *interosseous membrane* which runs between their *interosseous crests*. So situated, the membrane acts to divide the leg into anterior and posterior muscular compartments. The membrane's fibers course a lateralward and downward path from the tibia to the fibula and merge distally with the *interosseous* ligament of the distal tibiofibular joint (Fig. 15-2).

As a slender outrider to the tibia, the fibula experiences inordinate muscular stresses which tend to displace it distally. Because of the numerous muscles which attach to the fibula and adjacent membrane, the membrane's fiber orientation makes it capable of transferring some of the displacement stress from the fibula to the tibia. Thus the tibia, which is far more able to withstand these effects, can share the burden with the fibula.

The *proximal tibiofibular* joint is a diarthrodial joint of the plane or gliding type. It receives ligamentous reinforcement from *anterior* and *posterior* ligaments which cross the joint obliquely. They run lateralward and downward from the tibia to fibula in a manner similar to those of the

[1]J. R. Close, "Some Applications of the Functional Anatomy of the Ankle Joint," *Journal of Bone and Joint Surgery*, **33A** (1956), 761.

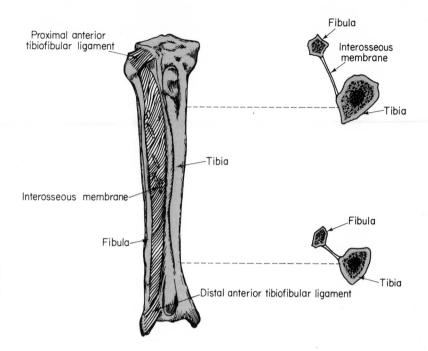

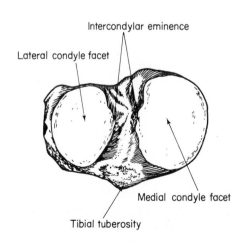

Figure 15–2. The interosseous membrane of the leg segment. Note the difference in its orientation between the leg bones in the proximal (closer to sagittal) and distal (closer to frontal) transverse sections.

distal joint as well as the fibers of the interosseous membrane. Although the joint is synovial, little or no motion is available except in association with the adjustments of the distal joint discussed above. In fact, this junction does not appear to have advanced functionally as far as its structural evolution might suggest.

THE KNEE JOINT

The position of the knee joint, approximately halfway between the hip and the foot, allows it to perform a most unique and important function. From an upright position, the mobility of the knee provides a mechanism for the precise adjustment of the height of the body above its supporting base. An example of its strategic position within the lower extremity identifies the knee joint as, perhaps, the single most important joint in the body. Certainly one could draw this conclusion from the vast amount of scientific study applied to its architecture and functions.

The proximal end of the tibia broadens considerably above its shaft to provide a plateau upon which the distal end of the femur may stand. Its smooth medial and lateral articular surfaces at the knee joint are of different shapes. Figure 15-3 indicates that both have longer anteroposterior dimensions than bilateral, with the lateral facet being more nearly circular in shape than the medial facet. The medial facet is mildly concave, while the lateral facet exhibits a mild bilateral concavity in conjunction with a mild anteroposterior convexity. Their borders are flattened to carry the *fibrocartilage menisci.*

Between the facets reside the attachment locations for the important, intra-articular ligaments and menisci. Figure 15-4 illustrates the knee junction from anterior and posterior views in which it is clear that the long

Figure 15–3. The superior surface of the tibia.

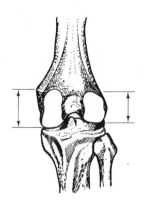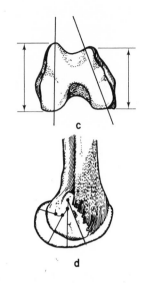

Figure 15–4. The knee joint architecture and special characteristics of the distal end of the femur. The mild indentation on the distal surface of the condyle in (*d*) is the point where the anterior border of the meniscus resides in complete extension of the knee joint.

axes of the two bones do not form a straight line. The condyles of the femur serve to enlarge the bony mass of the joint for weight bearing. Figure 15-4*d* illustrates the lateral femoral condyle, identifying the greater posterior protrusion with respect to its anterior surface. Careful inspection of the distal end of the femur shows that the medial and lateral femoral condyles differ in a number of respects which in large measure dictate the intricate movements which the joint may perform. Primary among these differences are (*1*) the lateral condyle has a greater anteroposterior dimension than the medial condyle (Fig. 15-4*c*); (*2*) the medial condyle has a larger polar dimension than its lateral counterpart (Fig. 15-4*b*); (*3*) the condyles are not parallel, the medial converging laterally from rear to front (Fig. 15-4*c*); and (*4*) the curvatures of their distal surfaces differ, the medial being somewhat more abruptly curved than the lateral condyle. In addition to differing from one another with respect to condyle curvature, neither is circular. The degree of curvature increases along the surface from the front to rear, as evidenced in Fig. 15-4*d* by the successively decreasing radii of curvature.

A large sesamoid bone, the *patella*, completes the bony structures of the knee joint. It is triangularly shaped with its apex pointing downward. Its anterior surface is gently curved to be somewhat convex in that direction. The posterior surface contains a divided articular area. Two facets, medial and lateral, articulate with the patellar surface of the femur. The patella offers anterior protection for the knee joint and, being embedded in the extensor tendon, is said to increase the tension angle for the knee extensors.

Joint Stability

Although both the tibia and femur demonstrate quite enlarged ends at the knee joint, because of the differing shapes of their condyles, only a small area of bony contact may occur. As a result, the knee joint must be considered to be unstable by bony arrangement through most of its movement range. Under these circumstances, the primary supporting structures must be the ligaments and muscles crossing the joint.

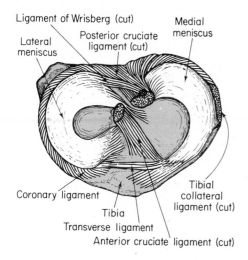

Figure 15–5. The intra-articular structures of the knee joint.

One means of improving the fit between the articulating bones is provided by the medial and lateral intra-articular fibrocartilages known as menisci. Figure 15-5 illustrates the minisci in positions atop the tibial condyles. Note that the lateral meniscus is more O-shaped than the medial, which is C-shaped to receive the longer *AP* articulating surface of the medial condyle. While the medial meniscus is less concave than the lateral, both are attached to the tibia around their edges by the *coronary* ligaments. In contrast to the medial meniscus, the lateral meniscus is not attached to the *fibular collateral* ligament of the knee and is, therefore, allowed a greater freedom of movement atop the lateral tibial condyle. The menisci are caused to migrate somewhat on their tibial plateaus in response to joint movements. In extension, they adjust forward, particularly the lateral meniscus, to provide a better fit for the less severely curved anterior condylar surfaces of the femur and to limit hyperextension owing to elastic opposition. Backward meniscus adjustment results in knee flexion.

The *tibial* and *fibular collateral* ligaments offer axial binding for the knee joint. Like the collaterals of the ankle joint, they are situated across the joint without inordinately hindering the swinging of the joint parts through a very wide range. The tibial collateral ligament (Fig. 15-6a) is of two parts: a deep posterior and a superficial anterior. The deeper reaches of the ligament adhere firmly to the medial meniscus. The ligament tends to limit abduction of the tibia on the femur and is taut in complete extension. The fibular collateral ligament is more in the shape of a cord and exhibits short- and long-fibered sections. It limits adduction of the tibia and is also taut in extension. The reason for the taut collaterals in complete extension may be found in Fig. 15-4*d*. As extension progresses, the distance between the axis of rotation and the joint surfaces increases to take up the slack in the ligaments. The anterior fibers of the ligaments are taut in complete flexion, where they may resist dislocation tendencies.

The *cruciate ligaments, anterior* and *posterior*, limit forward and backward displacements of the tibia on the femur, respectively. Their positions within the joint (Fig. 15-7) lead to the former becoming taut in extension and the latter in flexion. It is obvious that the cruciates as well as

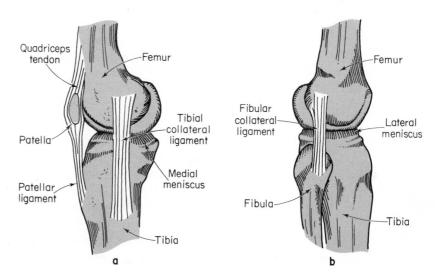

Figure 15–6. (*a*) Medial and (*b*) lateral views of the knee joint's collateral ligaments.

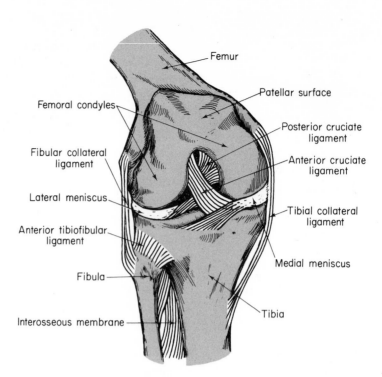

Femur

Femoral condyles

Patellar surface

Posterior cruciate ligament

Fibular collateral ligament

Anterior cruciate ligament

Lateral meniscus

Tibial collateral ligament

Anterior tibiofibular ligament

Medial meniscus

Fibula

Tibia

Interosseous membrane

Figure 15–7. An anterior view of the partially flexed knee joint where the cruciate ligaments are visible.

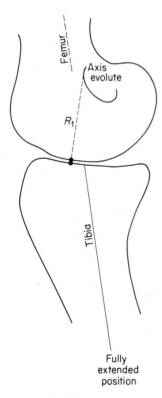

Femur

Axis evolute

R_1

Tibia

Fully extended position

Figure 15–8a

the other ligaments resist dislocation of the tibia from the femur. Because they cross within the joint, they tend to wind around each other somewhat in flexion and unwind in extension.

Anterior stabilization of the knee joint is primarily the responsibility of the *quadriceps femoris* muscle group and its associated connective structures. Spreading downward and away from the extensor tendon and lower ends of the muscle are the *medial* and *lateral retinacula*. Below the patella, the extensor tendon is named the *patellar* ligament. Contraction of the quadriceps musculature develops tension in these connective tissue structures to stabilize the joint and produce some upward migration of the patella in the course of knee extension.

→ *Stand on your right leg while allowing your left knee to hang extended without tensing the patellar ligament. Place your left thumb and index finger on the upper and lateral borders of the patella, respectively. Now forcefully contract the quadriceps and describe the movements of the patella in conjunction with the tendon. Draw a vector diagram of the forces operating as a result of this observation.*

Muscular stabilization is not limited to the anterior aspect of the joint. The fibular collateral ligament is aided by the actions of the *tensor fascia lata* and *gluteus maximus* through the *iliotibial tract*. Additional lateral stabilization is offered by the *biceps femoris* and *popliteus* tendons. The popliteus is approximately parallel to the posterior cruciate ligament in positions of knee flexion. Therefore it assists that ligament in resisting anterior displacement of the femur on the tibia in crouched or squatting positions. Medially, the *gracilis, sartorius*, and *semimembranosus* tendons assist the tibial collateral. Crossing the posterior aspect of the joint are the *hamstrings* group and the gastrocnemius to assist in reinforcing the posterior capsule wall. The ligament-muscle teamwork is fortunate because

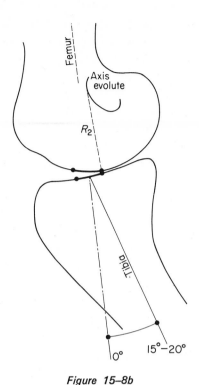

Figure 15–8b

the ligaments, by themselves, are not up to the task over extended periods of time without muscular assistance. The joint must be considered to be strong by ligamentous and muscular arrangement.

Joint Mobility

The knee is a condylar joint with two separated articular unions. As such, flexion and extension are available through about 135 deg. In addition, a certain percentage of normal knees can be hyperextended between 5 and 10 deg. Flexion is brought to a halt by soft tissue contact between the posterior aspects of the leg and thigh segments. These sagittally oriented movements are more complicated when one considers the internal action of the articulating surfaces. When this is done, it becomes clear that rolling, gliding, and transverse rotation movements are distinguishable also. In discussing these movements, the tibia will be employed as moving on a fixed femur. The student is encouraged, furthermore, to envision the reversed situation where the tibia is fixed in weight bearing with the femur moving on it.

The first combination of actions is best studied as viewed from the side with the joint in complete extension. Figure 15-8a illustrates the joint in that position, with the contact points marked on the two articular surfaces. The partially looped figure, an *evolute*, represents the path of the axis of rotation as successive points on the femoral condyle contact those

Figure 15–8. Internal action during 135° of knee flexion from complete extension.

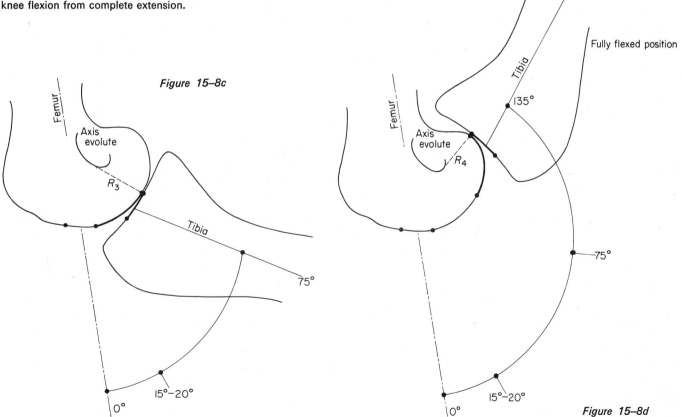

Figure 15–8c

Figure 15–8d

of the tibia as flexion progresses. Approximately the first 15–20 deg of flexion are involved with rolling action between the two articular surfaces (Fig. 15-8b). This conclusion is supported when the radii of curvature, R_1 and R_2, are seen to originate from approximately the same point on the evolute and are essentially of the same length. After 15 deg or so of flexion (Fig. 15-8c and d), the rolling motion between the surfaces smoothly disappears and is replaced by backward gliding. Consequently, the point of contact on the tibial surface remains almost constant from about 15 deg to nearly complete flexion. Some rolling action is said to begin once again during the last few degrees of flexion. Note that the concave articular surface of the tibia glides in the same direction as its roll. If the opposite were envisioned, the convex femoral surface moving on the concave tibia, the femur would be seen to glide forward, opposite to that of its roll.

With the knee fully extended, the anterior cruciate ligament is taut. In response to the force of the primary knee flexor muscles ($\mathbf{F}_T$ in Fig. 15-9a), two immediate actions occur. Because of the large stabilizing component, $\mathbf{F}_{sc}$, exhibited by the flexor muscles, the tibia is pressed upward against the femoral condyles. A similar upward force component is established through the anterior cruciate as the joint attempts to open anteriorly. The small rotatory component, $\mathbf{F}_{rc}$, is effective in producing the early rolling action between the two tightly held surfaces. This rolling action tends to open the joint space anterior to the condylar contact point, which increases the tension in the anterior cruciate. Since the femur is fixed, this tension may be shown as being directed upward and backward,

Figure 15–9. Force description of the beginning of knee joint flexion in (*a*) and extension in (*b*).

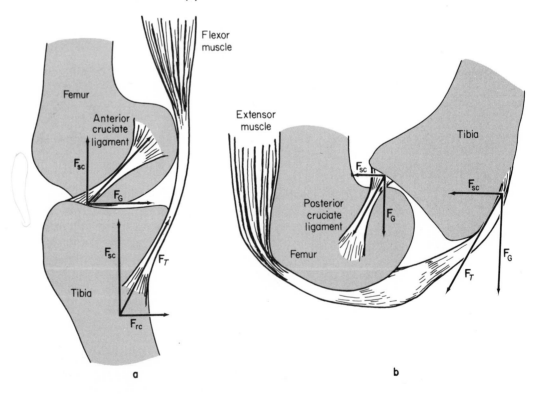

thus producing a significant gliding tendency force, F_G. When the tension in the ligament will allow no further rolling, gliding begins and is then continued as the rotatory component of the flexor muscles increases with the reduction of the joint angle.

Knee extension may be considered to be essentially the reverse of this process, where the posterior cruciate acts to initiate forward gliding of the tibia on the femur after limited forward rolling. The patellar ligament (Fig. 15-9b) is situated in complete flexion so that it nearly parallels the posterior cruciate. Its tension and that of the posterior cruciate pull the surfaces together to produce the early, limited rolling. Later, forward gliding of the tibia carries the tibia toward terminal extension. As this point is approached, increasing tension in the anterior cruciate, as well as the development of a formidable stabilizing force component by the powerful knee extensor muscles, reestablishes the rolling mode. The axis of rotation has moved forward somewhat and upward a great deal during the extension movement, which causes the collateral ligaments to become taut and bring the extension to a halt. In the position illustrated in the figure, gravity produces sufficient torque to carry out these extension movements.

→ *Describe these movements with the tibia fixed vertically under a rotating femur.*

During the final stages of knee extension, beginning slowly at 30 deg and developing maximally within the final 10 deg, a transverse rotation of the tibia occurs. It may be considered an outward rotation of the tibia relative to the fixed femur or an inward rotation of the femur on the fixed tibia. The lateral meniscus presents a shorter and deeper concavity for the lateral femoral condyle than is the case for the medial side. Consequently, as knee extension nears its completion, the shorter articular portion of the femur's lateral condyle tends to reach its terminal extension position before its medial counterpart. The resistance met produces a pivoting reaction which is similar to that experienced when one wheel of a two-wheeled grocery carriage or lawn spreader binds or is stopped by an obstruction. That is, the free wheel pivots around the fixed wheel, causing the entire device to veer sharply in the direction of the fixed wheel. Since the tibia glides and rolls in the same direction, the earlier lateral binding causes the medial condyle to swing outward.

The rotation amounts to about 12 deg about a polar axis located near the center of the lateral tibial condyle, as illustrated in Fig. 15-10. The outward rotation of the tibia in terminal extension is known as *locking* rotation, which brings the joint into the close-packed position. When the knee begins to flex from its locked position, the tibia must rotate inwardly, which is known as *unlocking* rotation. It does so rapidly in the early part of the rolling phase and appears to be actively motivated by the action of the popliteus muscle.

→ *Standing with your knees flexed slightly, examine the action of the knees as you extend and lock them. Is the locking rotation externally visible? If so, what surface changes indicate this action?*

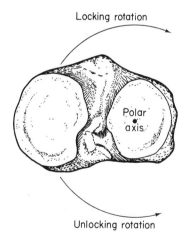

Locking rotation

Polar axis.

Unlocking rotation

Figure 15-10. Transverse rotations of the tibia in terminal extension (locking) and initial flexion (unlocking) movements of the knee joint.

When the knee joint is flexed, rotations of the leg on the thigh are available. As knee flexion progresses, the joint is released from its ligamentous tensions. With the knee flexed, 90 deg, inward and outward rotation excursions may reach 50 to 60 deg. They appear to occur primarily between the menisci and the tibia, with outward rotation from the midposition exceeding inward rotation in magnitude. When the joint is locked, such rotations are eliminated by the tight ligaments and maximal surface conformities between the femoral condyles and the underlying meniscus and tibial surfaces.

→ *Experiment with these rotations, both passively and actively, and referring to Muscle Chart 2, list the muscles which contribute to each rotation.*

The muscles crossing the knee joint are an interesting combination of one- and two-joint types. Both of the primary flexor and extensor groups of the knee include each type. The values of such an arrangement are found in the reduction of the number of muscles required to perform the recognized movements and the coordination of muscular action in pure synergy. For example, if individual, one-joint muscles were required for every movement at each joint of the body, considerable bulk would be added and a rather large increase in energy expenditure requirements would accrue. It appears that the large number of two-joint muscles of the thigh significantly reduces the energy demands in moving the massive lower limbs because of their abilities to efficiently transfer their contractile forces across more than one joint at a time. Hence, the hamstrings function to flex the knee as well as extend the hip; the *rectus femoris* extends the knee as well as flexes the hip; the *sartorius* and *gracilis* assist in flexing the knee and the hip.

In contrast to the advantages of two-joint muscles, at least one disadvantage is worthy of mention. That disadvantage is the rather large magnitudes of distensibility which are required if both joints crossed are carried to their extremes simultaneously. For example, the tension in the rectus femoris must be formidable in sprinting when the trailing extremity demonstrates considerable amounts of knee flexion and hip extension while undergoing contraction to bring that limb forward in the next stride (Fig. 15-11a). Conversely, the hamstrings must suffer the same sort of tension stress when a hurdler's leading limb demonstrates concurrent hip flexion and nearly complete knee extension (Fig. 15-11b). Considering the time intervals available in such running events for a muscle to relax and distend through such a wide range, it is not difficult to understand the number of muscle injuries which plague athletes, particularly the hamstrings. It is not difficult also to marvel at the remarkable abilities of two-joint muscles when they are properly trained through full ranges of motion.

With the forceful action of the *vasti* to produce knee extension concentrically and to control externally motivated knee flexion eccentrically, the thigh musculature is amply endowed to perform pure synergy functions. For example, if the hamstrings were called into action to assist in forceful hip extension, a significant amount of tension would be applied across the

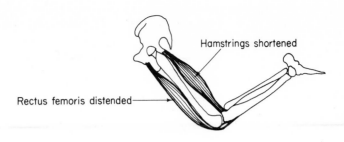

Hamstrings shortened

Rectus femoris distended

Trailing extremity
in
sprinting

a

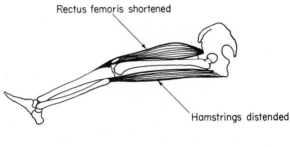

Rectus femoris shortened

Hamstrings distended

Leading extremity
in
hurdling

b

Figure 15–11. Two-joint muscle lengths of the (*a*) trailing limb in sprinting, and (*b*) the leading limb in hurdling.

knee joint as well to produce knee flexion. If the desired outcome excluded this concurrent knee flexion, the vasti could act as pure synergists to rule out or neutralize the knee flexion tendencies.

→ *Describe a possible pure synergy arrangement for the opposite of the situation just discussed, that is, hip flexion without concurrent knee extension. Upon examining the illustrations of the muscles of the quadriceps group in Muscle Chart 2, describe how the tendency for the patella to be displaced laterally may be counteracted muscularly by a medially directed force component, an example of component synergy.*

Muscle Chart 2: Leg, Knee Joint, Thigh

| Muscle | Attachments | | Innervation |
	Origin	Insertion	
I. The Knee Joint Muscles			
A. Anterior Group			
1. Rectus femoris		Base of the patella as the quadriceps tendon, to continue to the tibial tuberosity as the patellar ligament	Femoral nerve
a. Anterior head	a. Anterior inferior iliac spine		
b. Posterior head	b. Groove superior to the brim of the acetabulum		
2. Vastus intermedius	Lateral and anterior surfaces of the proximal two thirds of the shaft of the femur	Base of the patella as the quadriceps tendon, to continue to the tibial tuberosity as the patellar ligament	Femoral nerve
3. Vastus medialis	Distal half of the intertrochanteric line, medial lip of linea aspera, and proximal part of the supracondylar line of the femur	Base of the patella as the quadriceps tendon, to continue to the tibial tuberosity as the patellar ligament	Femoral nerve
4. Vastus lateralis	Anterior and inferior borders of the greater trochanter, lateral aspect of the gluteal tuberosity, and proximal part of the linea aspera of the femur	Base of the patella as the quadriceps tendon, to continue to the tibial tuberosity as the patellar ligament	Femoral nerve
5. Sartorius	Anterior superior iliac spine and the notch inferior to it	Proximal part of the medial surface of the shaft of the tibia	Femoral nerve
B. Posterior Group			
1. Biceps femoris		Lateral side of the head of the fibula, lateral condyle of the tibia	
a. Long head	a. Tuberosity of the ischium		a. Tibial nerve
b. Short head	b. Lateral lip of the linea aspera		b. Peroneal nerve
2. Semimembranosus	Tuberosity of the ischium	Medial aspect of the medial condyle of the tibia	Tibial nerve
3. Semitendinosus	Tuberosity of the ischium	Proximal part of the medial surface of the shaft of the tibia	Tibial nerve

Extension of the knee joint;
flexion of the hip joint; may
assist in forward tilt of the
pelvis

Extension of the knee joint

Extension of the knee joint

Extension of the knee joint

Assists in flexion of the knee
joint, inward rotation of the
leg, flexion and abduction of
the hip joint, and outward
rotation of the thigh; may
assist in forward tilt of the
pelvis

a. and b. Flexion of the knee
joint

a. Extension of the hip joint;
assists in adduction of the
hip joint from abducted hip
positions, outward rotation
of the thigh with the hip
joint in extended positions,
and backward tilt of the
pelvis

Flexion of the knee joint;
assists in inward rotation of
of the leg; extension of the
hip joint; assists in adduction of the hip joint against
resistance and inward rotation of the thigh

Flexion of the knee joint;
assists in inward rotation of
the leg; extension of the hip
joint; assists in adduction of
the hip joint against resistance and inward rotation of
the thigh

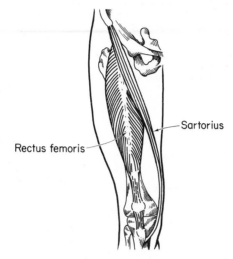

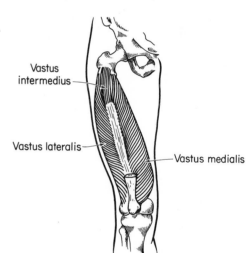

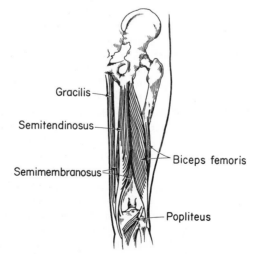

| Muscle | Attachments | | Innervation |
	Origin	Insertion	
4. Gastrocnemius	By two heads to the popliteal surface of the femur above the medial and lateral condyles	Forms the achilles tendon with the soleus to end on the middle part of the posterior surface of the calcaneus	Tibial nerve
5. Gracilis	Anterior margin of the inferior half of the symphysis pubis, inferior ramus of the pubis	Proximal part of the medial surface of shaft of the tibia	Obturator nerve
6. Popliteus	Lateral surface of the lateral condyle of the femur	Proximal one third of the posterior surface of the shaft of the tibia above the popliteal line	Tibial nerve

REFERENCES

Barnett, C. H. "Locking in the Knee Joint." *Journal of Anatomy* 87 (1953): 91.

Barnett, C. H.; Davies, D. V.; and MacConaill, M. A. *Synovial Joints: Their Structure and Mechanics.* Springfield, Ill.: Charles C. Thomas, Publisher, 1961.

Barnett, C. H., and Harding, D. "The Activity of Antagonist Muscles During Voluntary Movement." *Annals of Physical Medicine* 2 (1955): 290.

Barnett, C. H., and Richardson, A. "The Postural Function of the Popliteus Muscle." *Annals of Physical Medicine* 1 (1953): 177.

Basmajian, J. V. "Electromyography of Two-Joint Muscles." *Anatomical Record* 129 (1957): 371.

——— *Muscles Alive; Their Function Revealed by Electromyography.* 2d ed. Baltimore: The Williams & Wilkins Company, 1967.

Bierman, W., and Ralston, H. J. "Electromyographic Study During Passive and Active Flexion and Extension of the Knee of the Normal Human Subject." *Archives of Physical Medicine and Rehabilitation* 46 (1965): 71.

Brantigan, O. C., and Voshell, A. F. "The Mechanics of the Ligaments and Menisci of the Knee Joint." *Journal of Bone and Joint Surgery* 23 (1941): 44.

Brewerton, D. A. "The Function of the Vastus Medialis Muscle." *Annals of Physical Medicine* 2 (1955): 164.

Carpenter, A. "A Study of Angles in the Measurement of Leg Lift." *Research Quarterly* 9 (1938): 70.

Close, J. Robert. *Motor Function in the Lower Extremity.* Springfield, Ill.: Charles C. Thomas, Publisher, 1964.

Dempster, W. T. "The Range of Motion of Cadaver Joints: The Lower Limb." *University of Michigan Medical Bulletin* 23 (1956): 364.

Elftman, H. "Biomechanics of Muscle: With Particular Application to Studies of Gait." *Journal of Bone and Joint Surgery* 48-A (1966): 363.

——— "The Function of Muscles in Locomotion." *American Journal of Physiology* 125 (1939): 357.

——— "The Functional Structure of the Lower Limbs." In *Human Limbs and Their Substitutes*, edited by P. E. Klopsteg and P. D. Wilson. New York: McGraw-Hill Book Company, 1954.

Evans, F. Gaynor. *Stress and Strain in Bones.* Springfield, Ill.: Charles C. Thomas, Publisher, 1957.

Fenn, W. O. "Mechanical Energy Expenditure in Sprint Running as Measured by Moving Pictures." *American Journal of Physiology* 90 (1929): 343.

Fick, R. *Handbuch der Anatomie und Mechanik der Gelenke.* Jena, Germany: G. Fischer, 1910.

Actions

Assists in flexion of the knee joint; plantar flexion of the ankle joint

Assists in flexion of the knee joint and inward rotation of the leg; adduction of the hip joint, flexion of the hip joint from extended knee positions, and inward rotation of the thigh

Assists in flexion of the knee joint and inward rotation of the leg

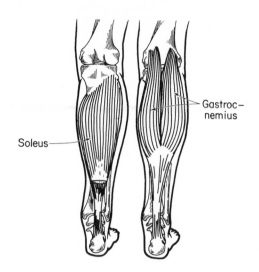

Fujikawa, K. "Functional Classification of Lower Limb Muscles." *Okajimas Folia Anatomica Japonica* 44 (1968): 383.

Haines, R. W. "A Note on the Action of the Cruciate Ligaments of the Knee Joint." *Journal of Anatomy* 75 (1941): 373.

Hall, Michael C. *The Locomotor System, Functional Anatomy.* Springfield, Ill.: Charles C. Thomas, Publisher, 1965.

Hall, W. L., and Klein, K. K. "The Man, the Knee and the Ligaments." *Medicina Dello Sport* 1 (1961): 500.

Hallen, L. G., and Lindahl, O. "The Lateral Stability of the Knee Joint." *Acta Orthopaedica Scandinavica* 36 (1965): 179.

—— "Muscle Function in Knee Extension." *Acta Orthopaedica Scandinavica* 38 (1967): 434.

—— "The 'Screw-Home' Movement in the Knee Joint." *Acta Orthopaedica Scandinavica* 37 (1966): 97.

Haxton, H. A. "A Comparison of the Action of Extension of the Knee and Elbow Joints in Man." *Anatomical Record* 93 (1945): 279.

Houtz, S. J., and Fischer, F. J. "An Analysis of Muscle Action and Joint Excursion During Exercise on a Stationary Bicycle." *Journal of Bone and Joint Surgery* 41-A (1959): 123.

Houtz, S. J.; Lebow, M. J.; and Beyer, F. R. "The Influence of Posture on the Strength of the Knee Flexor and Extensor Muscles." *Journal of Applied Physiology* 11 (1957): 475.

Jonsson, B., and Steen, B. "Function of the Gracilis Muscle." *Acta Morphologica Neerlando-Scandinavica* 6 (1966): 325.

Joseph, J., and Nightengale, A. "Electromyography of Muscles of Posture: Leg Muscles in Males." *Journal of Physiology* 117 (1952): 484.

—— "Electromyography of Muscles of Posture: Leg and Thigh Muscles in Women, Including the Effects of High Heels." *Journal of Physiology* 132 (1956): 465.

Kaplan, E. B. "Factors Responsible for the Stability of the Knee Joint." *Bulletin of the Hospital for Joint Diseases* 18 (1957): 51.

—— "The Iliotibial Tract." *Journal of Bone and Joint Surgery* 40-A (1958): 817.

—— "Some Aspects of Functional Anatomy of the Human Knee Joint." *Clinical Orthopedics* 23 (1962): 18.

Kendall, Henry O., and Kendall, Florence P. *Muscles, Testing and Function.* Baltimore: The Williams & Wilkins Company, 1949.

King, O. "The Function of Semilunar Cartilages." *Journal of Bone and Joint Surgery* 18 (1936): 1069.

Klein, K. K. "The Deep Squat Exercise as Utilized in Weight Training for Athletics and its Effect on the Ligaments of the Knee." *Journal of the Asso-*

ciation of Physical and Mental Rehabilitation 15 (1961): 6.

───── "The Knee and the Ligaments." *Journal of Bone and Joint Surgery* 44-A (1962): 1191.

Klissouras, V., and Karpovich, P. V. "Electrogoniometric Study of Jumping Events." *Research Quarterly* 38 (1967): 41.

Last, R. J. "The Popliteus Muscle and the Lateral Meniscus; with a Note on the Attachment of the Medial Meniscus." *Journal of Bone and Joint Surgery* 32-B (1950): 93.

Levens, A. S.; Berkeley, C. E.; and Inman, V. T. "Transverse Rotation of the Segments of the Lower Extremity in Locomotion." *Journal of Bone and Joint Surgery* 30-A (1948): 859.

Lombard, W. P., and Abbott, F. M. "The Mechanical Effects Produced by the Contraction of Individual Muscles of the Thigh of the Frog." *American Journal of Physiology* 20 (1907): 1.

MacConaill, M. A. "The Movements of Bones and Joints: IV. The Mechanical Structure of Articulating Cartilage." *Journal of Bone and Joint Surgery* 33-B (1951): 251.

Mathur, P. D.; McDonald, J. R.; and Ghormley, R. K. "A Study of the Tensile Strength of the Menisci of the Knee." *Journal of Bone and Joint Surgery* 31-A (1949): 650.

Merrifield, H. H. "An Electromyographic Study of the Gluteus Maximus, the Vastus Lateralis and the Tensor Fasciae Latae." *Dissertation Abstracts* 21 (1961): 1833.

Miwa, N.; Tanaka, T.; and Matoba, M. "Electromyography in Kinesiologic Evaluations: Subjects on Two Joint Muscle and the Relation Between the Muscular Tension and Electromyogram." *Journal of the Japanese Orthopaedic Association* 36 (1963): 1025.

Morton, Dudley J., and Fuller, Dudley D. *Human Locomotion and Body Form.* Baltimore: The Williams & Wilkins Company, 1952.

Pocock, G. S. "Electromyographic Study of the Quadriceps During Resistive Exercise." *Physical Therapy* 43 (1963): 427.

Prost, J. H. "Bipedalism of Man and Gibbon Compared Using Estimates of Joint Motion." *American Journal of Physical Anthropology* 26 (1967): 135.

Quiring, Daniel P., and Warfel, John F. *The Extremities.* Philadelphia: Lea & Febiger, 1967.

Saaf, J. "Effects of Exercise on Adult Articular Cartilage." *Acta Orthopaedica Scandinavica* 7 Suppl. (1950): 7.

Shinno, N. "Statico-Dynamic Analysis of Movement of the Knee. V. Analysis of Knee Function in Ascending and Descending Stairs." *Tokushima Journal of Experimental Medicine* 15 (1968): 53.

Shute, C. C. D. "The Geometry and Kinematics of the Knee Joint." *Journal of Anatomy* 90 (1956): 586.

Sinning, W. E., and Forsyth, H. L. "Lower-Limb Actions While Running at Different Velocities." *Medicine and Science in Sports* 2 (1970): 28.

Smith, J. W. "The Act of Standing." *Acta Orthopaedica Scandinavica* 23 (1953): 159.

───── "Observations on the Postural Mechanism of the Human Knee Joint." *Journal of Anatomy* 90 (1956): 236.

Sparger, Celia. *Anatomy and Ballet: A Handbook for Teachers of Ballet.* London: Adam & Charles Black, Ltd., 1965.

Steindler, A. "Locomotor Mechanics and Operation." *American Society of Mechanical Engineers Transactions* 67 (1945): 167.

Walmsley, R. "The Development of the Patella." *Journal of Anatomy* 74 (1940): 360.

───── "The Vertical Axes of the Femur." *Journal of Anatomy* 67 (1933): 284.

Williams, M., and Lissner, H. R. "Biomechanical Analysis of Knee Function." *Physical Therapy Review* 43 (1963): 93.

───── *Biomechanics of Human Motion.* Philadelphia: W. B. Saunders Company, 1962.

16

Thigh, Hip Joint, Pelvic Girdle

THE THIGH SEGMENT

The thigh segment joins the leg and trunk segments. Its shape, which is primarily the result of two-joint muscles, is that of a truncated cone which increases its diameter as the hip is approached from below. It is the site of some of the strongest muscles in the entire body. Since the thigh resides between two very mobile joints of the lower limb, it is involved in postural maintenance as well as body locomotion.

The Thigh Bone

This segment contains a single bone, the *femur*, which is both bowed and twisted in the adult. It is the longest and strongest bone of the human body. Figure 16-1 illustrates anterior and posterior views of the femur with the important bony landmarks designated.

Near its distal end are found the *medial* and *lateral epicondyles*, the latter being the more diminutive of the two. The anterior surface of the shaft is smooth and rounded, while its posterior surface is marked by several prominent ridges which identify demarcation points between muscle attachments and add to the strength of the bone. The femur's shaft

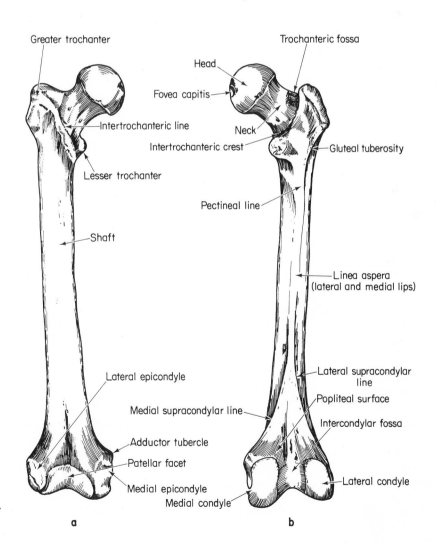

Figure 16–1. (*a*) Anterior and (*b*) posterior views of the femur.

a   b

231

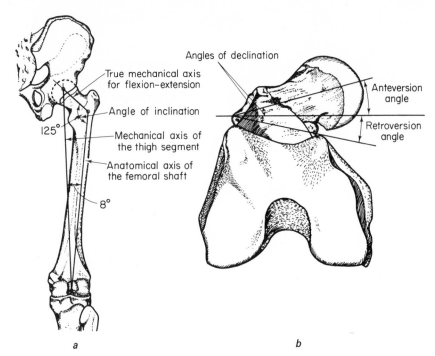

Figure 16–2. (a) Femoral relationships within the thigh segment in a vertical position. (b) Declination angle relationships of the femur as viewed from below the condyles.

a

b

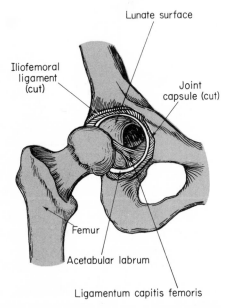

Figure 16–3. The disarticulated hip joint.

is bowed anteriorly to a marked degree and, in most cases, bowed laterally to a lesser degree.

The *gluteal tuberosity*, a continuation of the *lateral lip* of the *linea aspera*, is quite. rough, as befits the attachment point for a muscle as powerful as the *gluteus maximus*. Above the medial lip is the *pectineal line*, which merges with the base of the *lesser trochanter* proximally. Between the *lesser* and *greater trochanters* is an elevated, curved bony collar called the *intertrochanteric crest*. Its counterpart on the anterior surface is the *intertrochanteric line*, which is not nearly so prominent. Leading to the rounded, hemispherical, femoral *head* is the *neck*, which forms an angled junction with the shaft, which averages about 125 deg.

As made clear in Chapter 15, the thigh segment is not situated vertically under the trunk in standing, but angles from medial to lateral along its length as it courses upward from the knee. With the femur's sagittal and frontal bowing and offset shaft, it is subject to considerable bending stresses in weight-bearing positions. As the femoral heads are bilaterally separated by a rather large distance, symmetrical support of the trunk from below is distributed between the two lower extremities. When the feet are together in standing, the mechanical axis of the thigh segment slants slightly outward also from knee to hip. The mechanical axis then passes nearly vertically from the center of the knee to the center of the femoral head.

The true mechanical axis of hip flexion-extension and hyperextension runs from the femoral head laterally and downward through the neck of the femur (Fig. 16-2a). Thus the angle formed by the intersection of the true axis of the head and neck and the anatomical axis of the femoral shaft is designated the *angle of inclination*. When the angle of inclination markedly exceeds 125 deg, the condition is named *coxa valga*. When it is markedly less than 125 deg it is termed *coxa vara*.

The shaft of the femur is twisted so that the head and neck axis protrudes forward somewhat from the shaft axis. Figure 16-2b illustrates this phenomenon from below the femoral condyles, viewing upward along the femoral shaft. This angulation is called the *angle of declination* and may vary widely from person to person. It averages about 12 deg normally and is termed the *anteversion* angle. If the anteversion angle is considered to be a positive angle, negative angles, called *retroversion* angles, show the head and neck of the femur to protrude backward from the femoral shaft.

THE HIP JOINT

The head of the femur articulates with the acetabulum of the hip bone to form the hip joint. This union is of the ball and socket type, with the femoral head fitting well into the acetabular socket. The plane of the rim of the acetabulum, when viewed from the anterior, faces forward, downward, and outward. Its articular surface does not cover the entire socket but is limited to most of its circular margin to form the horseshoe-like *lunate surface* (Fig. 16-3).

Articular cartilage covers the entire head of the femur except for the *fovea capitis*, and when centrally seated in the acetabulum, it extends beyond the acetabular rim in all directions. Thus a union is formed which is suited for mobility as well as stability. The structural nature of the joint in its position near the body's center dictates that its mobility functions are subordinate to its stability functions.

Joint Stability

The depth of the acetabulum is increased by the fibrocartilage, *acetabular labrum* (Fig. 16-3), which encircles its rim. It then acts as a collar for the articular margins of the femoral head, which improves the fit between the two articular surfaces of the joint and tends to hold the head firmly in its socket. Within the joint, a condition of negative pressure or suction is established when the femoral ball is forceably pulled away from its seat. The reduced pressure within the enlarged capsular volume then allows outside atmospheric pressure to apply effective inward-directed holding forces. Therefore the already strong bony arrangement of the hip joint is augmented by these secondary mechanisms.

The ligamentous support of the joint and its capsule is formidable. The strongest of these hip joint ligaments, and for that matter, of the entire body, is the *iliofemoral* ligament. As can be seen in Fig. 16-4a, it crosses anteriorly to the joint from the *anterior inferior iliac spine* to attach along the entire length of the intertrochanteric line of the femur. It is formed in the shape of an inverted Y; hence it is often called the Y ligament. Its position with respect to the joint marks it as an anterior stabilizer which limits hyperextension. Since hyperextension of the hip may be produced by the backward rotation of the pelvis on the femoral heads, the iliofemoral ligament is involved in the maintenance of trunk-to-thigh alignment in standing. Consequently, it is sometimes termed a postural ligament. The combination of fiber directions across the joint leads to limitation of

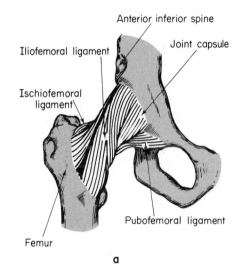

Anterior inferior spine

Iliofemoral ligament

Joint capsule

Ischiofemoral ligament

Pubofemoral ligament

Femur

a

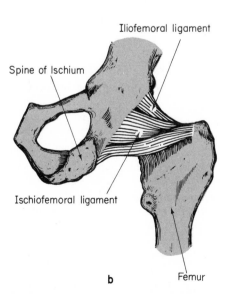

Iliofemoral ligament

Spine of Ischium

Ischiofemoral ligament

Femur

b

Figure 16–4. (*a*) Anterior and (*b*) posterior views of the hip joint ligaments.

outward rotation in flexion and inward rotation in extension and hyper-extension.

The *ischiofemoral* ligament crosses the posterior aspect of the joint to function as a posterior stabilizer. As its fibers course laterally (Fig. 16-4b), they twist upward and forward over the joint. It limits hyperextension owing to the wrap-around course across the joint. In addition, inward rotation in extension is checked and abduction is limited in common with the *pubofemoral* ligament. The pubofemoral ligament crosses the joint anteriorly and inferiorly and is said to limit outward rotation in flexion.

Muscular stabilization adds to the strength of the hip joint. The hamstrings and the gluteus maximus may act as posterior stabilizers when imbalances cause the pelvis to roll excessively on the femoral heads. The *iliopsoas* group acts as an anterior stabilizer to check excessive tendencies for the pelvis to roll backward on the femoral heads. Its downward-pulling action is essentially parallel with gravity, which it assists in pressing the joint surfaces together to further the stability of the joint.

When upright standing is supported by both lower limbs, little lateral or medial stabilization is required. However, when the standing weight is borne on one limb, tendencies to fall to either side must be overcome. The *gluteus medius* and *minimus* act as lateral stabilizers to resist the tilting of the pelvis toward the unsupported side. This muscular action is not sufficient to maintain whole-body balance and is accompanied by a shifting of the weight of the body over the supporting limb as the other limb is pressed away and lifted. The medial stabilizers, the three *adductors*, *pectineus*, and *gracilis*, act to hold the thigh under the pelvis or to tilt the unsupported side of the pelvis downward when lateral tilting past the point of balance over the supporting limb is excessive.

→ *Stand with your feet placed comfortably and palpate the lateral stabilizers below the iliac crests. Now gently sway from side to side so that the body weight is shifted from one limb to the other. Do you notice any muscular activity?*

Joint Mobility

The hip joint allows motion of a wide variety. The axis of rotation for flexion-extension and hyperextension courses through the femoral head and neck, as noted earlier. The head of the femur then pivots in the acetabulum in concert with the swinging of the shaft.

→ *Take an ordinary paper clip and straighten its two outer curves, leaving the inner curve intact. Adjust the straightened section to form an angle of approximately 125 deg with the curved inner section, as shown in Fig. 16-5. The straightened section may then represent the shaft of the femur with the head and neck represented by the shorter, curved section. Now place the tip of the curved section into the depression formed between the thumb, index, and middle fingers. Swing the "shaft" forward and backward to simulate flexion and extension and examine the rotation of the "head" between the finger tips. Simulate the other movements available at the normal hip joint and pay particular attention to thigh inward and outward rotations and the multiple gyrations involved in circumduction.*

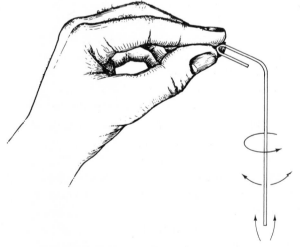

Figure 16–5. The use of a paperclip in simulating femoral movements at the hip joint.

Flexion from the anatomical position can be carried through approximately 120 deg if the knee joint is flexed. This movement of the thigh is brought to a halt as the result of contact with the abdomen and contractile insufficiency. With the knee extended, the hamstrings generally limit the flexion range to about 90 deg. After returning from flexion, about 15 deg of hyperextension may be produced. The magnitude of hyperextension is often thought to be considerably greater because of the trunk segment's ability to hyperextend. As noted earlier, this movement is restricted by the iliofemoral ligament. While these movements appear to be simple, they are not. For example, hip flexion is generally accompanied by some abduction and outward rotation, while extension is generally accompanied by inward rotation and adduction.[1]

When abduction is produced singly, it may be carried through about 45 deg but may vary considerably from person to person. The return from abduction is checked by the other limb. If the hip is flexed slightly to allow the adducting limb to bypass the obstruction, about 30 deg of additional adduction is possible.

→ *Using the redesigned paper clip as before, demonstrate these movements.*

As can be seen, the head and neck axis is tilted upward and downward, respectively, for abduction and adduction. The range of transverse abduction varies considerably between individuals and particularly between the sexes, from less than 45 deg to as high as 60 deg.

→ *Do men or women show the greater mobility, and can you offer any structural reasons for such a difference?*

Rotations vary with the degree of hip flexion, being about 45 deg for outward and inward when the hip is flexed, 90 deg. When the hip is in complete extension, outward rotation generally exceeds inward rotation, being about 45 and 35 deg, respectively.

→ *Describe the sweeping movements of the head and neck axis of the femur during these rotations. Also describe these movements as compared with those of the femoral shaft during circumductions. Carefully describe their respective cone tracings in terms of how they are oriented to one another. If you can, observe these movements on an articulated skeleton as well.*

As noted in Chapter 15, a number of muscles serve both the hip and knee joints. Muscle Chart 3 details the motivating functions of the muscles, and it will be noted that multiple actions are abundant. For instance, the iliopsoas group is both a hip flexor and thigh outward rotator; the gluteus maximus is an extensor and outward rotator; the adductors motivate inward rotation as well as the movement represented by their name. The action of the two-joint muscles bear some additional consideration at this point.

[1]Michael C. Hall, *The Locomotor System—Functional Anatomy* (Springfield, Ill.: Charles C Thomas, Publisher, 1965), p. 314.

Of particular importance is the muscle tension phenomenon known as *tendinous action*. As noted earlier, when a two-joint muscle contracts, tension is disposed to producing movements at both joints unless halted by a synergist or some obstructing mechanism. The hamstrings group presents an example in which great tension is developed when the hip is flexed maximally while the knee is fully extended. In fact, the more sedentary habits of adults appear to render this long muscle group less able to extend through wide ranges of concurrent hip flexion and knee extension. As a result, the hamstrings may act as if it were a tendon, in which case it transfers tension forces passively rather than by active contraction.

> → *To provide an example of hamstrings tendinous action, sit on a table near its edge so that one limb is extended along its surface while the other is placed on the floor for lateral support. When sitting in this position with the hip flexed to about 90 deg, some people will begin to feel the effects of the taut hamstrings, particularly across the back of the knee. As you proceed with hip flexion, the hamstrings gradually become less and less able to continue to distend. This is evident in the rise of discomfort experienced.*

Muscle Chart 3:   Thigh, Hip Joint, Pelvic Girdle

| Muscle | Attachments | | Innervation |
	Origin	Insertion	
I. The Hip Joint Muscles			
A. The Anterior Group			
1. Iliopsoas			
a. Iliacus	a. Superior two thirds of the iliac fossa and the ala of the sacrum	a. Lateral side of the tendon of the psoas major to end at the lesser trochanter of the femur	a. Femoral nerve
b. Psoas major	b. Transverse processes of all the lumbar vertebrae, sides of the bodies, and intervertebral disks of the last thoracic and all of the lumbar vertebrae	b. Lesser trochanter of the femur	b. A branch from the lumbar plexus
2. Rectus femoris			
a. Anterior head	a. Anterior inferior iliac spine	Base of the patella as the quadriceps tendon, to continue to the tibial tuberosity as the patellar ligament	Femoral nerve
b. Posterior head	b. Groove superior to the brim of the acetabulum		
3. Sartorius	Anterior superior iliac spine and the notch inferior to it	Proximal part of the medial surface of the shaft of the tibia	Femoral nerve

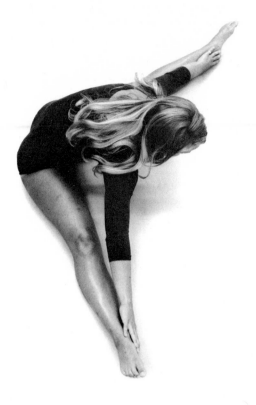

The muscle is, essentially, acting as a tendon to transfer hip flexion forces to the knee joint passively. Depending on one's normal flexibility limits, the knee joint will be unlocked and forced upward from the table top into flexion, thus relieving the tension stresses in the hamstrings.

→ *Try the same maneuver with varying positions of the ankle joint and attempt to describe the occurrences.*

Similar actions occur in exercises involving bending over to touch the floor while keeping the knees extended. The tendency toward knee flexion is a natural consequence which is gradually overcome as flexibility ranges are increased through training programs and should not be forced inordinately. That tendinous action need not cause undue concern is evident in the marked flexibilities demonstrated by gymnasts, hurdlers, and dancers, an example of which is provided in Fig. 16-6. Note that within this extreme position, the ankles may be plantar-flexed maximally as well.

Figure 16–6. Photo of a gymnast demonstrating an extreme example of hip joint and lower extremity flexibility.

Actions

a. Flexion of the hip joint; outward rotation of the thigh; assists in forward tilt of the pelvis

b. Flexion of the hip joint; outward rotation of the thigh; deepens the lumbar lordosis; assists in forward tilt of the pelvis

Flexion of the hip joint; may assist in forward tilt of the pelvis; extension of the knee joint

Assists in flexion and abduction of the hip joint, outward rotation of the thigh; may assist in forward tilt of the pelvis; assists in flexion of the knee joint and inward rotation of the leg

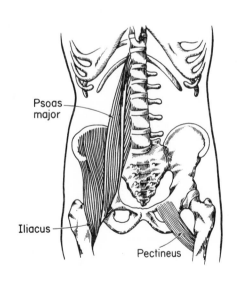

Psoas major

Iliacus

Pectineus

(continued)

Muscle	Attachments		Innervation
	Origin	Insertion	
B. The Medial Group			
1. Adductor brevis	Outer surface of the inferior ramus of the pubis	Proximal half of the linea aspera of the femur	Obturator nerve
2. Adductor longus	Anterior part of the pubis below the crest	Medial lip of the middle one third of the linea aspera of the femur	Obturator nerve
3. Adductor magnus	Small section of the inferior ramus of the pubis, inferior ramus of the ischium, inferior part of the ischial tuberosity	Complete length of the linea aspera, medial supracondylar line, and the adductor tubercle of the femur	Obturator and sciatic nerves
4. Gracilis	Anterior margin of the inferior half of the symphysis pubis, inferior ramus of the pubis	Proximal part of the medial surface of the shaft of the tibia	Obturator nerve
5. Pectineus	Pectineal line of the pubis	Pectineal line of the femur	Femoral nerve
C. The Lateral Group			
1. Gluteus medius	Outer surface of the ilium between the posterior and anterior gluteal lines	Lateral surface of the greater trochanter of the femur	Superior gluteal nerve
2. Gluteus minimus	Outer surface of the ilium between the anterior and inferior gluteal lines	The anterior border of the greater trochanter of the femur	Superior gluteal nerve
3. Tensor fasciae latae	Anterior part of the iliac crest and outer part of the anterior superior iliac spine	Iliotibial tract of the fascia lata of the thigh	Superior gluteal nerve

Adduction of the hip joint; transverse adduction of the hip joint from flexed hip positions; assists in flexion of the hip joint and inward rotation of the thigh

Adduction of the hip joint; transverse adduction of the hip joint from flexed hip positions; assists in flexion of the hip joint and inward rotation of the thigh

Assists in adduction of the hip joint against resistance, transverse adduction of the hip joint from flexed hip positions, flexion of the hip joint, and inward rotation of the thigh; lower portion may assist in extension of the hip joint from flexed hip positions

Assists in adduction of the hip joint, flexion of the hip joint with the knee joint extended; flexion of the knee joint, and inward rotation of the leg

Adduction of the hip joint; assists in flexion of the hip joint, transverse adduction of the hip joint from flexed hip positions, and inward rotation of the thigh

Abduction of the hip joint; assists in transverse abduction of the hip joint from flexed hip positions, and inward rotation of the thigh; stabilizes the pelvis against lateral tilt to the opposite side in single-limb standing

Abduction of the hip joint; assists in transverse abduction of the hip joint from flexed hip positions, and inward rotation of the thigh; stabilizes the pelvis against lateral tilt to the opposite side in single-limb standing

Assists in flexion and adduction of the hip joint and inward rotation of the thigh; may assist in extension of the knee joint and outward rotation of the leg through the iliotibial tract

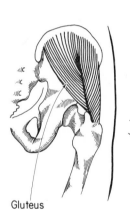

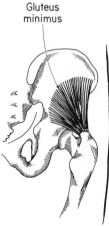

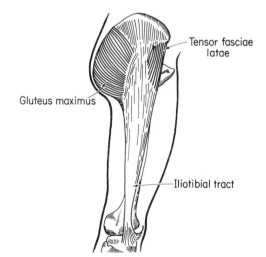

(*continued*)

| Muscle | Attachments | | Innervation |
	Origin	Insertion	
D. The Posterior Group			
1. Gluteus maximus	Superior gluteal line and crest of the ilium, the posterior surface of the lower sacrum, and the lateral border of the coccyx	Iliotibial tract and the gluteal tuberosity of the femur	Inferior gluteal nerve
2. Biceps femoris		Lateral side of the head of the fibula, lateral condyle of the tibia	
a. Long head	a. Tuberosity of the ischium		a. Tibial nerve
b. Short head	b. Lateral lip of the linea aspera		b. Peroneal nerve
3. Semimembranosus	Tuberosity of the ischium	Medial aspect of the medial condyle of the tibia	Tibial nerve
4. Semitendinosus	Tuberosity of the ischium	Proximal part of the medial surface of the shaft of the tibia	Tibial nerve
5. Quadratus femoris	Ischial tuberosity	Vertically centered on and below the intertrochanteric crest of the femur	Nerve to the quadratus femoris
6. Obturator externus	External surfaces of the rami of the pubis, ramus of the ischium, and the obturator membrane	Trochanteric fossa of the femur	Obturator nerve
7. Obturator internus	Ilium below the auricular surfaces, internal surface of the superior and inferior rami of the pubis, ramus of the ischium, and the obturator membrane	Medial surface of the greater trochanter of the femur	Nerve to the obturator internus
8. Gemellus inferior	Ischial tuberosity	Joins the tendon of the obturator internus	Nerve to the quadratus femoris

Extension of the hip joint against resistance; outward rotation of the thigh; upper fibers assist in transverse abduction of the hip joint against resistance in flexed hip positions; assists in backward tilt of the pelvis; may act to brace the lateral aspect of the knee joint through the iliotibial tract

a. Extension of the hip joint; assists in adduction of the hip joint from abducted hip positions, outward rotation of the thigh in extended hip positions, and backward tilt of the pelvis

a. and b. Flexion of the knee joint; may assist in outward rotation of the leg

Extension of the hip joint; assists in adduction of the hip joint against resistance, and inward rotation of the thigh; flexion of the knee joint; assists in inward rotation of the leg and in backward tilt of the pelvis

Extension of the hip joint; assists in adduction of the hip joint against resistance, and inward rotation of the thigh; flexion of the knee joint; assists in inward rotation of the leg and in backward tilt of the pelvis

Outward rotation of the thigh; may assist in adduction of the hip joint and extension and transverse abduction of the hip joint from flexed hip positions

Outward rotation of the thigh; may assist in adduction of the hip joint and extension and transverse abduction of the hip joint from flexed hip positions

Outward rotation of the thigh; may assist in extension and transverse abduction of the hip joint from flexed hip positions

Augments the actions of the obturator internus

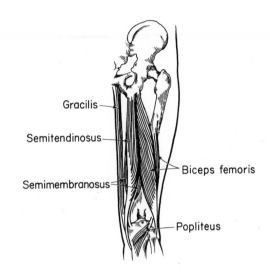

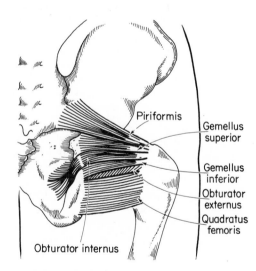

| | Attachments | | |
Muscle	Origin	Insertion	Innervation
9. Gemellus superior	Outer surface of the spine of the ischium	Joins the tendon of the obturator internus	Nerve to the obturator internus
10. Piriformis	Anterior surface of the sacrum, upper border of the greater sciatic notch, and the sacrotuberous ligament	Superior border of the greater trochanter of the femur	Nerve to the piriformis

REFERENCES

Ahlback, S., and Lindahl, O. "Sagittal Mobility of the Hip Joint." *Acta Orthopaedica Scandinavica* 34 (1964): 310.

Barnett, C. H.; Davies, D. V.; and MacConaill, M. A. *Synovial Joints, Their Structure and Mechanics.* Springfield, Ill.: Charles C. Thomas, Publisher, 1961.

Basmajian, J. V. "Electromyography of Postural Muscles." In *Biomechanical Studies of the Musculo-Skeletal System,* edited by F. G. Evans. Springfield, Ill.: Charles C Thomas, Publisher, 1961.

——— "Electromyography of Two-Joint Muscles." *Anatomical Record* 129 (1957): 371.

——— "Man's Posture." *Archives of Physical Medicine and Rehabilitation* 46 (1965): 26.

——— *Muscles Alive; Their Function Revealed by Electromyography.* 2d ed. Baltimore: The Williams & Wilkins Company, 1967.

Bassett, David L. *A Stereoscopic Atlas of Human Anatomy.* Portland, Ore.: Sawyer's Inc., 1955.

Boscoe, A. R. "The Range of Active Abduction and Lateral Rotation at the Hip Joint of Men." *Journal of Bone and Joint Surgery* 14 (1932): 325.

Close, J. Robert. *Motor Function in the Lower Extremity.* Springfield, Ill.: Charles C. Thomas, Publisher, 1964.

Crane, L. "Femoral Torsion and its Relation to Toeing-in and Toeing-out." *Journal of Bone and Joint Surgery* 41-A (1959): 421.

Cureton, T. K. "Mechanics and Kinesiology of the Crawl Flutter Kick." *Research Quarterly* 1 (1930): 87.

Dempster, W. T. "The Range of Motion of Cadaver Joints: The Lower Limb." *University of Michigan Medical Bulletin* 23 (1956): 364.

Denham, R. A. "Hip Mechanics." *Journal of Bone and Joint Surgery* 41-B (1959): 550.

deVries, H. A. "A Cinematographical Analysis of the Dolphin Swimming Stroke." *Research Quarterly* 30 (1959): 413.

——— "Evaluation of Static Stretching Procedures for Improvement of Flexibility." *Research Quarterly* 33 (1962): 230.

Dickinson, R. V. "The Specificity of Flexibility." *Research Quarterly* 39 (1968): 792.

Elftman, H. "The Functional Structure of the Lower Limbs." In *Human Limbs and Their Substitutes,* edited by P. E. Klopsteg and P. D. Wilson. New York: McGraw-Hill Book Company, 1954.

Fischer, F. J., and Houtz, S. J. "Evaluation of the Function of the Gluteus Maximus Muscle: An Electromyographic Study." *American Journal of Physical Medicine* 47 (1968): 182.

Flint, M. M. "An Electromyographic Comparison of the Function of the

Augments the actions of the
  obturator internus

Outward rotation of the thigh;
  may assist in transverse
  abduction of the hip joint
  from flexed hip positions

Iliacus and the Rectus Abdominus Muscles. A Preliminary Report."
  Physical Therapy 45 (1965): 248.

—— "Flexibility of Hip-Trunk, Trunk Strength, and Posture Related to
  Gravity Line Test." *Research Quarterly* 35 (1964): 141.

Frankel, Victor H. *The Femoral Neck.* Springfield, Ill.: Charles C Thomas,
  Publisher, 1960.

Frost, H. M. *The Laws of Bone Structure.* Springfield, Ill.: Charles C Thomas,
  Publisher, 1964.

Fujikawa, K. "Functional Classification of Lower Limb Muscles." *Okajimas
  Folia Anatomica Japonica* 44 (1968): 383.

Grant, C. Boileau. *An Atlas of Anatomy.* 5th ed. Baltimore: The Williams &
  Wilkins Company, 1962.

Gratz, C. M. "Tensile Strength and Elasticity Tests on Human Fascia Lata."
  Journal of Bone and Joint Surgery 13 (1941): 334.

Hall, Michael C. *The Locomotor System, Functional Anatomy.* Springfield, Ill.:
  Charles C Thomas, Publisher, 1965.

Houtz, S. J. "Influence of Gravitational Forces on Function of Lower Extremity
  Muscles." *Journal of Applied Physiology* 19 (1964): 999.

Houtz, S. J., and Fischer, F. J. "An Analysis of Muscle Action and Joint
  Excursion During Exercise on a Stationary Bicycle." *Journal of Bone and
  Joint Surgery* 41-A (1959): 123.

Inman, V. T. "Functional Aspects of the Abductor Muscles of the Hip." *Journal
  of Bone and Joint Surgery* 29-A (1947): 607.

Jonsson, B., and Steen, B. "Function of the Gracilis Muscle." *Acta Morphologica
  Neerlando-Scandinavica* 6 (1966): 325.

Joseph, J. *Man's Posture; Electromyographic Studies.* Springfield, Ill.: Charles C
  Thomas, Publisher, 1960.

Joseph, J., and Williams, P. L. "Electromyography of Certain Hip Muscles."
  Journal of Anatomy 91 (1957): 286.

Kaplan, E. B. "The Iliotibial Tract." *Journal of Bone and Joint Surgery* 40-A
  (1958): 817.

Karlsson, E., and Jonsson, B. "Function of the Gluteus Maximus Muscle; An
  Electromyographic Study.'' *Acta Morphologica Neerlando-Scandinavica* 6
  (1965): 161.

Keagy, R. D.; Brumlick, J.; and Bergan, J. J. "Direct Electromyography of the
  Psoas Major Muscle in Man." *Journal of Bone and Joint Surgery* 48-A
  (1966): 1377.

Kingsley, P. C., and Olmstead, K. L. "A Study to Determine the Angles of
  Anteversion of the Neck of the Femur." *Journal of Bone and Joint Surgery*
  30-A (1948): 745.

Klopsteg, Paul E., and Wilson, Philip D., eds. *Human Limbs and Their Substitutes.* New York: McGraw-Hill Book Company, 1954.

Koch, J. C. "The Laws of Bone Architecture." *American Journal of Anatomy* 21
  (1917): 177.

Kummer, B. "Gait and Posture Under Normal Conditions, With Special
  Reference to the Lower Limbs." *Clinical Orthopedics* 25 (1962): 32.

LaBan, M. M.; Raptou, A. D.; and Johnson, E. W. "Electromyographic Study
  of Function of Iliopsoas Muscle." *Archives of Physical Medicine and Rehabilitation* 46 (1965): 676.

Levens, A. S.; Berkeley, C. E.; and Inman, V. T. "Transverse Rotation of the
  Segments of the Lower Extremity in Locomotion." *Journal of Bone and Joint
  Surgery* 30-A (1948): 859.

Lombard, W. P., and Abbott, F. M. "The Mechanical Effects Produced by the
  Contraction of Individual Muscles of the Thigh of the Frog." *American
  Journal of Physiology* 20 (1907): 1.

MacConaill, M. A. "Joint Movements." *Physiotherapy* (November, 1964): 359.

—— "Mechanical Anatomy of Motion and Posture." In *Therapeutic Exercise.*
  2d ed., edited by S. Licht. New Haven, Conn.: Elizabeth Licht, Publisher,
  1961.

Markee, J. E.; Logue, J. T.; Williams, M.; Stanton, W. B.; Wrenn, R. A.; and Walker, L. B. "Two-Joint Muscles of the Thigh." *Journal of Bone and Joint Surgery* 37-A (1955): 125.

Marsk, A. "Studies on Weight-Distribution Upon the Lower Extremities in Individuals Working in a Standing Position." *Acta Orthopaedica Scandinavica* 27, Supplement XXI (1958).

Mathews, D. K.; Shaw, V.; and Bohnen, M. "Hip Flexibility of College Women as Related to Length of Body Segments." *Child Development Abstracts and Bibliography* 32 (1958): 85.

Mathews, D. K.; Shaw, V.; and Woods, J. B. "Hip Flexibility of Elementary School Boys as Related to Body Segments." *Research Quarterly* 30 (1959): 297.

May, W. W. "Relative Isometric Force of the Hip Abductor and Adductor Muscles. *Physical Therapy* 48 (1968): 845.

Mendler, H. M. "Relationships of Hip Abductor Muscles to Posture." *Physical Therapy* 44 (1964): 98.

Merrifield, H. H. "An Electromyographic Study of the Gluteus Maximus the Vastus Lateralis and the Tensor Fasciae Latae." *Dissertation Abstracts* 21 (1961): 1833.

Michele, Arthur A. *Iliopsoas*. Springfield, Ill.: Charles C. Thomas, Publisher, 1962.

Milch, H. "The Measurement of Pelvi-Femoral Motion." *Anatomical Record* 140 (1961): 135.

Murray, M. P., and Sepic, S. B. "Maximum Isometric Torque of Hip Abductor and Adductor Muscles." *Physical Therapy* 48 (1968): 1327.

Mustard, W. T. "Iliopsoas Transfer for Weakness of Hip Abductors." *Journal of Bone and Joint Surgery* 34-A (1952): 647.

Nachemson, A. "Electromyographic Studies of the Vertebral Portion of the Psoas Muscle." *Acta Orthopaedica Scandinavica* 37 (1966): 177.

Pick, J. W.; Stack, J. K.; and Anson, B. J. "Measurements on the Human Femur: II. Lengths, Diameters, and Angles." *Quarterly Bulletin of the Northwestern University Medical School* 17 (1943): 121.

Rasch, Philip J., and Burke, Roger K. *Kinesiology and Applied Anatomy*. 3rd ed. Philadelphia: Lea & Febiger, 1967.

Roberts, W. H. "The Locking Mechanism of the Hip Joint." *Anatomical Record* 147 (1963): 321.

Schneider, M. "The Effect of Growth on Femoral Torsion." *Journal of Bone and Joint Surgery* 45-A (1963): 1439.

Slocum, D. B., and Bowerman, W. "The Biomechanics of Running." *Clinical Orthopedics* 23 (1962): 39.

Sobotta, Johannes. *Atlas of Human Anatomy*, edited by Frank H. J. Figge. Vol. 1. *Skeleton, Ligaments, Joints, and Muscles*. New York: Hafner Publishing Company, Inc., 1968.

Steindler, Arthur. *Kinesiology of the Human Body*. Springfield, Ill.: Charles C Thomas, Publisher, 1955.

Tobin, W. J. "The Internal Architecture of the Femur and its Clinical Significance." *Journal of Bone and Joint Surgery* 37-A (1955): 57.

Troup, J. D.; Hood, C. A.; and Chapman, A. E. "Measurements of the Sagittal Mobility of the Lumbar Spine and Hips." *Annals of Physical Medicine* 9 (1968): 308.

Walmsley, T. "The Vertical Axes of the Femur." *Journal of Anatomy* 67 (1933): 284.

Wheatley, M. D., and Jahnke, W. D. "Electromyographic Study of the Superficial Thigh and Hip Muscles in Normal Individuals." *Archives of Physical Medicine* 32 (1951): 508.

Williams, M., and Wesley, W. "Hip Rotator Action of the Adductor Longus Muscle." *Physical Therapy Review*. 31 (1951): 90.

17

Pelvic Girdle, Vertebral Column, Head–Neck

The trunk segment is the most extensive of the body. Within it are numerous specialized structures, some of which are not essential to the present discussions of human motion. Attention will be paid to those structures which make available the body's primary movements. Within the trunk, the *pelvic girdle* and the *vertebral column* in this chapter, and the *shoulder girdle* in Chapter 18, will receive detailed attention. Since the vertebral column is not limited to the trunk segment, the movements and structures of the *head-neck* segment are included in this chapter.

Bones of the Pelvic Girdle

The pelvis is composed of the two hip bones and the *sacrum* to form a distinct but irregular bony ring. The two hip bones form more than two thirds of the pelvic ring to join anteriorly, but require the wedge-shaped sacrum to close the posterior aspect. The combination of the hip bones is technically known as the *pelvic girdle*, a term which would appear to be better suited to the description of the entire bony ring. That is how the term will be applied in this text. This structure is stronger in man, relative to his own size, than corresponding girdles of other animals.

When the articulated skeleton is viewed in its upright position, the pelvic basin of bone is seen to be tipped forward somewhat upon its rounded femoral supports. The more prominent hips of the female figure are due to a broader pelvic girdle, although the bones are less massive than those of the male pelvis. Consequently, the bony ring of the female is obviously better suited to act as a floor for the carriage of a developing infant as well as an adequate birth canal during parturition.

Figure 17-1 illustrates two views of the right hip bone, with the important bony landmarks identified. Three distinct but fused bones are involved in the adult: the *ilium*, *ischium*, and *pubis*. Their mutual point of union is located in the acetabulum and has been included in the lateral view. The ilium is then located above its two neighbors, which form the aperture known as the *obturator foramen*. The *crest* and the *anterior superior spine* of the ilium may be palpated laterally and anteriorly, respectively, on the trunk at points somewhat below the waistline. The *ischial tuberosities* are palpable also when seated because they protrude downward through the muscle mass upon which we sit. The anterior edge of the *crest* of the pubis becomes prominent when the hip is fully extended.

The ischium makes up the posteroinferior segment of the perimeter of the obturator foramen. Coursing downward from the acetabulum, the prominent ischial tuberosity offers a common origin for the hamstrings muscle group. Below this point, the *ramus* of the ischium courses forward and inward to join the pubis bone. The pubis makes up the anteroinferior segment of the perimeter of the obturator foramen. Its *inferior ramus* continues in the direction of the ischial ramus to join with its opposite member at the *symphasis pubis*. Coursing laterally and slightly upward from the crest of the pubis to the acetabulum is the *superior ramus*. If the two inferior pubic rami are viewed anteriorly, they form an angle opening

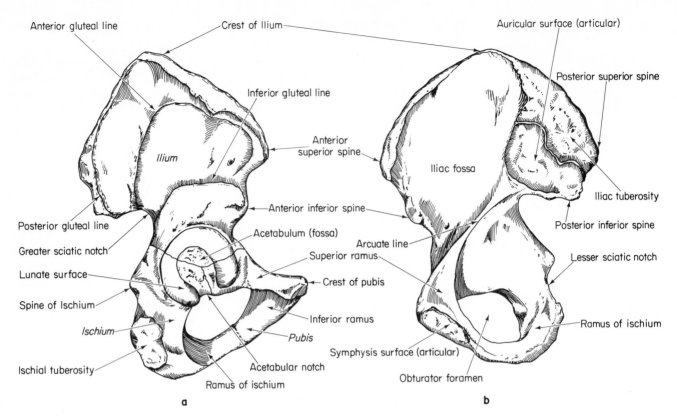

Figure 17–1. (a) Lateral and (b) medial views of the right hip bone.

Labels in figure (a):
Anterior gluteal line
Crest of Ilium
Inferior gluteal line
Ilium
Anterior superior spine
Posterior gluteal line
Acetabulum (fossa)
Greater sciatic notch
Superior ramus
Anterior inferior spine
Lunate surface
Crest of pubis
Spine of Ischium
Inferior ramus
Ischium
Pubis
Ischial tuberosity
Acetabular notch
Ramus of ischium
a

Labels in figure (b):
Auricular surface (articular)
Posterior superior spine
Iliac fossa
Iliac tuberosity
Posterior inferior spine
Arcuate line
Lesser sciatic notch
Ramus of ischium
Symphysis surface (articular)
Obturator foramen
b

downward, the *pubic arch*, which is generally on the order of 70 deg for males and 90 deg for females. When viewing the superior pubic rami from above, the rearward-opening angle formed at the pubic junction is again larger for the female.

The ilium exhibits two broad surfaces for muscle attachments. The outer surface, often called the *gluteal surface*, provides spacious concave areas for the gluteus medius and minimus muscles whose margins are bordered by the *gluteal lines*. The *posterior gluteal line* represents the anterior attachment border for the gluteus maximus muscle. The concave inner surface of the ilium is called the *pelvic surface* and contains the *iliac fossa*, the attachment site of the important *iliacus* muscle of the iliopsoas group.

Following the *arcuate line* upward and backward, two dissimilar surfaces are noted. The first, the *auricular surface*, is the surface which articulates with the sacrum. It receives its name from the fact that it is shaped like an ear and is covered with articular cartilage. Above this surface is a roughened area known as the *iliac tuberosity*. As such, it supports the attachment of important ligaments and muscles of the back.

The borders of the ilium are most irregular, forming two anterior and two posterior spines. Its crest offers an upper surface which contains inner and outer lips for the attachment of the muscular layers of the abdomen. Below the *posterior inferior spine* resides a deep indentation, the *greater*

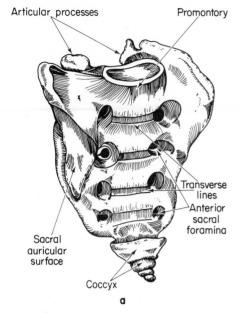

Articular processes — Promontory

Transverse lines

Anterior sacral foramina

Sacral auricular surface

Coccyx

a

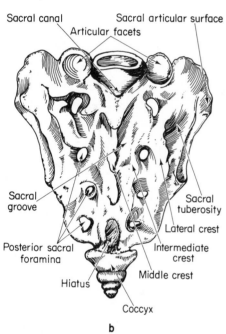

Sacral canal — Sacral articular surface

Articular facets

Sacral groove

Posterior sacral foramina

Sacral tuberosity

Lateral crest

Intermediate crest

Middle crest

Hiatus

Coccyx

b

Figure 17–2. (*a*) Anterolateral and (*b*) posterior views of the sacrum and coccyx.

sciatic notch, which acts as a passageway for important vessels and nerves passing from the trunk segment into the thigh area.

Figure 17-2 illustrates two views of the sacrum and *coccyx*. The five fused sacral vertebrae are evident in Fig. 17-2*a*, while Fig. 17-2*b* clearly denotes its triangular shape. The sacrum fits into the pelvic girdle between the auricular surfaces of the two hip bones and is said to be wedged in place because downward displacement is severely restricted. The anterior or *pelvic surface* is quite concave and presents four transverse lines which separate the five vertebral bodies. At the lateral terminations of these lines are the four sacral *foramina*, which function as important nerve and vessel passageways. Along the anterior, superior border of the uppermost vertebra is the *promontory* of the sacrum. The articular surfaces of the sacrum are also called auricular surfaces because they match those of the hip bones.

The posterior sacral surface is convex and not as broad as the anterior surface. Three longitudinal crests are evident: the *middle*, *intermediate*, and *lateral*. Between the middle and intermediate crests is a shallow groove which serves as a muscle attachment site for the *multifidus*. The fifth sacral vertebra is incomplete posteriorly to form an aperture known as the *sacral hiatus*. Two *superior articular processes* are shown which join with the fifth lumbar vertebra. They are positioned to face backward and inward. Between them is located the upper end of the *sacral canal*. This surface of the sacrum may be palpated.

The Pelvic Joints

It is important to recognize that the pelvic girdle is not designed to allow movement between its parts. Indeed, it is so rigid structurally that movements are restricted to the girdle as a whole under most gross movement conditions. The fusion of the three segments of the hip bones, the extremely tight *sacroiliac* joints, plus the junction between the pubes offer a structure which sacrifices mobility for stability.

The *pubic symphysis* (Fig. 17-3*a*) is classified as an amphiarthrodial joint which is slightly movable. Between the adjoining symphysis surfaces is the fibrocartilage, *interpubic disk*, providing interosseous binding. Directly below this junction along the pubic arch is the thick *arcuate pubic* ligament, while the *superior pubic* ligament binds the joint from above. The result is a joint of weak bony arrangement, made stable by ligamentous and cartilaginous arrangement.

The *sacroiliac* joints are stable by both bony and ligamentous arrangements. They are difficult to classify because they show characteristics of diarthrodial as well as synarthrodial joints. The position held by the sacrum between the two ilia and its shape contribute significantly to the stability of these joints. The sacral wedge, with its narrow end facing downward, rests between the similarly oriented auricular surfaces of the ilia. Being broader above than below, downward displacement of the sacrum is obviated. The prominent iliac tuberosities pose a barrier to posterior displacements. However, there is no outstanding bony impediment for anterior displacement of the sacrum. Consequently, displacement in this direction must be resisted by ligamentous binding.

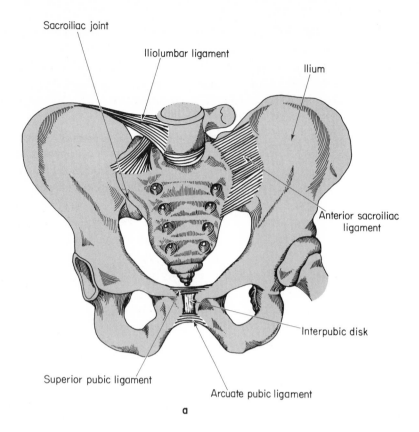

Sacroiliac joint

Iliolumbar ligament

Ilium

Anterior sacroiliac ligament

Interpubic disk

Superior pubic ligament

Arcuate pubic ligament

a

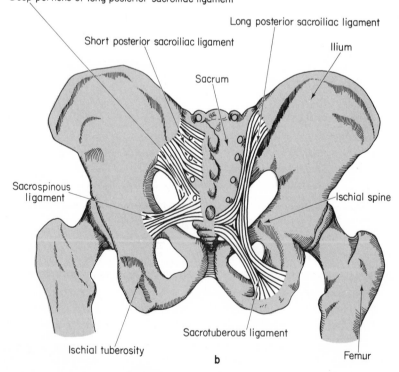

Deep portions of long posterior sacroiliac ligament

Long posterior sacroiliac ligament

Short posterior sacroiliac ligament

Ilium

Sacrum

Sacrospinous ligament

Ischial spine

Ischial tuberosity

Sacrotuberous ligament

Femur

b

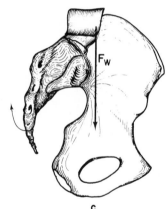

F_W

c

Figure 17–3. (*a*) Anterior and (*b*) posterior views of the important ligaments of the pelvic girdle. In (*c*), the sacral rotation tendency is illustrated.

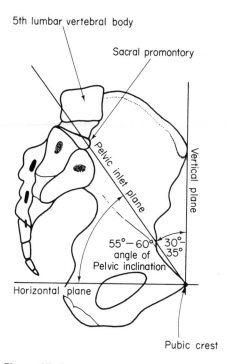

5th lumbar vertebral body

Sacral promontory

Pelvic inlet plane

Vertical plane

55°–60°
angle of
Pelvic inclination

30°/
35°

Horizontal plane

Pubic crest

Figure 17–4

Figure 17-3*a* illustrates the *anterior sacroiliac* ligament which provides the primary anterior stabilization of the joint. Figure 17-3*b* illustrates the *short* and *long posterior sacroiliac* ligaments. Not shown is a third ligament, the *interosseous sacroiliac* ligament, which adds to the binding. Of particular importance to sacroiliac stability is the weight of the upper body, which passes anterior to the center of the sacrum in erect standing. As a result, the sacrum (Fig. 17-4*c*) is continually acted upon to rotate to a more horizontal position within the pelvic girdle. Three ligaments are situated to resist this rotation tendency. The backward and upward rotation of the lower sacrum is checked by the *sacrotuberous* and *sacrospinous* ligaments (Fig. 17-3*b*). The downward and forward rotation tendency of the sacral promontory is checked by the *iliolumbar* ligament (Fig. 17-3*a*).

Pelvic Girdle Mobility

In addition to the transfer of upper-body weight from the trunk segment to the lower extremities, the pelvic girdle may rotate above the fixed thigh segments, within the trunk. In the upright standing position, the pelvic girdle is situated as shown in Fig. 17-4. The anterior superior iliac spines are very nearly contained in a plane which is directly above the pubic crests. If a line is then constructed to run from the pubic crest through the sacral promontory, it will be contained in the *pelvic inlet plane* to form an angle of about 30 deg with the vertical plane. The angle formed between the inlet plane and a horizontal plane at the pubic crest then approaches 60 deg and is called the *angle of pelvic inclination*.

Muscles acting to form force couples may produce rotations about the bilateral axis through the femoral heads (Fig. 17-5*a*). Figure 17-5 (*b* and *c*) illustrates the rotations known as *forward* and *backward tilts*, respectively. The former allows the larger movement range from the neutral position. If the habitual position of the pelvic girdle is one of forward tilt, it is considered a poor postural position which can lead to low-back pain. It results in an increase in the angle of pelvic inclination. Backward tilt reduces the inclination angle and is often used to relieve the discomfort associated with postures of forward tilt. Its range of movement is more limited because of iliofemoral ligament resistance. Muscles which may

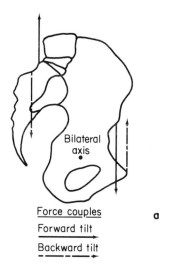

Bilateral axis

Force couples **a**

Forward tilt

Backward tilt

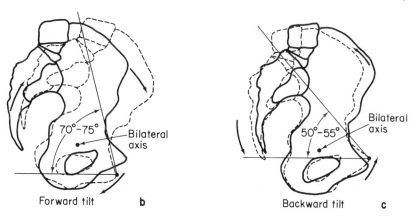

70°–75°

Bilateral axis

Forward tilt **b**

Bilateral axis

50°–55°

Backward tilt **c**

Figure 17–5. Force couple action to produce forward and backward tilting of the pelvic girdle.

contribute to forward tilt are the primary hip flexors, such as the iliopsoas group and the rectus femoris, and the deep back muscles plus the *quadratus lumborum*. Backward tilt force couple action may be provided by the abdominal wall muscles anteriorly with the gluteus maximus and hamstrings posteriorly.

→ *Place your thumbs along the iliac crests and your fingers along the anterior borders of the pelvis and demonstrate forward and backward tilts. Demonstrate these movements in front of a mirror so that you may see the involvement of adjacent segments.*

Limited ranges of *lateral tilting* may be accomplished also. This is particularly true in walking when the weight of the body is shifted laterally over the supporting hip. Viewing the pelvic girdle from the front, force couple muscular action may pull downward-outward on one rim of the pelvis while an upward-inward force is applied to the opposite rim. For example, the right hip abductors (lateral stabilizers) may contract to maintain a level pelvis when the right limb is supporting the body's weight by itself. Concurrent contractions of the left quadratus lumborum, lateral abdominals, and deep back muscles act to elevate the opposite rim. This lateral tilting may be palpated during walking and is designated as to direction in terms of which rim exhibits the shorter radius of rotation. Hence, the movement just described is termed lateral tilt to the right because the right pelvic rim exhibits the shorter radius from the hip joint center of rotation. In addition, some transverse rotations to the left and right are available.

It is of importance to remember that all pelvic movements necessitate changes in the vertebral column directly above. That is, forward and backward tilts increase and decrease, respectively, the natural lumbar curve, while lateral tilts tend to bow the lumbar region of the column to the side opposite the elevated pelvic rim. Transverse pelvic rotations are accompanied by vertebral column rotations in the same directions. Moreover, most large-magnitude vertebral column and hip joint movements involve pelvic girdle adjustments. In this way, coordinated interactions between multiples of body segments may be accomplished. The two lower limbs may move in ways which are essentially independent of each other and still be coordinated with the movements of the flexible trunk segment, as is typified at the moment of take-off in high jumping (Fig. 17-6).

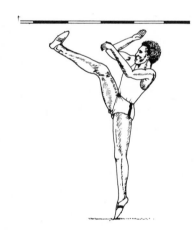

Figure 17–6

→ *Describe the adjustments required of the pelvic girdle and two thigh segments as demonstrated in Fig. 17-6.*

THE VERTEBRAL COLUMN

The vertebral column is a unique structure which performs many different functions. In layman's terminology, it is the backbone, a term which has obvious validity with respect to position in the body, but offers little help in structural and movement matters. Fortunately, the vertebral column is not a single bone, as the layman's term implies, but an amazing stack of individual, irregular bones which are flexibly connected, one above the other. We have become acquainted with the column's lower end in the previous sections. Two of the column's subsections or regions, the sacrum and coccyx, consist of nine separate vertebrae early in life. In adulthood, the five upper vertebrae are fused to form the sacrum, while the remaining four become the coccyx. Because of their rigid structural incorporation into the pelvic girdle, our concerns for them in this section will be limited to the sacrum's upper aspect, which articulates with the fifth lumbar vertebra.

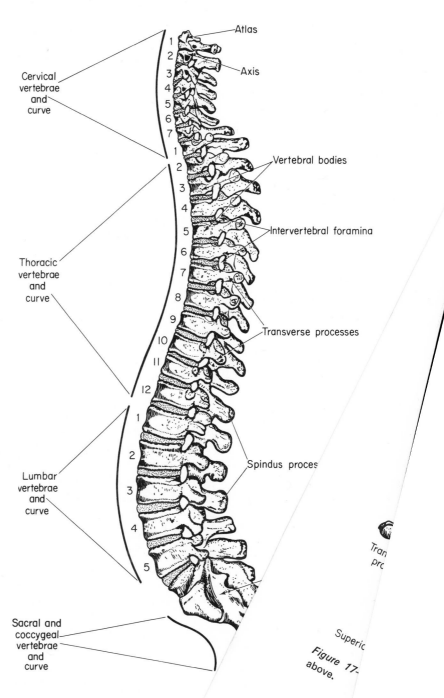

Figure 17–7. The adult vertebral column and its four anteroposterior curves.

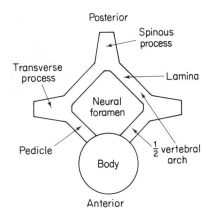

Figure 17–8. The gross parts of vertebrae in diagrammatic form.

Viewed from the side (Fig. 17-7), the adult vertebral column presents four anteroposterior curves. The adult column differs markedly from that in early, fetal life, which is C-shaped, convex to the posterior. The first anteroposterior curve in the adult is the *sacral kyphosis*, which is concave to the anterior and includes both the sacrum and the coccyx. The lumbar region presents an opposite curvature, concave to the posterior, which is known as the *lumbar lordosis*. As an infant begins to maintain vertical postures, the curve develops. Above the lumbar region, the column reverts to a kyphosis in the *thoracic* region which is much like that of the fetus. It courses from the twelfth thoracic vertebra to the center of the second thoracic vertebra. From this point upward, the column again reverts to the opposite curvature, the *cervical lordosis*. Late in fetal life the cervical curve begins to form concave to the posterior. Crawling and sitting actions of the young infant make the curve more pronounced.

Examination of the vertebral column in the figure makes it evident that one of the reasons for the development of the curves is related to unequal growth of the anterior and posterior borders of the *vertebral bodies*. They are somewhat thicker anteriorly than posteriorly in the lumbar and cervical regions and the opposite in the thoracic region. Hall refers to this unequal dimension relationship as wedging of the vertebrae.[1] When viewed from the side, the gravity line passes in such a way as to increase each of the curves above the sacrum. It runs posterior to the center of the lumbar bodies, anterior to the thoracic bodies, and, again, slightly posterior to the cervical bodies. Consequently, vertical compression forces produce increased curvatures which are generally balanced in front of and behind the gravity line.

Structure of the Lumbar, Thoracic, and Cervical Vertebrae

A typical vertebra consists of several fused parts, as presented in diagrammatic form in Fig. 17-8. The generally cylindrical vertebral body begins anteriorly. From its posterior face, two *pedicles* or pillars project backward. They, in turn, join a pair of *laminae*, which course backward and together to close a bony ring, which is called the *vertebral* or *neural foramen*. At the laminae junction arises the *spinous process*, which is directed posteriorly. Each pedicle-lamina pair forms one half of the *vertebral arch* and supports a *transverse process*. *Articular processes* arise near the pedicle-lamina junctions. These elevated areas contain smooth facets which articulate with those of vertebrae below and above. Thus there is a set of inferior and superior articular processes, four in all.

Regional variations in vertebrae structure provide a means of individual identification. Figure 17-9 illustrates the *third lumbar* vertebra as being typical of that region. The lumbar bodies are more massive than are those of other regions. Each shows a greater bilateral than anteroposterior dimension. The long transverse processes are slender and project horizontally. The spinous process is broad and heavy. The articular processes are

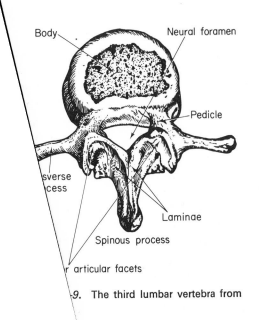

.9. The third lumbar vertebra from

[1]Michael C. Hall, *The Locomotor System—Functional Anatomy* (Springfield, Ill.: Charles C Thomas, Publisher, 1965), p. 472.

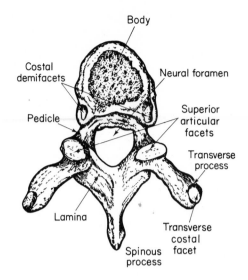

Figure 17–10. The sixth thoracic vertebra from above.

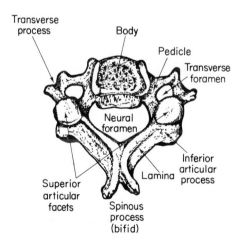

Figure 17–11. The fourth cervical vertebra from above.

quite prominent. The superior facets are concave and face slightly upward and backward, but particularly inward. The inferior facets are convex and reverse those directions to face slightly downward and forward, but particularly outward. Thus the facet joints in the lumbar region are very nearly oriented in the sagittal plane. The neural foramen is large and triangular in shape, which is in keeping with vertebral regions with the greatest mobility. The *intervertebral disks* in the lumbar region are quite thick.

Figure 17-10 illustrates the *sixth thoracic* vertebra as being typical of that region. In comparison to the lumbar vertebrae, the thoracic bodies are smaller and exhibit very similar bilateral and anteroposterior dimensions. On the sides of the bodies, near the junction with the pedicles, there are a pair of articular facets which receive the heads of the ribs. These are designated *costal demifacets* because they are incomplete. For an articulating pair of thoracic vertebrae in the central part of this region, an upper and lower demifacet with the intervertebral disk combine to form a complete reception area for the head of a rib. The first, tenth, eleventh, and twelfth thoracic bodies contain complete upper facets for rib head reception. The transverse processes are long and thick and are directed backward and laterally. Their broadened ends present articular facets for the *tubercles* of the ribs, which generally face forward and outward. This is the case for the upper ten thoracic vertebrae. Numbers eleven and twelve have no costal facets on their transverse processes.

The spinous process is long with a triangular cross section. It is directed obliquely downward and backward in the central section so that it overlaps the one below. The upper and lower vertebrae do so to a much lesser degree, thus exhibiting their transitional nature. The articular facets in the central section are flat and nearly of a frontal orientation. The superior facets face slightly upward and outward, but particularly backward. As expected, the inferior facets are directed oppositely. The neural foramen is circular in shape and smaller than in the lumbar vertebrae. The thoracic intervertebral disks are thin when compared to those of the lumbar region.

The head-neck segment contains the cervical vertebrae of the column, the uppermost of which articulates with the skull at the *atlantoöccipital* joint. Figure 17-11 illustrates the *fourth cervical* vertebra as being typical of the third through sixth vertebrae. It can be seen that the body is small with a flat posterior aspect. Its wider side-to-side dimension is terminated in elevated lips on its superior surface. The pedicles sweep nearly laterally to form unusual transverse processes. Each contains a *transverse foramen* which serves to transmit nerves and vessels and terminates in two *tubercles*, the *anterior* and *posterior*. The articular processes are short and heavy. The flattened superior facets face upward and backward and slightly inward. The inferior facets are oppositely directed. The spinous process is rather short and *bifid* or separated into two, generally unequal tubercles. The neural foramen is triangular in shape and is large.

The first and second cervical vertebrae are atypical and are named the *atlas* and *axis*, respectively. Figure 17-12 illustrates the axis, showing a body of a peculiar shape. Rising vertically from it is a tooth-like projection

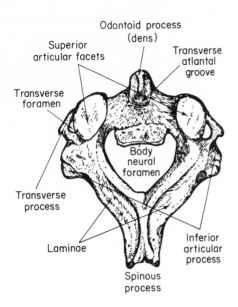

Figure 17–12. The second cervical vertebra, the axis, from above.

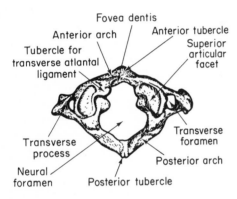

Figure 17–13. The first cervical vertebra, the atlas, from above.

known as the *odontoid process* or *dens*, which is mildly constricted at its base to form a neck. The anterior aspect of the dens contains an articular facet which joins the anterior arch of the atlas. The transverse processes exhibit a single tubercle as well as a transverse foramen which faces upward and outward. The mildly convex superior articular facets face upward and outward and are nearly circular. The inferior facets are located farther to the posterior and resemble those of the typical vertebrae of the cervical region in that they are oval and face downward, forward, and slightly outward. The spinous process is massive and is bifid at its posterior termination. The neural foramen is large and triangular.

The uppermost vertebra, the atlas, is characterized by the absence of a body and a spinous process (Fig. 17-13). The dens of the axis represents the body of the atlas, which in development becomes fused with the body of the axis. In place of the body is the *anterior arch*, which is faceted on its posterior aspect to receive the articular facet of the dens. Two well-formed tubercles serve as attachments for the *transverse atlantal* ligament, which holds the dens in contact with the anterior arch. This ligament courses behind the dens, residing in the transverse groove on its posterior surface. Two *alar* ligaments connect the dens to the nonarticular part of the *occipital condyles*.

The *posterior arch* completes the bony ring of the atlas and ends in a *posterior tubercle*. Transverse processes are in evidence with their transverse foramina. The bases of the transverse processes are named the *lateral masses*, the sites of the articular facets. The superior facets are large and prominently concave. They tilt upward, inward, and slightly backward. They are shaped to receive the occipital condyles of the occipital bone. Their anterior ends converge medially somewhat. The inferior facets are nearly circular and face downward and inward to articulate with the axis.

The occipital condyles are convex areas which face downward with articular surfaces placed somewhat laterally to meet with the articular concavities of the atlas. The atlantoöccipital junction incorporates these condylar surfaces as if they were the inferior facets of still another vertebra.

Vertebral Column Stability

Separating the vertebral bodies are the intervertebral disks, which vary in size to match the functions required of them in their individual locations. It has been estimated that about one fourth of the total length of the column is due to their presence. Each disk is firmly attached to the opposed bony surfaces of the vertebral bodies. The connection is to a layer of hyaline cartilage covering the upper and lower body surfaces. As such, these cartilage layers serve rather like a floor and ceiling for each disk.

Forming the disk's circumference is a tough ring of crossing, fibrous tissue layers known as the *annulus fibrosus*. Peripheral fibers attach around the circumference to the vertebral bodies. Contained within this ring is a soft, pulpy substance which is very mobile. It is known as the *nucleus pulposus*, and when the disk is under compression stress, it flattens, pressing

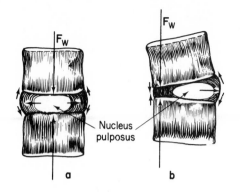

F_W F_W

Nucleus
pulposus

a   b

Figure 17–14. Balanced (*a*) and off-center (*b*) compression force effects on the intervertebral disk.

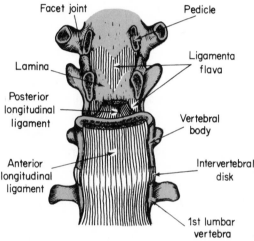

Facet joint   Pedicle

Lamina   Ligamenta flava

Posterior longitudinal ligament   Vertebral body

Anterior longitudinal ligament   Intervertebral disk

1st lumbar vertebra

Figure 17–15

radially against the annulus in all directions (Fig. 17-14*a*). When the pressure is removed, the natural elasticity of both components provide for a rapid return to their original shapes. Consequently, their combined action within the disk is to offer considerable stability and shock absorption control between each vertebrae pair. With age, progressive changes occur to narrow the intervertebral space as the result of dehydration and an increase in fibrous content of the disk. Hence, the disk cannot cushion the shocks as well as in youth, which is partially responsible for the gradual loss of standing height as age advances.

In addition to the disk connections, the vertebral bodies are bound together by *anterior* and *posterior longitudinal* ligaments. Dense longitudinal fibers, forming a broad, strong, anterior band, course from the sacrum to the occipital bone (Fig. 17-15). The posterior longitudinal ligament courses along the posterior aspect of the vertebral bodies within the neural foramen. It extends from the axis to the sacrum, forming broader sections over and connecting to the intervertebral disks and narrowing over the vertebral bodies. These ligaments offer important support to the vertebral column, particularly along its anterior aspect. In hyperextension of the column, the anterior ligament performs a splinting action along the column.

The laminae and their processes are connected by various ligaments. For example, the spinous processes are connected through the *supraspinal* and *interspinal* ligaments. The latter run between the upper border of one spinous process to the lower border of that above. The former runs the length of the column from the sacrum to the seventh cervical vertebra along the tips of the spinous processes. From the seventh cervical vertebra to the occipital bone, this ligament is known as the *ligamentum nuchae*. The *ligamenta flava* connect the laminae of adjacent vertebrae. They cross the interlaminar spaces from the sacrum to the axis. This tissue consists predominantly of elastic fibers which are said to provide for the conservation of muscular energy in supporting upright postures. The *intertransverse* ligaments are also in evidence, running between transverse processes, which completes the connections of adjacent vertebral arches except the pedicles. Therefore the *intervertebral foramina* are clear for the passage of spinal nerves from the column to the periphery (see Fig. 17-7), and a remarkable degree of stability is obtained along the posterior aspects of the column.

In standing postures, very little muscular stabilization of the column is required. Certainly, muscular effort is noted when marked imbalances occur. As trunk flexion and hip flexion commence, the extensive *erector spinae* muscle group and the *multifidus* become active eccentrically to control the forward-downward movement of the massive trunk and head-neck complex. Otherwise, a loss of control could be disastrous. However, when these flexions near their terminations in standing, the back muscles become quiescent and the support function is transferred to the ligaments of the column. Muscles which affect the position of the pelvis above the stabilized lower limbs may assist in vertebral column stability. Those coursing downward from the trunk would include the iliopsoas group, the glutii, and the abdominals; refer to Muscle Chart 3 for details.

Vertebral Column Mobility

The movements of the vertebral column are the result of the combined actions of the intervertebral disk joints and the facet joints. The disk joint movements result from the shifting of the disk substance in response to compression forces. Since the nucleus pulposus is essentially incompressible, off-center, wedging compression causes it to be squeezed in the direction of the open side (see Fig. 17-14*b*). This may occur in any direction since the disk is symmetrical in shape. In addition, rotations of the vertebral bodies upon each other may be carried through rather limited ranges as the annulus fibrosus provides twisting resistance. The facet joints allow gliding movements to occur over their surfaces. Of particular importance is the orientation of these surfaces in the three regions of the column. Because of the structurally complex nature of the vertebral column, compound movements are the rule. This is particularly true of rotations and lateral flexions.

Lumbar Region Mobility

The lumbar disks are thick, while the articular facets approach the sagittal plane. This combination allows flexion, extension, hyperextension, and lateral flexion. Rotation is very limited owing to the orientation of the articular facets. With one facet facing inwardly and the other outwardly, transverse rotations about a polar axis centered within the vertebral body, whether or not they are the result of muscular effort or accompany lateral flexions, would simply cause the facets to press against each other. The mobility in this region is greatest in the vicinity of the lower vertebrae and decreases upon moving upward toward the thoracic region. However, lateral flexion tends to be the least limited where the lumbar and thoracic regions join.

The *lumbosacral* joint differs from the other lumbar joints primarily because of the prominent *anterior lumbosacral angle*, opening 15–20 deg forward and downward (Fig. 17-16). Thus the intervertebral disk is wedge-shaped to fill the interbody space. A strong tendency for the fifth lumbar vertebra to slide forward must be overcome by the supporting ligaments. The articular facets joining the sacrum and the fifth lumbar vertebra are oriented more frontally than above and provide a blend of movements, including rotation, which adapts the joint to both vertebral column and pelvic requirements.

The lumbar lordosis may be markedly altered by pelvic tilting. The *posterior lumbosacral angle* responds to forward and backward pelvic tilts by being decreased by the former and increased by the latter.

→ *Referring again to Figs. 17-4 and 17-5, what are the effects of the changing angles of pelvic inclination on the lumbar lordosis and lumbosacral angles? To illustrate, lie down (supine) on a flat, rigid surface. After achieving a comfortable position, slide your hands under the arch formed beneath the lumbar region. In some individuals the opening will be large, while in others it will be slight. Now, tilt the pelvis backward, keeping the hips and knees extended. Note how the curvature decreases.*

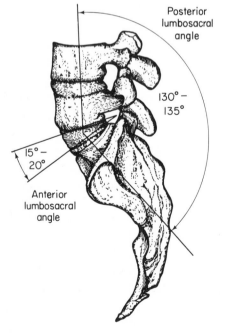

Posterior lumbosacral angle

130° – 135°

15° – 20°

Anterior lumbosacral angle

Figure 17–16. The lumbosacral junction.

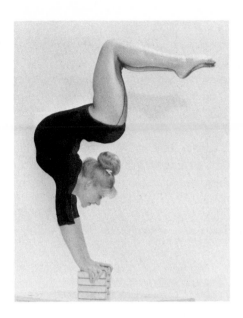

Figure 17–17. A remarkable example of vertebral column flexibility. (By permission of Mrs. Mary Jane Scanlan Logan, the performer.)

Next, after relaxing to the original supine position, flex the hips and knees, drawing the heels toward the buttocks. What is the outcome? Explain the structural and kinetic bases for this occurrence. Discuss the consequences of exercises such as sit-ups and leg-raisers on the low back and pelvic areas.

Thoracic Region Mobility

As mentioned earlier, the disks in this region are thin. Tilting movements between the vertebral bodies are therefore limited somewhat. The special provisions required for the thoracic rib cage tend to provide an additional limitation to movement. Although flexion and extension are available, hyperextension is particularly resisted by the overlapping spinous processes and the articular facets which are nearly frontally oriented. Since the superior facets face slightly upward as well as backward, flexion produces an upward sliding of their inferior mates over them. This motion is finally restricted by the thoracic cage, as is most of any tendency toward lateral flexion. The blending of structural features of the lower thoracic and upper lumbar vertebrae allows for a smooth transition of movement functions. Figure 17-17 points up a remarkable example of vertebral column hyperextension flexibility in which it is obvious that the last two thoracic junctions are involved in attaining this extreme position.

Rotation is free in the thoracic region but is not extensive or pure in that some lateral flexion accompanies it. These slight, accompanying lateral flexions are always in the same direction as the rotation. That is, rotation to the right is accompanied by slight, right lateral flexion. This characteristic holds true throughout the vertebral column. Likewise, when lateral flexion is imposed upon the column, some rotation is always evident. This outcome is passive in nature and depends on the positions of the articular facets and the nature of curved structures. The thoracic rotation is possible because, in addition to facing backward and slightly upward, the superior facets face slightly outward. When viewed from above, they approximate circumferential segments of a conical surface about a polar axis through the vertebral body. The inferior facets may then glide transversely over them.

The combination of rotation and lateral flexion is usually explained upon the basis of the difficulties encountered when attempting to bend a curved rod when the plane of the bending is perpendicular to the plane of the original curves. The outcome always includes a resultant twisting or rotation about the rod's longitudinal axis. Although the vertebral column is not a solid rod, all of its natural curves are of a single plane, and perpendicular, lateral flexions produce concurrent rotations. In the thoracic region, which is always concave to the anterior, the rotation accompanying lateral flexion directs the vertebral body toward the convex side of the lateral curve. This is known as *convex-side rotation*. Active rotations produced by the rotator muscles are, therefore, *concave-side rotations* because the vertebral body moves toward the concave side of the accompanying lateral flexion.

Thoracic lateral flexions and rotations are position-dependent. That is, with the trunk in the erect position, lateral flexions and their accompanying rotations are situated near the thoracolumbar junction and underlying lumbar region. The lower thoracic region is only mildly involved. If lateral flexion is performed while the trunk is hyperextended, there is virtually no involvement in the thoracic region, the hyperextension effectively locking the facet joints. If lateral flexion is initiated during trunk flexion, the thoracic region is involved, but at a higher level, near the eighth thoracic vertebra. The facet joints are no longer locked, and rotation directs the vertebral bodies to the convex side of the lateral curve. The approximate combined ranges of thoracic and lumbar movements are flexion-extension, 85 deg; hyperextension, 30 deg; lateral flexion, 28 deg; and rotation to the left or right, 38 deg.

→ *With the assistance of a friend, see if these figures can be verified.*

Cervical Region Mobility

The ability to rotate the vertebral column improves as the upper regions are involved. In the cervical region, the disks are again quite thick, resulting in enhanced interbody tilting. Furthermore, the articular facets provide little obstruction to the common movements so that flexion-extension and hyperextension movements are accompanied by some gliding of the vertebral bodies in those directions. Lateral flexion and rotation are free and again occur in combination. In this region, most rotations move the vertebral bodies to the concave side of the lateral flexion curve. The area of the fourth and fifth cervical vertebrae allow the greatest flexion-extension-hyperextension range. Circumduction of the head-neck segment is available to a prominent degree.

The two uppermost vertebrae, the axis and atlas, combine to provide a unique platform for the skull. Two joints, the *atlantoaxial* and the *atlantoöccipital*, provide the mechanisms for rotation, flexion-extension, hyperextension, and slight lateral flexion. Rotations are the primary movements of the atlantoaxial joint. The peg-like dens represents the site of the polar axis about which the head and atlas pivot. The axis may rotate below the atlas, which causes the dens to pivot within the osteofibrous ring of the atlas. The articular facets of the atlantoaxial joint do not fit together well, which allows slight gliding to occur during flexion-extension and hyperextension. As rotation progresses, the two alar ligaments tend to wind around the dens until their resulting tensions bring the movement to a halt at about 45 deg in either direction from center. The ability to rotate the body beneath the head is particularly important in such maneuvers as "spotting" in dance and free exercise so that rapid spinning movements do not result in inordinate dizziness and loss of balance and movement control.

The condylar, atlantoöccipital joint provides for flexion-extension and hyperextension primarily. In addition, some slight lateral flexion can be identified. The atlantal sockets are not parallel but converge anteriorly. Note the commonality between this joint and the knee joint.

→ *Would you expect some gliding as well as rolling?*

Flexion-extension can be carried through about 10 deg, while hyper-extension proceeds another 25 deg or so. Combining all the separate motions within the cervical region, flexion-extension and hyperextension amount to about 40 deg, lateral flexion of about 40 deg to each side, and rotation of about 90 deg in each direction.

Combined Columnar Mobilities

Movements between pairs of vertebrae are quite small in magnitude. It is the combination of such movements along the entire vertebral column which provides for the gross movements which are so readily observed. Muscular mechanisms in the trunk and head-neck segments are arranged to allow numerous movement combinations as well as the relatively pure. Although the usual descriptions of individual muscle actions are presented in Muscle Chart 4, there appears to be little justification for establishing numerous subdivisions of action. These paired muscles work together to provide most of the movements of the column. It is clear that most of the muscles are situated to perform unified flexions, extensions, and hyper-extensions. Because they are attached to a generally cylindrical structure, they may also contribute to lateral flexions and rotations.

An important consideration in the study of vertebral column move-ments is the location, direction, and length of the muscles. For the most part, the short muscles of the back are the deepest, with the intermediate in length lying between them and the long superficial group. The deep multifidus points up an example of lateral-to-medial fiber arrangement. Since its action tends to motivate the spinous process levers, rotation directs the vertebral bodies to the side opposite the active fibers. When both sides are active, the opposing rotations are neutralized. Conversely, the *splenius cervicis* and *splenius capitis*, particularly, demonstrate medial-to-lateral fiber arrangements. Hence, unilateral action of these muscles tends to rotate the vertebral bodies and head to the same side. Acting bilaterally, extension and hyperextension result because opposing, secon-dary movements are ruled out. Obviously, the vertebral column presents almost limitless opportunities for synergic action.

→ *What is the general fiber direction for the arboreal,* erector spinae *group?*

The abdominal musculature is also present in layers and in bilateral pairs. The outer three, the *internal* and *external obliques* and *rectus abdominis*, are situated to operate in trunk flexion, particularly in the lumbar region. Lateral flexions and rotations are also performed, and therefore synergy is abundant. As noted by Jensen and Schultz, the right and left external oblique pair can cooperate in a sit-up exercise to flex the trunk.[2] Acting singly, each has a lateral flexion and rotation func-tion. Balanced bilateral contraction rules out the opposite-side rotations and same-side lateral flexions. Similarly, if nearly pure lateral flexion to

[2]Clayne R. Jensen and Gordon W. Schultz, *Applied Kinesiology* (New York: McGraw-Hill Book Company, 1970), p. 37.

the left were desired from an erect starting position, concurrent flexion, hyperextension, and rotation tendencies would have to be neutralized.

→ *Using Muscle Chart 4 to assist you, identify the muscles which could be involved to produce left lateral flexion and describe the synergic actions performed. Then do the same for trunk and head-neck rotation to the right. Pay particular attention to the* sternocleidomastoid *when describing head-neck movements and do not limit your consideration to anterior or posterior muscle groups. Can you visualize eccentric muscular contributions to the control of movements motivated by gravity?*

Since the muscle layers of the trunk and head-neck spread over more than one region of the vertebral column, it is to be expected that actions in one region would be accompanied by similar actions in adjacent regions. For example, because the range of rotation movements generally increases from the sacrum upward to the head, maximal rotation of the entire vertebral column results in a "winding-up" action. Reversing the direction of rotation first unwinds the column and proceeds to wind it up again in the other direction. Similarly, it is not wise to artificially separate the muscular actions of the lower extremities and the vertebral column. In

Muscle Chart 4: *Pelvic Girdle, Vertebral Column, Head–Neck*

| *Muscle* | Attachments | | *Innervation* |
	Origin	*Insertion*	
I. The Hip Joint Muscles			
A. The Anterior Group			
1. Iliopsoas			
a. Iliacus	a. Superior two thirds of the iliac fossa and the ala of the sacrum	a. Lateral side of the tendon of the psoas major to end at the lesser trochanter	a. Femoral nerve
b. Psoas major	b. Transverse processes of all the lumbar vertebrae, sides of the bodies and intervertebral disks of the last thoracic and all of the lumbar vertebrae	b. Lesser trochanter of the femur	b. A branch from the lumbar plexus
2. Rectus femoris			
a. Anterior head	a. Anterior inferior iliac spine	Base of the patella as the quadriceps tendon, to continue to the tibial tuberosity as the patellar ligament	Femoral nerve
b. Posterior head	b. Groove superior to the brim of the acetabulum		

standing postures and in locomotion, trunk and head-neck adjustments are constantly being enacted to properly balance the column and stabilize the head for its important perceptions.

Here is an example of interrelated, adjacent segment action for study and analysis. It should graphically point out the overlapping roles played by the muscles.

→ *Have a subject, dressed in swimming briefs, lie on a firm table in the prone position. Adjust his position so that his knees pass beyond the table's edge with contact occurring about 2 in. above the patella. Instruct the subject to flex both knees through 90 deg or at least to the vertical position and examine the thigh-hip joint-trunk complex for concurrent activity. Now place your hands over his ankles, and while he attempts to repeat the flexion maneuver, apply a small resistance only. Repeat the procedure again with added resistance. As these trials progress through increasing resistances to the flexions, you will begin to notice obvious thigh, hip joint, and trunk involvement to alter the original lying posture. Describe these movements and their magnitude changes as the resistance increases. Is there evidence of tendinous action of the two-joint muscles? Is there marked pelvic tilting? What compensatory movements are evident in the lumbar region of the trunk? In what way is lever action contributing to these adjustments?*

Actions

---

a. Assists in forward tilt of the pelvis; flexion of the hip joint; outward rotation of the thigh

b. Assists in forward tilt of the pelvis; deepens the lumbar lordosis; flexion of the hip joint; outward rotation of the thigh

May assist in forward tilt of the pelvis; flexion of the hip joint; extension of the knee joint

---

(*continued*)

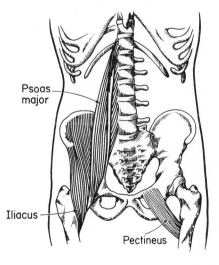

Sartorius

Rectus femoris

Psoas major

Iliacus

Pectineus

| Muscle | Attachments | | Innervation |
	Origin	Insertion	
B. The Medial Group			
1. Adductor brevis	Outer surface of the inferior ramus of the pubis	Proximal half of the linea aspera of the femur	Obturator nerve
2. Adductor longus	Anterior part of the pubis below the crest	Medial lip of the middle third of the linea aspera of the femur	Obturator nerve
3. Adductor magnus	Small section of the inferior ramus of the pubis, inferior ramus of the ischium, inferior part of the ischial tuberosity	Complete length of the linea aspera, medial supracondylar line, and the adductor tubercle of the femur	Obturator sciatic nerves
4. Pectineus	Pectineal line of the pubis	Pectineal line of the femur	Femoral nerve
C. The Lateral Group			
1. Gluteus medius	Outer surface of the ilium between the posterior and anterior gluteal lines	Lateral surface of the greater trochanter of the femur	Superior gluteal nerve
2. Gluteus minimus	Outer surface of the ilium between the anterior and interior gluteal lines	The anterior border of the greater trochanter of the femur	Superior gluteal nerve
D. The Posterior Group			
1. Gluteus maximus	Superior gluteal line and crest of the ilium, the posterior surface of the lower sacrum, and the lateral border of the coccyx	Iliotibial tract and the gluteal tuberosity of the femur	Inferior gluteal nerve

Adduction of the hip joint; transverse adduction of the hip joint from flexed hip positions; assists in flexion of the hip joint, and inward rotation of the thigh

Adduction of the hip joint; transverse adduction of the hip joint from flexed hip positions; assists in flexion of the hip joint, and inward rotation of the thigh

Assists in adduction of the hip joint against resistance, transverse adduction of the hip joint from flexed hip positions, flexion of the hip joint, and inward rotation of the thigh; lower portion may assist in extension of the hip joint from flexed hip positions

Adduction of the hip joint; assists in flexion of the hip joint, transverse adduction of the hip joint from flexed hip positions, and inward rotation of the thigh

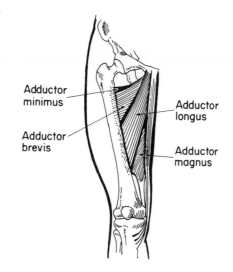

Stabilizes the pelvis against lateral tilt to the opposite side in single-limb standing; abduction of the hip joint; assists in transverse abduction of the hip joint from flexed hip positions, and inward rotation of the thigh

Stabilizes the pelvis against lateral tilt to the opposite side in single-limb standing; abduction of the hip joint; assists in transverse abduction of the hip joint from flexed hip positions, and inward rotation of the thigh

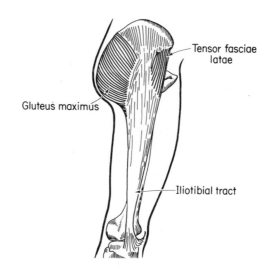

Assists in backward tilt of the pelvis; extension of the hip joint against resistance; outward rotation of the thigh; upper fibers assist in transverse abduction of the hip joint against resistance in flexed hip positions

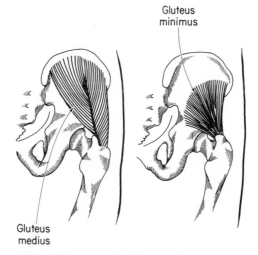

263   *Pelvic Girdle, Vertebral Column, Head-Neck*

| Muscle | Attachments | | Innervation |
	Origin	Insertion	
2. Biceps femoris a. Long head	a. Tuberosity of the ischium	Lateral side of the head of the fibula, lateral condyle of the tibia	a. Tibial nerve
b. Short head	b. Lateral lip of the linea aspera		b. Peroneal nerve
3. Semimembranosus	Tuberosity of the ischium	Medial aspect of the medial condyle of the tibia	Tibial nerve
4. Semitendinosus	Tuberosity of the ischium	Proximal part of the medial surface of the shaft of the tibia	Tibial nerve

II. The Trunk and Head-Neck Muscles

A. The Abdominal Group

Muscle	Origin	Insertion	Innervation
1. Rectus abdominis	Crest of the pubis and the ligaments covering the ventral surface of the symphysis pubis	The cartilage of the 5th, 6th, and 7th ribs	Seventh through 12th intercostal nerves
2. External abdominal oblique	Lower borders of the lower eight ribs by tendinous slips	Anterior half of the iliac crest, crest of the pubis, and the linea alba	Eighth through 12th intercostal and the iliohypogastric and ilioinguinal nerves

a. Assists in backward tilt of the pelvis; extension of the hip joint; assists in adduction of the hip joint from abducted hip positions, and outward rotation of the thigh in extended hip positions

a. and b. Flexion of the knee joint

Assists in backward tilt of the pelvis; extension of the hip joint; assists in adduction of the hip joint against resistance, and inward rotation of the thigh; flexion of the knee joint; assists in inward rotation of the leg

Assists in backward tilt of the pelvis; extension of the hip joint; assists in adduction of the hip joint against resistance, and inward rotation of the thigh; flexion of the knee joint; assists in inward rotation of the leg

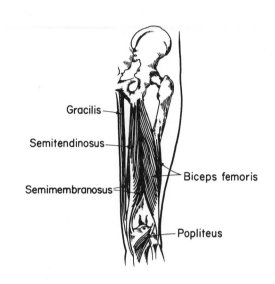

Gracilis

Semitendinosus

Semimembranosus

Biceps femoris

Popliteus

Combined: Flexion of the trunk; backward tilt of the pelvis; assists in tensing the abdominal wall

Individual: Assists in lateral flexion of the trunk to the same side

Combined: Flexion of the trunk; assists in backward tilt of the pelvis; assists in tensing the abdominal wall

Individual: Lateral flexion of the trunk to the same side; rotation of the trunk to the opposite side

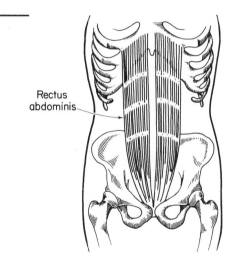

Rectus abdominis

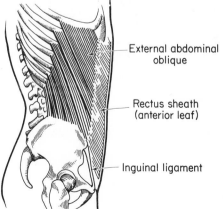

External abdominal oblique

Rectus sheath (anterior leaf)

Inguinal ligament

| | Attachments | | |
Muscle	Origin	Insertion	Innervation
3. Internal abdominal oblique	Lateral half of the inguinal ligament, anterior two thirds of the crest of the ilium, and the thoracolumbar fascia	Inferior borders of the cartilage of the lower three or four ribs and the linea alba	Eighth through 12th intercostal and the iliohypogastric and ilioinguinal nerves
4. Transversus abdominis	Lateral third of the inguinal ligament, anterior three-fourths of the inner lip of the iliac crest, cartilage of the lower six ribs, thoracolumbar fascia	Linea alba	Seventh through 12th inter-costals, the iliohypogastric, and the ilioinguinal nerves
5. Quadratus lumborum	Iliolumbar ligament and the iliac crest	Inferior border of the last rib	Twelfth thoracic and 1st lumbar nerves

B. Posterior Back and Neck Group—Layer I

1. Erector spinae (Sacrospinalis)

a. Iliocostalis lumborum	a. Posterior aspect of the sacrum, iliac crest, spinous processes of the lumbar vertebrae and the 11th and 12th thoracic vertebrae	a. Inferior borders of the lower six or seven ribs	a. Spinal nerves
b. Iliocostalis thoracis	b. Upper borders of the angles of the lower six ribs	b. Upper borders of the angles of the first six ribs and the transverse process of the 7th cervical vertebra	b. Spinal nerves
c. Iliocostalis cervicis	c. Upper borders of the angles of the 3rd, 4th, 5th, and 6th ribs	c. Transverse processes of the 4th, 5th, and 6th cervical vertebrae	c. Spinal nerves
d. Longissimus thoracis	d. Posterior surface of the transverse processes of the lumbar vertebrae and the lumbocostal aponeurosis	d. The tips of the transverse processes of all the thoracic vertebrae and the lower nine or ten ribs medial to their angles	d. Spinal nerves
e. Longissimus cervicis	e. Transverse processes of the upper four or five thoracic vertebrae	e. Transverse processes of the 2nd through 6th cervical vertebrae	e. Spinal nerves

Actions

Combined: Flexion of the trunk; assists in tensing the abdominal wall

Individual: Lateral flexion and rotation of the trunk to the same side

Assists in tensing the abdominal wall; compresses the abdominal contents

Combined: Stabilization of the lumbar region of the vertebral column; may assist in forward tilt of the pelvis

Individual: Assists in lateral flexion of the trunk to the same side

a. Combined: Extension and hyperextension of the trunk; forward tilt of the pelvis

Individual: Lateral flexion and rotation of the trunk to the same side

b. Combined: Extension and hyperextension of the trunk; forward tilt of the pelvis

Individual: Lateral flexion and rotation of the trunk to the same side

c. Combined: Extension and hyperextension of the upper trunk and neck regions

Individual: Lateral flexion and rotation of the upper trunk and neck regions to the same side

d. Combined: Extension and hyperextension of the trunk

Individual: Lateral flexion and rotation of the trunk to the same side

e. Combined: Extension and hyperextension of the upper trunk and neck regions

Individual: Lateral flexion and rotation of the upper trunk and neck regions to the same side

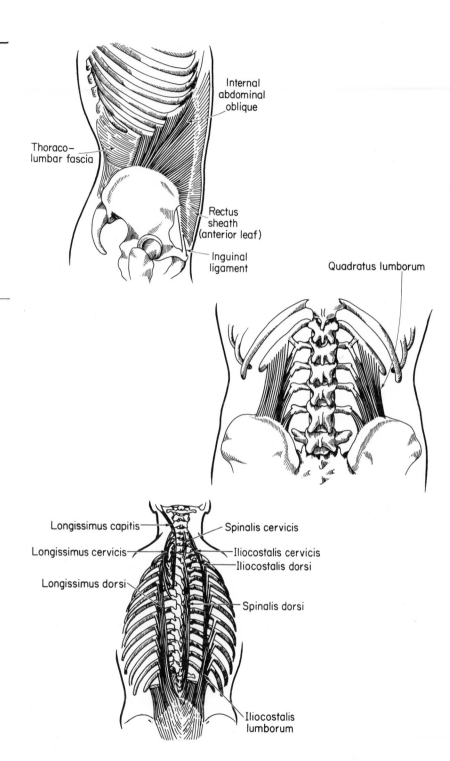

Internal abdominal oblique

Thoraco-lumbar fascia

Rectus sheath (anterior leaf)

Inguinal ligament

Quadratus lumborum

Longissimus capitis

Longissimus cervicis

Longissimus dorsi

Spinalis cervicis

Iliocostalis cervicis

Iliocostalis dorsi

Spinalis dorsi

Iliocostalis lumborum

| Muscle | Attachments | | Innervation |
	Origin	Insertion	
f. Longissimus capitis	f. Transverse processes of the upper four or five thoracic vertebrae, articular processes of the last four cervical vertebra	f. Mastoid process	f. Spinal nerves
g. Spinalis thoracis	g. Spinous processes of the first two lumbar and the last two thoracic vertebrae	g. Spinous processes of the upper thoracic vertebrae	g. Spinal nerves
h. Spinalis cervicis	h. Ligamentum nuchae and the spinous process of the 7th cervical vertebrae	h. Spinous process of the axis	h. Spinal nerves
2. Splenius cervicis	Spinous processes of the 3rd through 6th thoracic vertebrae	Transverse processes of the upper two or three cervical vertebrae	Middle and lower cervical spinal nerves
3. Splenius capitis	Ligamentum nuchae and the spinous processes of the 7th cervical and first three or four thoracic vertebrae	Superior nuchal line of the occipital bone and the mastoid process of the temporal bone	Middle and lower cervical spinal nerves

C. The Posterior Back and Neck Group—Layer II

Muscle	Origin	Insertion	Innervation
1. Multifidus	Posterior aspect of the sacrum and iliac crest, transverse processes of the lumbar and thoracic vertebral articular processes of the 4th through 7th cervical vertebrae	All spinous processes from the last lumbar vertebra to the axis	Spinal nerves
2. Rotatores	Transverse processes of all the vertebrae from the sacrum to the axis	Spinous processes of the next two vertebrae above the origin	Spinal nerves
3. Semispinalis thoracis	Transverse processes of the 6th through 10th thoracic vertebrae	Spinous processes of the upper four through the lower two cervical vertebrae	Spinal nerves
4. Semispinalis cervicis	Transverse processes of the first five or six thoracic vertebrae	The spinous processes of the axis through the 5th cervical vertebrae	Spinal nerves
5. Semispinalis capitis	Transverse processes of the first six thoracic and the 7th cervical vertebrae, articular processes of the 4th through 6th cervical vertebrae	Between the superior and inferior nuchal lines of the occipital bone	Spinal nerves

f. Combined: Extension and hyperextension of the upper trunk region and the head-neck segment

Individual: Lateral flexion and rotation of the head-neck to the same side

g. Combined: Extension and hyperextension of the upper trunk

Individual: Lateral flexion of the upper trunk to the same side

h. Combined: Extension and hyperextension of the neck

Individual: Lateral flexion and rotation of the neck to the same side

Combined: Assists in extension and hyperextension of the neck

Individual: Lateral flexion of the neck to the same side

Combined: Extension and hyperextension of the head-neck segment

Individual: Lateral flexion and rotation of the head-neck to the same side

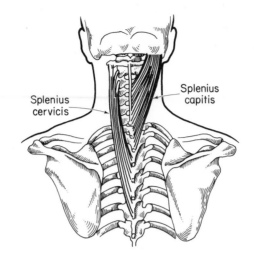

Splenius cervicis

Splenius capitis

Combined: Extension and hyperextension of the trunk and neck; assists in forward tilt of the pelvis

Individual: Assists in lateral flexion and rotation of the trunk and neck regions to the opposite side

Combined: Extension and hyperextension of the trunk and neck

Individual: Assists in rotation of the trunk and neck to the opposite side

Combined: Extension and hyperextension of the upper trunk

Individual: Lateral flexion and rotation of the upper trunk to the opposite side

Combined: Extension and hyperextension of the upper trunk and neck regions; assists in supporting the head in standing

Individual: Lateral flexion and rotation of the upper trunk and neck regions to the opposite side

Combined: Extension and hyperextension of the head-neck segment; assists in supporting the head in standing

Individual: Assists in lateral flexion of the head-neck segment to the same side

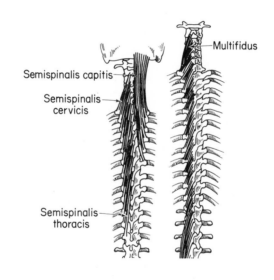

Multifidus

Semispinalis capitis

Semispinalis cervicis

Semispinalis thoracis

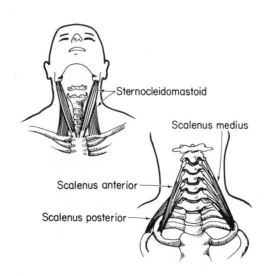

Sternocleidomastoid

Scalenus medius

Scalenus anterior

Scalenus posterior

(continued)

Muscle	Attachments		Innervation
	Origin	Insertion	
D. The Anterior Neck Group			
1. Scaleni (anterior, medius, posterior)	First and 2nd ribs	Transverse processes of the 2nd through 7th cervical vertebrae	Cervical spinal nerves
2. Sternocleidomastoid	Upper part of the manubrium of the sternum, anterior superior border of the medial third of the clavicle	Mastoid process	Spinal part of the accessory nerve and branches from the 2nd and 3rd cervical nerves

REFERENCES

Asmussen, E., and Klausen, K. "Form and Function of the Erect Human Spine." *Clinical Orthopedics* 25 (1962): 55.

Barnett, C. H. "The Structure and Function of Fibrocartilage Within Vertebral Joints." *Journal of Anatomy* 88 (1954): 363.

Bartelink, D. L. "The Role of Abdominal Pressure in Relieving the Pressure on the Lumbar Intervertebral Discs." *Journal of Bone and Joint Surgery* 39-B (1957): 718.

Basmajian, J. V. "Electromyography of Postural Muscles." In *Biomechanical Studies of the Musculo-Skeletal System*, edited by F. G. Evans. Springfield, Ill.: Charles C Thomas, Publisher, 1961.

———— "Man's Posture." *Archives of Physical Medicine and Rehabilitation* 46 (1965): 26.

———— *Muscles Alive; Their Function Revealed by Electromyography.* 2d ed. Baltimore: The Williams & Wilkins Company, 1967.

Bearn, J. G. "The Significance of the Activity of the Abdominal Muscles in Weight Lifting." *Acta Anatomica* 45 (1961): 83.

Brown, L. T. "The Mechanics of the Lumbosacral and Sacroiliac Joints." *Journal of Bone and Joint Surgery* 19 (1937): 770.

Campbell, E. J. M. "An Electromyographic Study of the Role of the Abdominal Muscles in Breathing." *Journal of Physiology* 117 (1952): 222.

Cave, A. J. E. "On the Occipito-atlanto-axial Articulation." *Journal of Anatomy* 68 (1934): 416.

Clayson, S. J.; Newman, I. M.; Debevec, D. F.; Anger, R. W.; Skowland, H. V.; and Kottke, S. J. "Evaluation of Mobility of Hip and Lumbar Vertebrae of Normal Young Women." *Archives of Physical Medicine* 43 (1962): 1.

Colachis, S. C.; Worden, R. E.; Bechtol, C. O.; and Strohm, B. R. "Movement of the Sacroiliac Joint in the Adult Male: Preliminary Report." *Archives of Physical Medicine and Rehabilitation* 44 (1963): 490.

David, H.; Hamley, E. J.; and Saunders, G. R. "Electromyographic and Cinematographic Analysis of Spinal Extension Under Stress." *Journal of Physiology* 200 (1969): 4P.

Davies, D. V. "Aging Changes in Joints." In *Structural Aspects of Aging*, edited by G. H. Bourne. New York: Hafner Publishing Company, Inc., 1961.

Davis, P. R. "Human Lower Lumbar Vertebrae: Some Mechanical and Osteological Considerations." *Journal of Anatomy* 95 (1961): 337.

———— "The Medial Inclination of the Human Thoracic Intervertebral Articular Facets." *Journal of Anatomy* 93 (1959): 68.

———— "Posture of the Trunk During the Lifting of Weights." *British Medical Journal* 5114 (1959): 87.

Davis, P. R.; Troup, J. D. G.; and Burnard, J. H. "Movements of the Thoracic

Combined: Assists in flexion of the head-neck segment
Individual: Assists in lateral flexion of the head-neck segment to the same side

Combined: Flexion of the head-neck segment
Individual: Lateral flexion and rotation of the head-neck segment to the opposite side

and Lumbar Spine When Lifting: A Chronocylophotographic Study." *Journal of Anatomy* 99 (1965): 13.

Defibaugh, J. J. "Measurement of Head Motion: Part I. A Review of Methods of Measuring Joint Motion." *Physical Therapy* 44 (1964): 157.

——— "Measurement of Head Motion: Part II. An Experimental Study of Head Motion in Adult Males." *Physical Therapy* 44 (1964): 163.

Evans, F. G., and Lissner, H. R. "Biomechanical Studies on the Lumbar Spine and Pelvis." *Journal of Bone and Joint Surgery* 41-A (1959): 278.

Evans, F. G.; Lissner, H. R.; and Patrick, L. M. "Acceleration-Induced Strains in the Intact Vertebral Column." *Journal of Applied Physiology* 17 (1962): 405.

Ferlic, D. "The Range of Motion of the 'Normal' Cervical Spine." *Bulletin of the Johns Hopkins Hospital* 110 (1962): 59.

Fineman, S.; Boreili, F. J.; Rubenstein, B. M.; Epstein, H.; and Jacobson, H. G. "The Cervical Spine: Transformation of the Normal Lordotic Pattern into a Linear Pattern in the Neutral Posture. A Roentgenographic Demonstration." *Journal of Bone and Joint Surgery* 45 (1963): 1179.

Fischer, F. J., and Houtz, S. J. "Evaluation of the Function of the Gluteus Maximus Muscle: An Electromyographic Study." *American Journal of Physical Medicine* 47 (1968): 182.

Flint, M. M. "Abdominal Muscle Involvement During the Performance of Various Forms of Sit-Up Exercise." *American Journal of Physical Medicine and Rehabilitation* 44 (1965): 224.

——— "An Electromyographic Comparison of the Function of the Iliacas and the Rectus Abdominis Muscles. A Preliminary Report." *Physical Therapy* 45 (1965): 248.

——— "Flexibility of Hip-Trunk, Trunk Strength and Posture Related to Gravity Line Test." *Research Quarterly* 35 (1964): 141.

——— "Lumbar Posture: A Study of Roentgenographic Measurement and the Influence of Flexibility and Strength." *Research Quarterly* 34 (1963): 15.

Flint, M. M., and Diehl, B. "Influence of Abdominal Strength, Back Extensor Strength and Trunk Strength Balance Upon Antero-Postero Alignment of Elementary School Girls." *Research Quarterly* 32 (1961): 490.

Flint, M. M., and Gudgell, J. "Electromyographic Study of Abdominal Muscular Activity During Exercise." *Research Quarterly* 36 (1965): 29.

Floyd, W. F., and Silver, P. H. S. "Electromyographic Study of Patterns of Activity of the Anterior Abdominal Wall Muscles in Man." *Journal of Anatomy* 84 (1950): 132.

——— "Function of Erectores Spinae in Flexion of the Trunk." *Lancet* 1 (1951): 133.

——— "The Function of the Erectores Spinae Muscles in Certain Movements and Postures in Man." *Journal of Physiology* 129 (1955): 184.

Fountain, F. P.; Minear, W. L.; and Allison R. D. "Function of Longus Colli and Longissimus Cervicis Muscles in Man." *Archives of Physical Medicine and Rehabilitation* 47 (1966): 665.

Fox, M. G., and Young, O. G. "Placement of the Gravity Line in Anteroposterior Posture." *Research Quarterly* 25 (1954): 277.

Francis, C. C. "Dimensions of the Cervical Vertebrae." *Anatomical Record* 122 (1955): 603.

Goss, Charles Mayo, ed. *Gray's Anatomy of the Human Body.* 28th ed. Philadelphia: Lea & Febiger, 1966.

Grant, C. Boileau. *An Atlas of Anatomy.* 5th ed. Baltimore: The Williams & Wilkins Company, 1962.

Hadley, L. A. "Anatomico-Roentgenographic Studies of the Posterior Spinal Articulations." *American Journal of Roentgenology, Radium Therapy and Nuclear Medicine* 86 (1961): 27.

Hall, Michael C. *The Locomotor System: Functional Anatomy.* Springfield, Ill.: Charles C. Thomas, Publisher, 1965.

Hawley, Gertrude. *The Kinesiology of Corrective Exercise.* 2d ed. Philadelphia: Lea & Febiger, 1949.

Hellebrandt, F. A.; Riddle, K. S.; Larson, E. M.; and Fries, E. C. "Gravitational Influences on Postural Alignment." *Physiotherapy Review* 22 (1942): 143.

Hirsch, C. "The Reaction of Intervertebral Discs to Compression Forces." *Journal of Bone and Joint Surgery* 37-A (1955): 1189.

Holtze, I. "Aid for Teaching Pelvic Tilt." *Physical Therapy Review* 43 (1963): 114.

Horton, W. G. "Further Observations on the Elastic Mechanism of the Intervertebral Disc." *Journal of Bone and Joint Surgery* 40-B (1958): 552.

Jensen, Clayne R., and Schultz, Gordon W. *Applied Kinesiology.* New York: McGraw-Hill Book Company, 1970.

Joseph, J. *Man's Posture, Electromyographic Studies.* Springfield, Ill.: Charles C. Thomas, Publisher, 1960.

Joseph, J., and McCall, I. "Electromyography of Posterior Vertebral Muscles." *Journal of Anatomy* 94 (1960): 285.

Keagy, R. D.; Brumlick, J.; and Bergan, J. J. "Direct Electromyography of the Psoas Major Muscle in Man." *Journal of Bone and Joint Surgery* 48-A (1966): 1377.

Kendall, Henry O., and Kendall, Florence P. *Muscles, Testing and Function.* Baltimore: The Williams & Wilkins Company, 1949.

Knapp, M. E. "Function of the Quadratus Lumborum." *Archives of Physical Medicine* 32 (1951): 505.

Kottke, F. J., and Mundale, M. A. "Range of Mobility of the Cervical Spine." *Archives of Physical Medicine and Rehabilitation* 40 (1959): 379.

LaBan, M. M.; Raptou, A. D.; and Johnson, E. W. "Electromyographic Study of Function of Iliopsoas Muscle." *Archives of Physical Medicine and Rehabilitation* 46 (1965): 676.

Lipetz, S., and Gutin, B. "An Electromyographic Study of Four Abdominal Exercises." *Medicine and Science in Sports* 2 (1970): 35.

Logan, G. A., and McKinney, W. C. "The Serape Effect." *Journal of Health, Physical Education, Recreation* 41 (1970): 79.

Lucas, D. B., and Bresler, B. "Stability of the Ligamentous Spine." Technical Report Series II, no. 40. University of California Biomechanics Laboratory, 1960.

MacConaill, M. A., and Basmajian, J. V. *Muscles and Movement, A Basis for Human Kinesiology.* Baltimore: The Williams & Wilkins Company, 1969.

Massey, Benjamin H.; Manson, Frank R.; Freeman, Harold W.; and Wessel, Janet A. *The Kinesiology of Weight Lifting.* Dubuque, Iowa: William C. Brown Company, Publishers, 1959.

Michele, Arthur A. *Iliopsoas*. Springfield, Ill.: Charles C Thomas, Publisher, 1962.

Milch, H. "The Measurement of Pelvi-Femoral Motion." *Anatomical Record* 140 (1961): 135.

Mitchell, G. A. G. "The Lumbosacral Junction." *Journal of Bone and Joint Surgery* 16 (1934): 233.

Morris, J. M.; Benner, G.; and Lucas, D. B. "An Electromyographic Study of the Intrinsic Muscles of the Back in Man." *Journal of Anatomy* 96 (1962): 509.

Morris, J. M.; Lucas, D. B.; and Bresler, B. "Role of the Trunk in Stability of the Spine." *Journal of Bone and Joint Surgery* 43-A (1961): 327.

Nachemson, A. "Electromyographic Studies of the Vertebral Portion of the Psoas Muscle." *Acta Orthopaedica Scandinavica* 37 (1966): 177.

Partridge, M. J., and Walters, C. E. "Participation of the Abdominal Muscles in Various Movements of the Trunk in Man." *Physical Therapy Review* 39 (1959): 791.

Pauly, J. E. "An Electromyographic Analysis of Certain Movements and Exercises: I. Some Deep Muscles of the Back." *Anatomical Record* 155 (1966): 223.

Quiring, Daniel P., and Warfel, John H. *The Head, Neck, and Trunk*. 2d ed. Philadelphia: Lea & Febiger, 1960.

Raper, A. J.; Thompson, W. T.; Shapiro, W.; and Patterson, J. S. "Scalene and Sternomastoid Muscle Function." *Journal of Applied Physiology* 21 (1966): 497.

Rasch, Philip J., and Burke, Roger K. *Kinesiology and Applied Anatomy*. 3rd ed. Philadelphia: Lea & Febiger, 1967.

Sheffield, F. J. "Electromyographic Study of the Abdominal Muscles in Walking and Other Movements." *American Journal of Physical Medicine* 41 (1962): 142.

Silver, P. H. S. "Direct Observation of Changes in Tension in the Supraspinous and Interspinous Ligaments During Flexion and Extension of the Vertebral Column in Man." *Journal of Anatomy* 88 (1954): 550.

Solonen, K. A. "The Sacro-iliac Joint in the Light of Anatomical Roentgenological and Clinical Studies." *Acta Orthopaedica Scandinavica* 27 Suppl. (1957).

Steen, B. "The Function of Certain Neck Muscles in Different Positions of the Head With and Without Loading of the Cervical Spine." *Acta Morphologica Neerlando-Scandinavica* 6 (1966): 301.

Steindler, Arthur. *Kinesiology of the Human Body*. Springfield, Ill.: Charles C. Thomas, Publisher, 1955.

Swearingen, J. J. "Determination of Centers of Gravity of Man." *Federal Aviation Agency Report* 62-14 (1962): 37.

Troup, J. D.; Hood, C. A.; and Chapman, A. E. "Measurements of the Sagittal Mobility of the Lumbar Spine and Hips." *Annals of Physical Medicine* 9 (1968): 308.

Walters, C. E., and Partridge, M. J. "Electromyographic Study of the Differential Action of the Abdominal Muscles During Exercises." *American Journal of Physical Medicine* 36 (1957): 259.

Weisl, H. "The Articular Surfaces of the Sacro-Iliac Joint and Their Relation to the Movements of the Sacrum." *Acta Anatomica* 22 (1954): 1.

——— "The Ligaments of the Sacro-Iliac Joint Examined with Particular Reference to Their Function." *Acta Anatomica* 20 (1954): 201.

——— "The Movements of the Sacro-Iliac Joint." *Acta Anatomica* 20 (1955): 80.

Wells, Katharine F. *Kinesiology*. 4th ed. Philadelphia: W. B. Saunders Company, 1966.

Wiles, P. "Movements of the Lumbar Vertebrae During Flexion and Extension." *Proceedings of the Royal Society of Medicine* 28 (1935): 647.

Winter, F. W. "Mechanics of the Tuck Position in Executing the Forward Three and One-Half Somersault." *Athletic Journal* 45 (1965): 19.

18

Shoulder Girdle, Shoulder Joint, Arm

The upper limb provides man with a unique mechanism to interact with his environment. In comparison with the lower limb, it is endowed with nearly limitless positioning abilities which are so very useful in adjusting the body to suit the environment or in adjusting the environment to suit the body. At the terminations of the upper limbs, the hands can carry out precise manipulations that range from the pianist's technique to scratching an itch near the center of one's back. The fact that this mechanism is attached to the upper-lateral part of the trunk segment illustrates its critical positioning in the body to gain the best advantage for building on the accumulated movements of the lower limbs and the trunk. In addition, its positioning with respect to the head allows for a visual sighting and aiming control which cannot be duplicated elsewhere in the body.

THE SHOULDER GIRDLE

For the purpose of studying the skeletal structure of the upper limb, it is divided into sections. The most proximal section is the *shoulder girdle*, which includes two pairs of bones which function within the trunk segment of the body. Its position in the shoulder areas of the trunk is similar to the epaulets worn on military uniforms which not only crown the point of the shoulder but course inward toward the neck. Like its pelvic counterpart, it, too, is incomplete posteriorly but is not completed by a bony structure.

The Bones of the Shoulder Girdle

A pair of *clavicle* and *scapula* bones join the *sternum* at its superior edges to form the shoulder girdle. Figure 18-1 illustrates their positions relative to the thorax. The left clavicle is shown from below and above in Fig. 18-2

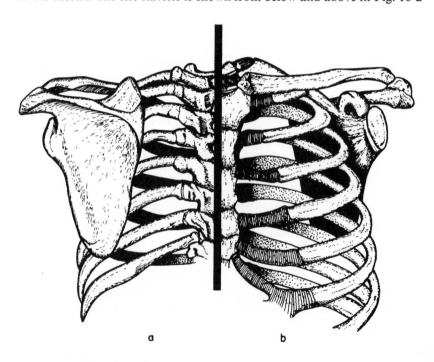

Figure 18–1. The bones of the shoulder girdle as viewed from (*a*) the posterior, and (*b*) the anterior.

a   b

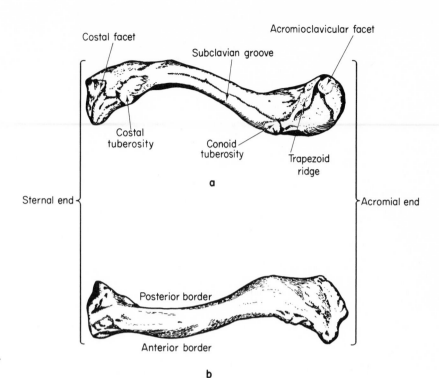

Costal facet

Subclavian groove

Acromioclavicular facet

Costal
tuberosity

Conoid
tuberosity

Trapezoid
ridge

a

Sternal end

Acromial end

Posterior border

Anterior border

b

Figure 18–2. (*a*) Superior and (*b*) inferior views of the left clavicle.

in which it presents a set of graceful curves in the form of a shallow letter S. Its *sternal end* (medial) is to the left, with the *acromial end* (lateral) to the right. It is broader laterally than medially and may be palpated over its entire length. The only bony connection of this incomplete girdle to the thorax is at its sternal end to the *manubrium* of the sternum and the cartilage of the first rib. Positioned somewhat horizontally between the thorax and the scapula, the clavicle acts as a strut which prevents the scapula from collapsing inward on the thorax, thus freeing the upper limb for unobstructed movement. In addition to providing anterior protection to underlying structures, the clavicle is a first-rate lever. Small movements at its sternal end are transformed into large movements at its acromial end, while large lateral movements are suitably reduced in magnitude at the medial, pivoting end.

The left scapula is illustrated in Fig. 18-3, showing its anterior and posterior surfaces. It is a spade-like bone which is suspended in muscle between strictly sagittal and frontal orientations. Three *borders*—the *vertebral, superior,* and *axillary*—are evident between three *angles*—the *superior, inferior,* and *lateral.* The anterior surface is broadly concave to offer the *subscapular fossa* for the attachment of the *subscapularis* muscle. The posterior surface is sectioned into the *infraspinatous* and *supraspinatous fossae* by the intervening scapular *spine.* Its continuation laterally, the *acromion,* overlooks the *glenoid fossa.* The *coracoid process* juts forward and then laterally. In addition to providing extensive surface areas for muscular attachments, the scapula serves as a multiple lever, its numerous angles and bony projections representing lever arms for scapular pivoting.

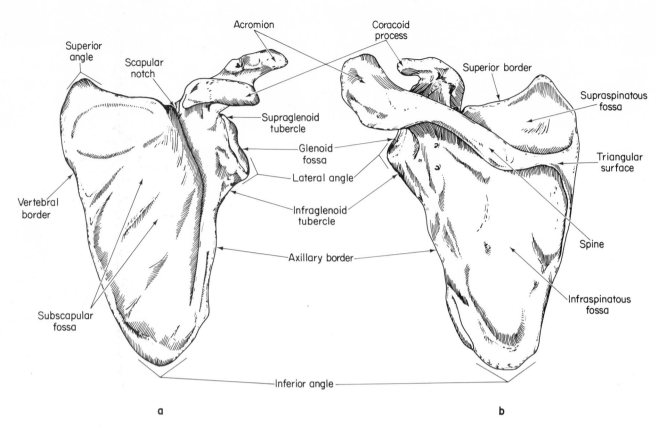

Figure 18–3. (a) Anteromedial and (b) posterolateral views of the left scapula.

The Shoulder Girdle Joints

Viewing the shoulder girdle from above identifies two *acromioclavicular angles* opening inward. From this vantage point (examine the shoulder girdle of an articulated skeleton from above), the *sternoclavicular* and *acromioclavicular* joints and their positions with respect to the thorax may be clearly seen, the former residing farther forward and inward than the latter. In addition to these true joints, a third articulation is commonly noted, the *scapulothoracic*. It is not a true joint but is of value when describing the movements of the scapula over the thorax.

The *sternoclavicular* joint's capsule contains two complete cavities separated by an intra-articular disk (Fig. 18-4). The disk attaches to the clavicle above and to the first costal cartilage below. It functions as an efficient shock buffer between the rather poorly mated joint surfaces. The joint is supported by several ligaments. The strong *anterior* and *posterior sternoclavicular* ligaments are directed obliquely downward and medially, preventing upward and lateral displacements of the clavicle from the small clavicular facet of the manubrium. The *interclavicular* ligament bridges the gap between the sternal ends of each clavicle. The *costoclavicular* ligament joins the clavicle with the first costal cartilage at the costal tuberosity. It, too, courses downward and medially and serves to limit excessive upward and forward movements of the clavicle. The joint is afforded little stability by bony arrangement but is strong because of its ligaments and intervening disk.

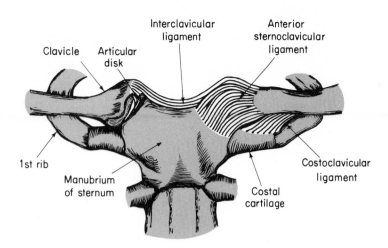

Figure 18-4. The sternoclavicular joint and its ligaments.

This joint provides for gliding movements which, externally, resemble the movements of a ball and socket joint. The clavicle can, therefore, be moved upward-downward and forward-backward and can be circumducted elliptically. Upward and downward movements are accompanied by rotation about the clavicle's long axis. When the clavicle is lifted sufficiently upward, its upper surface rolls somewhat to the posterior. When moved downward again, the rotation is reversed. Functionally, clavicular movements are dependent on the associated movements at the acromioclavicular and shoulder joints.

→ *To illustrate this, palpate the anterior border of one clavicle where its forward concavity begins. Shrug your shoulder up and down, forward and backward. Now circumduct the clavicle in both directions.*

The rotations about its long axis are usually beyond the sensitivity of palpation. By marking the skin anterior to and above the approximate center of clavicular pivoting (this is located somewhat lateral to the knobby sternal end) and a second pair of points along its length, one can estimate the angular range of the upward-downward and forward-backward movements.

The *acromioclavicular* joint obtains its primary stability from its ligamentous binding rather than from its bony architecture. Even so, the joint is generally weak and is therefore easily dislocated. The articular surfaces are situated so that forces applied to the lateral aspect of the acromion tend to drive it beneath the more elevated clavicle. In addition to the *superior* and *inferior capsular* ligaments, the primary resistance to such an outcome is provided by the strong, two-part *coracoclavicular* ligament (Fig. 18-5), which acts to transfer these scapular stresses to the clavicle and then to the sternoclavicular joint. Its two sections are known as the *conoid* and *trapezoid* ligaments. The clavicle is thus bound to the scapula at the coracoid process to form what is occasionally called the fibrous, *coracoclavicular* joint. The scapula is then said to hang from the clavicle. Residing beneath the joint is the *coracoacromial* ligament.

The scapula may move upon the clavicle at this joint, and may move with the clavicle as well when the acromioclavicular mobility is com-

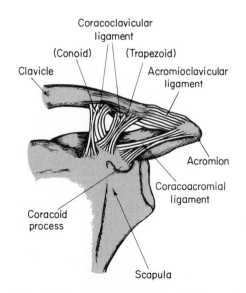

Figure 18-5. The acromioclavicular joint and its supporting ligaments.

pleted. Thus, movements beyond those where the scapula accompanies the clavicle are available. Shoulder girdle movements are customarily defined with respect to scapular movements, in which case it is necessary to point out again the inseparable nature of these movements from those of the sternoclavicular and shoulder joints. They are shoulder girdle

1. *Protraction* (abduction), which moves the scapula laterally in essentially the same line as is demonstrated by its superior border. Because the scapula hugs the curved rib cage during most of its movements, the resulting action is not limited to the frontal plane but resembles the movement of an open hand sliding around the surface of a basketball. Accordingly, the glenoid fossa would face more to the anterior than in its neutral position. With these circumstances in mind, it would appear that *protraction* may well be the more useful term for this movement, although abduction is in common usage.

2. *Retraction* (adduction), the return from protraction and a continuation of the motion beyond the neutral position toward the vertebral column. In the terminally retracted position, the glenoid fossa faces laterally, with the scapular plane approximating a frontal orientation.

3. *Elevation*, accomplished when the scapula moves upward without changing the orientation of its vertebral border. The movement involves the upward movement of the clavicle, which necessitates acromioclavicular adjustments to allow the scapula to rise without undue upward rotation.

4. *Depression*, the return from elevation, accompanied by downward movement of the clavicle. Depression beyond the neutral position is quite limited because further downward excursion by the clavicle is limited by the first rib.

5. *Upward rotation*, a movement which pivots the scapula so that the glenoid fossa is directed upwardly. Consequently, the inferior angle moves away from the vertebral column, while the vertebral border progressively forms a larger, downward-opening angle with the vertebral column. Upward rotation and protraction often accompany one another.

6. *Downward rotation*, the return from upward rotation. It may continue to a small extent beyond the neutral position. Downward rotation and retraction are commonly associated.

In addition to the primary movements described above, slight amounts of scapular *tilting* may occur. Tilting is characterized by the rotations of the scapula about its bilateral and polar axes. In the former, the inferior angle is lifted posteriorly away from the thorax so that a notable protrusion is visible externally. In the latter, the vertebral border is lifted away from the thorax. Both may occur simultaneously when reaching behind the back to touch the inferior angle of the opposite scapula.

→ *Try this in front of a mirror and determine why they occur together. Have a friend perform the movement so that you can examine the degree to which the scapula is tilted. You should be able to place your fingertips directly behind the vertebral border along most of its length. If the acromioclavicular joint were replaced by solid bone, how would shoulder girdle movements differ from those already discussed?*

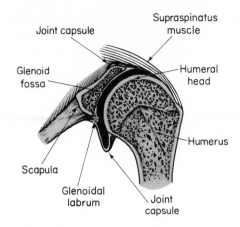

Figure 18–6. A frontal section through the shoulder joint.

The muscles which motivate shoulder girdle movements from proximal origins to shoulder girdle insertions are the *subclavius, serratus anterior*, and *pectoralis minor* anteriorly, and the *rhomboids, trapezius*, and *levator scapulae* posteriorly. The careful study of Muscle Chart 5 reveals that the combined actions of these muscles include many classic synergic and force couple operations. Numerous other muscles affect the positioning of the shoulder girdle and scapula in particular. However, they may be conveniently classified with respect to shoulder joint movements on the scapula, the subject of the subsequent section.

The rhomboids, levator scapulae, and trapezius all are positioned to exhibit retraction components. In addition, the rhomboids and levator scapulae exhibit elevation and downward rotation components. Examination of the fiber directions of the extensive trapezius shows that in addition to retraction, it may also assist in upward rotation of the scapula. The lower fibers are positioned to exhibit a useful depression component as well. If all of these force components were applied in unison, the result would be relatively pure retraction with mutual neutralization of the elevation-depression and upward-downward rotation components. If upward rotation were desired with other associated scapular movements reduced to a minimum, the upper and lower trapezius, levator scapulae, and lower portion of the serratus anterior would serve as the force couple mechanism. Synergic actions to rule out protraction and retraction result from trapezius and serratus anterior antagonism, while elevation and depression antagonism is evident also within the components of the three muscles.

→ *Limiting your choices of muscles to the six mentioned above, work out tentative muscle synergies and force couples for the remaining shoulder girdle movements which were defined above.*

THE SHOULDER JOINT

The union between the glenoid fossa of the scapula and the head of the *humerus* is an example of a ball and socket joint. In contrast to the hip joint, the shoulder joint sacrifices stability for a remarkable degree of mobility. Figure 18-6 illustrates a frontal section through the shoulder joint. It is evident that the glenoid fossa exhibits a considerably smaller surface area than does the humeral head, which is nearly a half sphere. In addition to the differing surface areas, the glenoid cavity is not curved nearly as abruptly as the humeral head. Consequently, the contact area between the two surfaces is usually rather small. The position of best fit (close-packed) is that of terminal abduction and outward rotation.

In common with the femur, the anatomical axis of the shaft of the humerus forms an angle (angle of inclination) with the true axis for flexion-extension of about 130 deg (Fig. 18-7). Differing from the normal femur, the head and neck axis deviates generally in retroversion. The amount of retroversion is variable from person to person and with age. The glenoid fossa faces outward from behind the thorax, angled about

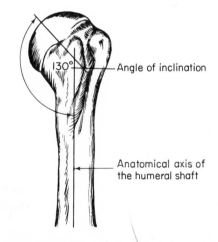

Figure 18–7. The relationship between humeral shaft and head.

equally between frontal and sagittal planes. In addition, it faces upward somewhat. Consequently, the two bones join in the natural side-hanging (pendant) position so that the medial epicondyle of the humerus is posterior to the lateral epicondyle.

→ *Examine your own arms to verify this arrangement. How does assuming the anatomical position from this relaxed position change this relationship?*

Joint Stability

The *glenoidal labrum* is connected to the rim of the glenoid fossa. While it deepens the shoulder socket somewhat, little if any contribution to additional stability accrues. The joint capsule, with its capsular, *glenohumeral* ligaments, provides an anteriorly reinforced but very loose sleeve around the joint. The capsule's inferior aspect includes a very loose fold (Fig. 18-6), which ensures adequate latitude for abduction movements to be carried throughout their great ranges. One ligament, the *coracohumeral*, is positioned to check outward rotation of the humerus and offer a suspension service to the humerus when it hangs unsupported from below. Obviously, by ligamentous arrangement, the shoulder joint is unstable. Refer to Fig. 18-8 for illustrations of these ligaments.

With limited bony and ligamentous stability available, the joint depends heavily on its musculature for the majority of its support. Of primary interest are the four muscles of the *rotator cuff* group, the *supraspinatus*, *infraspinatus*, *teres minor*, and *subscapularis*. Each inserts just beyond the humeral head, blending with the joint capsule and supporting the head by pulling it firmly into its socket. Because of its association with the joint capsule and its superior position over the joint, the supraspinatus is particularly effective in ruling out downward displacement of the humerus in concert with the passive coracohumeral ligament. The ability to suitably position the shoulder girdle to support the wide variety of arm segment movements must also be listed as serving the cause of joint stability; it will be discussed in the following section.

Joint Mobility

The movements of the shoulder joint are the same as those of the hip joint but with larger magnitudes. However, our primary interest is to describe the movements of the arm segment on the trunk, which is not limited to the shoulder joint. It appears clear that the movements of the shoulder girdle accompany those of the shoulder joint to position the glenoid fossa so that minimal inhibition of the proximal end of the humerus is afforded throughout. Also, the ability to reposition the scapula within a wide movement range allows it to be stabilized and act as a platform to anchor a number of the muscles which move the arm. The study of the composite movements of the shoulder complex (shoulder girdle plus shoulder joint) must draw attention to 11 muscles in addition to the 6 listed earlier as moving the shoulder girdle. The temporal relationships of the movements of the shoulder complex have been termed the *scapulohumeral rhythm*.

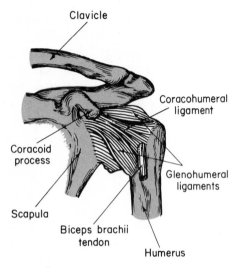

Clavicle

Coracohumeral ligament

Coracoid process

Glenohumeral ligaments

Scapula

Biceps brachii tendon

Humerus

Figure 18–8. An anterior view of the left shoulder joint and its capsular ligaments.

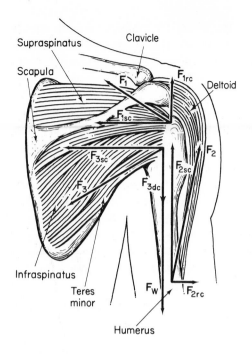

F_1 = Supraspinatus force

F_{1rc} = Supraspinatus rotatory component

F_{1sc} = Supraspinatus horizontal stabilizing component

F_2 = Deltoid force

F_{2rc} = Deltoid rotatory component

F_{2sc} = Deltoid stabilizing component

F_3 = Compound depressor cuff force

F_{3sc} = Depressor cuff horizontal stabilizing component

F_{3dc} = Depressor cuff dislocating component

F_W = Weight of the upper extremity

Figure 18–9. Force analysis about the shoulder joint as abduction begins from the pendant position.

As noted by Duvall, it is wise to use the relaxed, pendant position of the arm segment as the starting position for movement discussion rather than the anatomical position.[1] In this position, the opposing muscles are essentially at rest. From this position the average movements of the shoulder complex are seen to vary considerably from person to person, particularly favoring the female. Average ranges of flexion-extension occur over 160 to 170 deg. Hyperextension averages about 50 to 60 deg. Abduction can be carried through 170- to 180-deg ranges, with some individuals going substantially beyond. Adduction, with the shoulder slightly flexed so that the arm may pass in front of the trunk, may be carried about 50 deg beyond the pendant position. After the shoulder is flexed, 90 deg, transverse abduction is available through approximately 135 deg, with transverse adduction continuing beyond the starting position by about 50 deg. Inward and outward rotations have ranges of nearly 70 deg.

Two shoulder joint movements have been studied carefully with respect to associated shoulder girdle movements. They are shoulder flexion and abduction. Both of these movements may be generally classified as elevation and are therefore similar. In the early phases of shoulder abduction, the deltoid and supraspinatus muscles (Fig. 18-9) are active and increase their intensity as abduction progresses. The horizontally placed supraspinatus mildly arches over the humeral head to insert on the top of the greater tubercle. Its frontally oriented action, F_1, gives rise to a combination of abduction, F_{1rc}, and horizontal stabilization, F_{1sc}. The deltoid (only the middle deltoid is pictured) is much more vertically placed so that its early action, F_2, is characterized by a large, vertical stabilizing component, F_{2sc}, and a small rotatory (abduction) component, F_{2rc}. In combination, deltoid and supraspinatus contractions result in abduction and a very strong tendency to translate the humerus upward along its length, driving the upper surface of the joint into overlying structures.

Since the glenoid fossa faces somewhat upward in this pendant position, it offers little resistance to the upward movement which could result from F_{1rc} and F_{2sc}. It then becomes necessary to provide additional muscular action to stabilize more effectively the head of the humerus in the glenoid cavity. The three remaining rotator cuff muscles, the infraspinatus, teres minor, and subscapularis (not shown), contract synchronously to partially neutralize the upward translation and act as a secondary member of the abductory force couple. In combination with the weight of the limb, F_w, the dislocating component, F_{3dc}, is effective in its neutralizing task to the point where these three muscles are referred to as the *depressor cuff* group. Their action in ruling out the elevation tendencies of the abductors is an example of component synergy.

The combined horizontal stabilizing and depressing components, F_{1sc}, F_{3sc}, and F_{3dc}, of the rotator cuff muscles act to pin the articulating joint surfaces together, which allows the humeral shaft to pivot in abduction about its proximal end. Although F_2 and F_3 are not exactly parallel as illustrated, they represent the abductory force couple members. Intern-

[1]Ellen Neall Duvall, *Kinesiology, The Anatomy of Motion* (Englewood Cliffs, N.J.: Prentice-Hall, Inc., 1959), p. 169.

ally, the head of the humerus glides downward as abduction progresses to finally reach the position of maximal surface contact with the glenoid fossa. The opposing arm-rotation tendencies of the subscapularis and the infraspinatus-teres minor pair are essentially ruled out in helping synergy in the first half of the abduction range.

The first 30 deg of abduction and 60 deg of flexion have been termed "the setting phase" by Inman, Saunders, and Abbott because it appeared to them that these movement ranges were required generally for a stable relationship between the humeral head and scapula to be established.[2] The movements of the scapula on the thorax (scapulothoracic joint) during this phase are irregular from subject to subject and cannot be generalized with accuracy. Upon completion of the setting period, scapulothoracic-to-shoulder joint movements become consistent in a 1:2 ratio. Between 30 and 170 deg of abduction and 60 and 170 deg of flexion, each 15 deg of additional arm elevation is made up of 5 deg of scapular upward rotation and 10 deg of shoulder joint abduction or flexion.

From these figures, it is evident that for a complete 180 deg movement, total shoulder girdle involvement is limited to approximately 60 deg, while shoulder joint involvement may total as much as 120 deg. In addition, for complete abduction to be effected, outward rotation of the humerus must be accomplished to release the shoulder joint area from a building tension which interferes with the motion somewhat after 90 deg. Electromyographic evidence suggests that the neutralized rotation tendencies of the depressor cuff group are interrupted at about this point where the outward rotators obtain the advantage. Thus accomplished, no binding occurs.

→ *To demonstrate the nature of the binding encountered at about 90 deg of abduction, before starting the motion, inward rotate the arm segment completely. Now abduct the shoulder and note that the binding occurs while approaching 90 deg for men and usually somewhat later for women. Now rotate the segment outward and feel the resistance melt away.*

This preliminary inward rotation maneuver is often recognized by gymnasts, performing the iron cross on the still rings, to be of value in augmenting their other muscular efforts to resist falling between the ring supports. Because of the rigidity with which this binding may be enacted, it is important to instruct beginners in the danger of losing control while maintaining the inward rotated position.

The movements within the shoulder girdle during these limb movements are worthy of attention also. For example, of the 60 deg of scapulothoracic upward rotation available, about 40 deg or more are accomplished through elevation of the clavicle at the sternoclavicular joint. It begins early in abduction and obtains at a rate of about 4 deg of clavicular elevation for each 10 deg of shoulder abduction. The clavicular motion is nearly completed in the first 90 deg of shoulder abduction. The backward, axial rotation of the clavicle noted earlier begins after about 55 to 60 deg

[2]V. T. Inman, J. B. deC. M. Saunders, and L. C. Abbott, "Observations on the Functions of the Shoulder Joint," *Journal of Bone and Joint Surgery*, **XXVI**, No. 1 (1944): 9.

of abduction and continues evenly throughout the remaining range of movement. At the acromioclavicular joint, the remaining 20 deg of upward rotation are available. The movement is separated to occur partially in the first 30 deg of abduction, and again after 135 deg. It would appear that in the early portion of this movement, the scapula moves on the clavicle as far as it is able by ligamentous arrangement and joint surface congruity. The two bones then act as a unit, with upward rotation occurring primarily at the sternoclavicular joint. As the sternoclavicular elevation progresses toward its 40 deg limit, backward rotation commences to relieve the tension in the coracoclavicular ligament, thus allowing the scapula to complete its full 20-deg contribution to shoulder girdle upward rotation.

→ *Using Muscle Chart 5* (over), *make a list of the primary shoulder girdle movements, and with the aid of palpation and another person, itemize the shoulder joint muscles which bring them about. Then, identify common sport and athletic activities which depend heavily on these movements.*

Muscle	Origin	Insertion	Innervation
	Attachments		

I. The Shoulder Region Muscles

A. The Shoulder Girdle Group

Muscle	Origin	Insertion	Innervation
1. Levator scapulae	Transverse processes of the axis and atlas and the 3rd and 4th cervical vertebrae	Vertebral border of the scapula between the superior angle and the triangular surface of the scapular spine	Third and 4th cervical nerves
2. Pectoralis minor	Outer surfaces of the 3rd, 4th, and 5th ribs near their costal cartilage	Coracoid process of the scapula	Medial pectoral nerve
3. Rhomboids			
a. Major	a. Spinous processes of the 2nd, 3rd, 4th, and 5th thoracic vertebrae	a. The inferior part of the vertebral border of the scapula below the triangular surface	a. Dorsal scapular nerve
b. Minor	b. Ligamentum nuchae and the spinous processes of the 7th cervical and 1st thoracic vertebrae	b. The vertebral border of the scapula at the triangular surface	b. Dorsal scapular nerve
4. Serratus anterior	Outer surfaces of the first eight or nine ribs	Anterior surface of the vertebral border of the scapula including the inferior angles	Long thoracic nerve
5. Subclavius	First rib and its costal cartilage	Inferior surface of clavicle	Nerve to the subclavius
6. Trapezius			
a. Part I	a.–d. Nuchal line of the occipital bone, ligamentum nuchae, spinous processes of the 7th cervical and all the thoracic vertebrae	a. Posterior border of the lateral third of the clavicle	Spinal accessory nerve and branches from the 3rd and 4th cervical nerves
b. Part II		b. Upper surface of the acromion	
c. Part III		c. Upper border of the scapular spine	
d. Part IV		d. Scapular spine near the apex of the triangular surface	

B. The Shoulder Joint Group

Muscle	Origin	Insertion	Innervation
1. Coracobrachialis	Coracoid process of the scapula	Medial surface of the shaft of the humerus	Musculocutaneous nerve
2. Deltoid			
a. Anterior	a. Anterior border of the lateral third of the clavicle	a.–c. Deltoid tuberosity of the humerus	Axillary nerve
b. Middle	b. Superior surface and lateral margin of the acromion		
c. Posterior	c. Lower border of the scapular spine		

Elevation and downward rotation of the scapula; assists in retraction of the scapula

Depression, downward rotation, protraction, and upward tilt of scapula

a. and b. Elevation, downward rotation, and retraction of the scapula

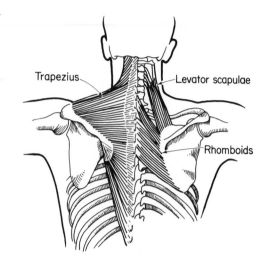

Protraction and upward rotation of the scapula

Depression and stabilization of the clavicle

a. Elevation of the scapula

b. Elevation and upward rotation of the scapula; assists in retraction of the scapula

c. Retraction of the scapula

d. Upward rotation and depression of the scapula; assists in retraction of the scapula

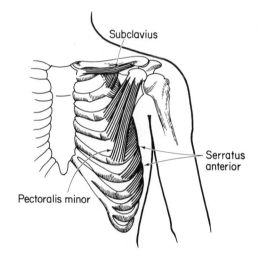

Assists in transverse adduction, flexion, and adduction of the shoulder joint

a. Flexion and transverse adduction of the shoulder joint; assists in inward rotation of the arm

b. Abduction of the shoulder joint

c. Extension and transverse abduction of the shoulder joint; assists in outward rotation of the arm

a.–c. Abduction of the shoulder joint in the plane of the scapula

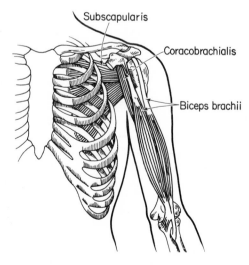

| | Attachments | | |
Muscle	Origin	Insertion	Innervation
3. Supraspinatus	Supraspinatous fossa of the scapula	Greater tubercle of the humerus	Suprascapular nerve
4. Infraspinatus	Medial two thirds of the infraspinatous fossa of the scapula	Greater tubercle of the humerus	Suprascapular nerve
5. Teres minor	Posterior surface of the axillary border of the scapula	Greater tubercle of the humerus	Axillary nerve
6. Subscapularis	Medial two thirds of the subscapular fossa of the scapula	Lesser tubercle of the humerus	Upper and lower subscapular nerves
7. Latissimus dorsi	Spinous processes of the lower six thoracic and all lumbar vertebrae, posterior surface of the sacrum, crest of the ilium, and the lower three ribs	Bicipital groove of the humerus	Thoracodorsal nerve
8. Pectoralis major	Medial half of the clavicle, anterior surface of the sternum, and from the cartilages of the upper six ribs	Crest of the greater tubercle of the humerus	Medial and lateral pectoral nerves
9. Teres major	Inferior angle of the posterior surface of the scapula	Crest of the lesser tubercle of the humerus	Lower subscapular nerve
10. Biceps brachii a. Short head b. Long head	a. Coracoid process of the scapula b. Supraglenoid tubercle of the scapula	Radial tuberosity of the radius	Musculocutaneous nerve
11. Triceps brachii a. Long head b. Lateral head c. Medial head	a. Infraglenoid tubercle of the scapula b. Posterior surface of the shaft of the humerus proximal to the radial groove c. Posterior surface of the shaft of the humerus distal to the radial groove	Proximal surface of olecranon of the ulna	Radial nerve

Abduction of the shoulder joint; stabilizes the humeral head in the glenoid fossa

Assists in transverse abduction of the shoulder joint; outward rotation of the arm; depression and stabilization of the humeral head in the glenoid fossa

Assists in transverse abduction of the shoulder joint; outward rotation of the arm; depression and stabilization of the humeral head in the glenoid fossa

Assists in transverse adduction of the shoulder joint; inward rotation of the arm; depression and stabilization of the humeral head in the glenoid fossa

Extension, hyperextension, and adduction of the shoulder joint; inward rotation of the arm; depression and retraction of scapula through the shoulder joint

Flexion, adduction, and transverse adduction of shoulder joint; inward rotation of the arm; depression and downward rotation of the scapula through the shoulder joint

Active in the maintenance of static arm positions; assists in extension of the shoulder joint in the backswing in walking

a. and b. Flexion of the shoulder joint; flexion of the elbow joint; supination of the forearm against resistance

b. Stabilizes the humeral head in the glenoid fossa

a. Extension and adduction of the shoulder joint

a.–c. Extension of the elbow joint

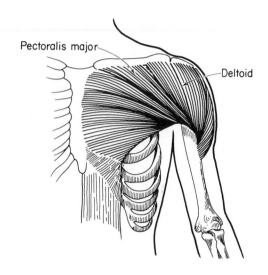

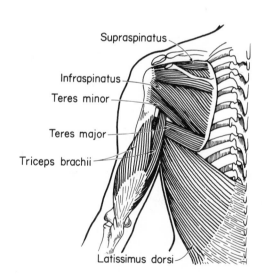

REFERENCES

American Academy of Orthopaedic Surgeons. *Joint Motion—Method of Measuring and Recording.* Chicago: The Academy 1965.

Barnett, C. H.; Davies, D. V.; and MacConaill, M. A. *Synovial Joints, Their Structure and Mechanics.* Springfield, Ill.: Charles C. Thomas, Publisher, 1961.

Basmajian, J. V. *Muscles Alive; Their Function Revealed by Electromyography.* 2d ed. Baltimore: The Williams & Wilkins Company, 1967.

Basmajian, J. V., and Bazant, F. J. "Factors Preventing Downward Dislocation of the Adducted Shoulder Joint." *Journal of Bone and Joint Surgery* 41-A (1959): 1182.

Bassett, David L. *A Stereoscopic Atlas of Human Anatomy.* Portland, Ore.: Sawyer's Inc., 1955.

Bateman, J. E. *The Shoulder and Environs.* St. Louis, Mo.: The C. V. Mosby Company, 1955.

Bearn, J. G. "An Electromyographic Study of the Trapezius, Deltoid, Pectoralis Major, Biceps and Triceps Muscles, During Static Loading of the Upper Limb." *Anatomical Record* 140 (1961): 103.

———— "Function of Certain Shoulder Muscles in Posture and in Holding Weights." *Annals of Physical Medicine* 6 (1961): 100.

Carlin, E. J. "Mechanics of the Shoulder Girdle." *American Journal of Occupational Therapy* 17 (1963): 49.

Clarke, H. H.; Irish, E. A.; Trzynka, G. A.; and Popowich, W. "Conditions for Optimum Work Output in Elbow Flexion, Shoulder Flexion, and Grip Ergography." *Archives of Physical Medicine & Rehabilitation* 39 (1958): 475.

Codman, E. A. *The Shoulder.* Boston: Thomas Todd, 1934.

Conway, A. M. "Movements at the Sternoclavicular and Acromioclavicular Joints." *Physical Therapy* 41 (1961): 421.

Coppock, P. E. "Relationship of Tightness of Pectoral Muscles to Round Shoulders in College Women." *Research Quarterly* 29 (1958): 139.

Dempster, W. T. "Mechanisms of Shoulder Movement." *Archives of Physical Medicine and Rehabilitation* 46 (1965): 49.

Duvall, E. N. "Critical Analysis of Divergent Views of Movement at the Shoulder Joint." *Archives of Physical Medicine and Rehabilitation* 36 (1955): 149.

———— *Kinesiology: The Anatomy of Motion.* Englewood Cliffs, N.J.: Prentice-Hall, Inc., 1959.

Elftman, H. "The Function of the Arms in Walking." *Human Biology* 11 (1939): 529.

Field, Ephraim J., and Harrison, Robert J. *Anatomical Terms: Their Origin and Derivation.* 2d ed. Cambridge: W. Heffer, 1947.

Gaughran, G. R. L., and Dempster, W. T. "Force Analyses of Horizontal Two-Handed Pushes and Pulls in the Sagittal Plane." *Human Biology* 26 (1956): 67.

Hermann, G. W. "An Electromyographic Study of Selected Muscles Involved in the Shot Put." *Research Quarterly* 33 (1962): 1.

Hogue, R. E. "Upper-Extremity Muscular Activity at Different Cadences and Inclines During Normal Gait." *Physical Therapy* 49 (1969): 963.

Inman, V. T. "The Shoulder as a Functional Unit." *Journal of Bone and Joint Surgery* 44-A (1962): 977.

Inman, V. T.; Saunders, J. B. deC. M.; and Abbott, LeR. C. "Observations on the Function of the Shoulder Joint." *Journal of Bone and Joint Surgery* 26 (1944): 1.

Kerwin, G. A.; Roseberg, B.; and Sneed, W. R. "Arthrographic Studies of the Shoulder Joint." *Journal of Bone and Joint Surgery* 39-A (1957): 1267.

Kitzman, E. W. "Baseball: Electromyographic Study of Batting Swing." *Research Quarterly* 35 (1964): 166.

Lewis, O. J. "The Coraco-Clavicular Joint." *Journal of Anatomy* 93 (1959): 296.

Logan, G. A., and McKinney, W. C. "The Serape Effect." *Journal of Health, Physical Education, Recreation* 41 (1970): 79.

Marmor, L.; Bechtol, C. O.; and Hall, C. B. "Pectoralis Major Muscle." *Journal of Bone and Joint Surgery* 43-A (1961): 81.

Mosterd, W. L., and Jongblued, J. "Analysis of the Stroke of Highly Trained Swimmers." *Arbeitsphysiologie* 20 (1964): 288.

Murray, M. P.; Sepic, S. B.; and Barnard, E. J. "Patterns of Sagittal Rotation of the Upper Limbs in Walking: A Study of Normal Men During Free and Fast Speed Walking." *Physical Therapy* 47 (1967): 272.

Provins, K. A. "Maximum Forces Exerted About the Elbow and Shoulder Joints on Each Side Separately and Simultaneously." *Journal of Applied Physiology* 7 (1955): 390.

Quiring, Daniel P., and Warfel, John F. *The Extremities.* Philadelphia: Lea & Febiger, 1967.

Reeder, T. "Electromyographic Study of the Latissimus Dorsi Muscle." *Physical Therapy* 43 (1963): 165.

Saha, A. K. "Zero Position of the Glenohumeral Joint: Its Recognition and Clinical Importance." *Annals of the Royal College of Surgeons of England* 22 (1958): 223.

Salter, N., and Darcus, H. D. "The Amplitude of Forearm and of Humeral Rotation." *Journal of Anatomy* 87 (1953): 407.

Scheving, L. E., and Pauly, J. E. "An Electromyographic Study of Some Muscles Acting on the Upper Extremity of Man." *Anatomical Record* 135 (1959): 239.

Sigerseth, P. O., and McCloy, C. H. "Electromyographic Study of Selected Muscles Involved in Movements of Upper Arm at the Scapulo-humeral Joint." *Research Quarterly* 27 (1956): 409.

Slater-Hammel, A. T. "Action Current Study of Contraction-Movement Relationships in the Golf Stroke." *Research Quarterly* 19 (1948): 164.

———— "An Action Current Study of Contraction-Movement Relationships in the Tennis Stroke." *Research Quarterly* 20 (1949): 424.

Slaughter, D. R. "Electromyographic Studies of Arm Movements." *Research Quarterly* 30 (1959): 326.

Steindler, Arthur. *Kinesiology of the Human Body.* Springfield, Ill.: Charles C. Thomas, Publisher, 1955.

Taylor, C. L., and Blaschke, A. C. "A Method for Kinematic Analysis of Motions of the Shoulder, Arm and Hand Complex." *Annals of the New York Academy of Science* 51 (1951): 1251.

VanLinge, B., and Mulder, J. D. "Function of the Supraspinatus Muscle and its Relation to the Supraspinatus Syndrome." *Journal of Bone and Joint Surgery* 45-B (1963): 750.

Whitley, J. D., and Smith, L. E. "Measurement of Strength of Adduction of the Arm in Various Positions." *Archives of Physical Medicine and Rehabilitation* 45 (1964): 326.

Wiedenbauer, M. M., and Mortensen, D. A. "An Electromyographic Study of the Trapezius Muscle." *American Journal of Physical Medicine* 31 (1952): 363.

Williams, Marian, and Lissner, Herbert R. *Biomechanics of Human Motion.* Philadelphia: W. B. Saunders Company, 1962.

Wright, Wilhelmine G. *Muscle Function.* New York: Hafner Publishing Company, 1962.

Yashmon, L. J., and Bierman, W. "Kinesiologic Electromyography, II. The Trapezius." *Archives of Physical Medicine* 29 (1948): 647.

———— "Kinesiologic Electromyography: III. The Biceps." *Archives of Physical Medicine* 30 (1949): 286.

19

Arm,
Elbow Joint,
Forearm

THE ARM SEGMENT

The arm segment contains the largest bone of the upper extremity, the *humerus*. At its proximal end, it articulates with the scapula to form the shoulder joint. At its distal end, it articulates with both of the forearm bones, forming the elbow joint. The arm and its musculature have received much attention as the symbol of muscular development and strength. So common is its name that it has become the layman's term for the entire upper extremity.

The Arm Bone

Figure 19-1 illustrates anterior and posterior views of the humerus. Its thick proximal end consists of the rounded *head*, which is joined to its shaft by a constricted section known as the *anatomical neck*. Lateral to this neck are two projections, the *greater* and *lesser tubercles*. The proximal surfaces of these tubercles are flattened for the insertions of the rotator cuff muscles. Running between the tubercles is an intermediate trench, which is called the *bicipital groove* because the tendon of the long head of the *biceps brachii* muscle courses within its medial and lateral crests.

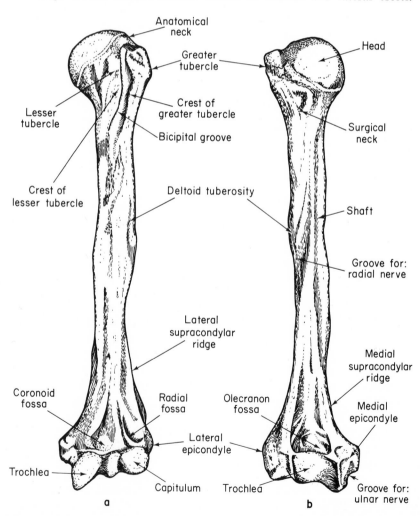

Figure 19–1. (*a*) Anterior and (*b*) posterior views of the left humerus.

Below the tubercles, the proximal end tapers into the *shaft* and is known as the *surgical neck* because fractures often occur at this point.

The upper end of the humeral shaft is rather circular in cross section. About half way down its length on its anterior surface, near its lateral border, is found the triangular projection, the *deltoid tuberosity*. Approaching the distal end, the shaft becomes flatter and broader bilaterally. This broadened area is bordered by *lateral* and *medial supracondylar ridges* which enlarge distally to form the *lateral* and *medial epicondyles*. The medial epicondyle is the more prominent, with its posterior surface containing a groove for the ulnar nerve.

→ *Flex your elbow to about a right angle and palpate this area behind the medial side of the joint. The ulnar nerve may be rolled beneath your fingers. Beware, too much pressure will set your "funny bone" to tingling, a consequence which is often less than humorous.*

Situated below the epicondyles is an articular surface of two parts, separated by a small ridge. The lateral section is rounded and is named the *capitulum*. It receives the proximal end of the *radius* bone at the elbow joint. Directly above the capitulum on the anterior surface is the *radial fossa*. Lateral to it is the *coronoid fossa*, which resides above the *trochlea*, the lateral section of the articular surface. The trochlea articulates singly with the *ulna* of the forearm segment at the elbow joint and from a posterior view is seen to be situated just below the *olecranon fossa*. The coronoid and olecranon fossae are separated from each other by a very thin bone layer which, in some cases, may be perforated to form what is known as the *supratrochlear foramen*. If such a foramen did not exist prior to preparation, the construction of artificial elbow joint hinge mechanisms for articulated skeletons invariably would create one.

As noted in Chapter 18, the humerus is twisted to a marked degree. When comparing the position of the humeral head with those of the epicondyles, a retroverted torsion angle is apparent (Fig. 19-2). The magnitude of the torsion varies considerably in adults to reside generally between 45 and 75 deg. In addition, the distal end of the humerus bends forward to form an angle with the shaft which opens distally to about 20 deg.

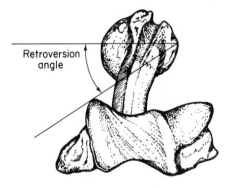

Figure 19–2. The retroversion angle of the humerus.

THE ELBOW JOINT

This intermediate joint of the upper extremity performs a function in common with the knee joint of the lower extremity. Its movements change the direct-line distance between the shoulder and hand just as the knee joint is capable of adjusting the distance between the hip and base of support in standing. The consequences of these seemingly routine distance adjustments are staggering when considered with respect to the habitual actions which depend on them. For instance, if the elbow were always locked in complete extension, the shoulder joint would carry the adjustments burden, and the common radius of its motions would be the length of the entire limb.

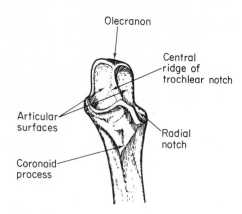

Figure 19–3. The trochlear notch of the left ulna which receives the trochlea of the humerus to form the humeroulnar joint.

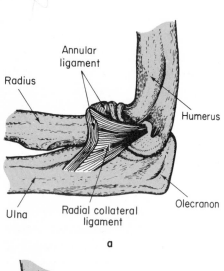

a

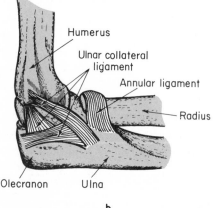

b

Figure 19–4. (a) Lateral and (b) medial views of the left elbow joint, showing its important ligaments.

→ *What would be the mechanism for properly situating the book you are reading to make reading comfortable? In what ways would our dinner table utensils be altered in shape, size, and function to be useful in feeding ourselves? What would be the results of having our elbow joints permanently fixed in complete flexion? Ponder these and similar situations, and the values of a mobile elbow joint mechanism will become abundantly clear.*

The distal end of the humerus is designed to articulate intimately with the ulna medially and with the radius to a less intimate degree laterally. The elbow joint capsule encloses three junctions, including the *proximal radioulnar* joint, which will be discussed in a later section of this chapter. The trochlea, which articulates with the *trochlear notch* of the ulna, is unusually shaped so that its longer medial aspect faces downward and laterally. Its surface then exhibits two curvatures: concave downward in the frontal plane and convex downward in the sagittal plane. The semi-circular, trochlear notch is divided vertically by a ridge (Fig. 19-3) which fits into the constricted channel of the trochlea and is bordered distally by the coronoid process and proximally by the olecranon process. This union within the elbow joint complex is often subclassified as the *humeroulnar* joint.

The capitulum is convex frontally and sagittally to form a half-sphere which faces more forward than downward. The proximal end of the radius is indented mildly to receive the capitulum. It is named the *fovea* and is covered with hyaline cartilage. This junction is often subclassified as the *humeroradial* joint.

Joint Stability

The elbow joint capsule is thin and loose to accommodate the wide range of motion possible in the joint. It is thickened laterally and medially to represent the *radial* and *ulnar collateral* ligaments, respectively. The radial collateral ligament is triangular in shape, with its apex being attached to the lateral epicondyle, coursing downward across the joint so that its base blends into the *annular* ligament which encircles the head of the radius (Fig. 19-4). In addition to reinforcing the joint capsule, it is placed to limit adduction displacement of the forearm on the arm.

The ulnar collateral ligament is also triangular in shape and is variously described by authorities. Its apex is attached to the medial epicondyle of the humerus with two prominent bands, angling downward and forward to the coronoid process in one case and downward and backward to the olecranon in the other. Prominent transverse fibers course between their distal attachments to form the base of the triangle. The area within these bands is usually closed by thin fibrous tissue. Its primary stability functions are the checking of abduction displacement and the reinforcement of the medial aspect of the capsule.

The collateral ligaments of the elbow joint offer another example of axial binding, as was the case for the ankle and knee joints. Again, forward and backward swinging motions are unrestricted. Although anterior and posterior capsular ligaments have been described, certainly little stability function is obtained from them. Consequently, anterior and posterior stabilization is relegated to the musculature. Referring to Muscle Chart 6, it is seen that numerous muscles cross the elbow joint and therefore offer forces for stabilization purposes.

It is the primary flexors (*brachialis*, *biceps brachii*, and *brachioradialis*) and extensors (*triceps brachii* and *anconeus*) which contribute most to the joint's stability in a manner similar to the flexors and extensors of the knee joint. However, their positions are reversed with respect to direction. In addition, a few of the muscles crossing the joint have fibrous attachments to the collateral ligaments, particularly the radial collateral, to add dynamic support. As a result of these structures, the elbow joint is quite stable.

Joint Mobility

Although the elbow joint complex contains three individual articulations, only the humeroulnar and humeroradial junction movements are included here. After the radioulnar joints of the forearm have been described, a discussion of the entire elbow complex mobility will be offered. When the elbow is fully extended in the anatomical position and viewed from the anterior, the long axes of the arm and forearm segments are not simple continuations of one another (Fig. 19-5). The obliquity of the trochlea and trochlear notch surfaces establishes a *carrying angle* which usually cants the forearm segment laterally below the arm. The angle formed varies with different individuals between 175 and 150 deg, opening laterally. When the elbow is flexed or the forearm is pronated, the obtuse carrying angle disappears.

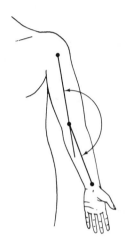

Figure 19–5. The carrying angle of the left arm-forearm segment combination.

→ *Examine these phenomena in your own upper limbs. The use of a mirror is very helpful. Note that the changing contour of the distal portion of the forearm in supination and pronation also contributes an illusory effect beyond that described above.*

The humeroulnar junction acts as a hinge joint with certain peculiarities because of its sellar surfaces. As noted above, very small amounts of abduction and adduction are allowed through the flexion-extension range of about 145 deg. The flexion component is checked by contact of forearm and arm soft tissue. Extension is probably limited by the muscles which cross the anterior aspect of the joint. Hyperextension is in evidence in some individuals, usually women, and is limited to rather small ranges of 10 to 20 deg.

→ *After fully supinating your forearm and hyperextending your wrist, place the heel of your hand on a table with the fingers curled over its edge. Fully extend the elbow by leaning your body weight onto it. Can you detect any hyperextension? Is it a passive function of the applied weight or can it be accomplished through active extensor contractions?*

The humeroradial junction is carried along with its medial mate in a circular gliding action of its proximal surface over the capitulum. Because the radius is tightly bound to the ulna, it shifts bilaterally on the capitulum in conjunction with ulnar abduction and adduction. When flexion is maximal, the coronoid process and radial head reside in their respective receptacles, the coronoid and radial fossae. Similarly, when extension is complete, the olecranon resides in the olecranon fossa. Each of these bony prominences is conveniently cushioned in its terminal position by fossae fat pads.

THE FOREARM SEGMENT

The forearm bears a resemblance to the leg segment in that it contains two separate bones and articulates with the terminal segment of the limb. Following the scheme of the upper limb architecture, the forearm differs markedly from the leg in terms of motion within the segment between the two bones. As a result, additional positioning abilities are afforded to the hand which may be added to those of the arm segment.

The Bones of the Forearm

Figure 19-6 illustrates anterior and posterior views of the radius and ulna of the left forearm, separated somewhat to facilitate identification.

Figure 19–6. (*a*) Anterior and (*b*) posterior views of the left radius and ulna.

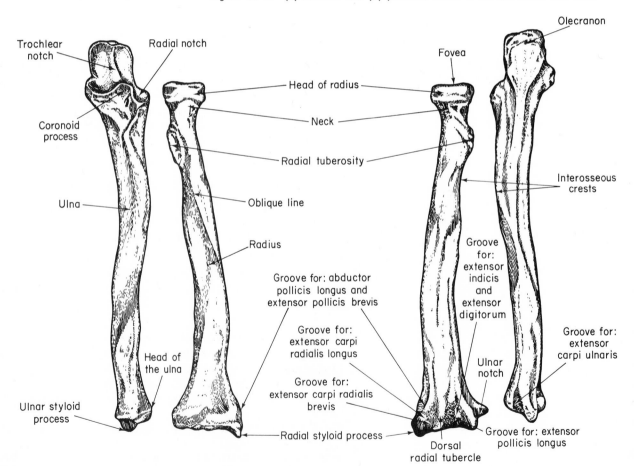

The ulna and radius lie parallel to each other and share a tendency to bow laterally, but at different levels. The ulna is medial to the radius and is more massive at its proximal end. This end exhibits a large, articular concavity, the *trochlear notch*, which is reciprocally shaped to join the trochlea of the humerus. The *olecranon* and the *coronoid process* are heavy bony eminences between which the trochlear notch resides. Each acts as a prominent attachment point for important muscles crossing the joint—the triceps brachii to the olecranon and the brachialis to the coronoid process. Located on the lateral side of the coronoid process is the *radial notch*, which receives the border of the radial *head*. Anterior and posterior borders of the coronoid support attachments of the circular, annular ligament.

The *shaft* of the ulna progressively becomes less massive as its distal end is approached. Its upper-end tendency to be convex laterally is supplanted by the opposite curvature along its lower half. The lateral border is known as the *interosseous crest*, which supports the ulnar attachment of the *interosseous membrane*. The distal end exhibits the *head of the ulna*, which articulates with the radius at the *distal radioulnar* joint, and the ulnar *styloid process*, which is easily palpated at the wrist.

The radius is the thumb-side bone of the forearm. Its proximal surface is indented shallowly (*fovea*) to receive the capitulum of the humerus. Articular cartilage courses downward beyond the borders of this surface in all directions to form an articular circumference for the head. Below the head, the radius constricts into the radial *neck*. Below the neck on the medial side, the *radial tuberosity* protrudes prominently. The important biceps brachii muscle inserts here, its tendon cushioned by a bursa. The interosseous crest begins just below the radial tuberosity and separates into anterior and posterior ridges which form the margins of the *ulnar notch*. The distal end of the radius broadens bilaterally and exhibits a number of grooves on its posterior face for muscle tendons crossing the wrist joint. The radial *styloid process* is a prolongation of the lateral border and may be easily palpated. The *carpal articular surface* is of two concave parts to receive the *scaphoid* and *lunate* bones of the hand.

The Radioulnar Joints of the Forearm

In contrast to the leg segment, the forearm is constructed to be internally flexible. The three radioulnar joints provide for most of that flexibility. The *proximal radioulnar* joint is located within the capsule of the elbow joint. The head of the radius is held against the radial notch by a nearly circular band of fibers known as the annular ligament. This ligament is shaped like an incomplete cup, with its lower fibers impinging inward to clasp the upper part of the radial neck. The head of the radius is then stabilized against lateral and distal displacements and is free to pivot within the fibrous ring. Providing the distal end of the radius is also free to rotate with its proximal end, supination and pronation result. It is clear that this proximal forearm joint is of the pivot classification.

Coursing between the interosseous crests of the ulna and radius is the interosseous membrane, and the resulting fibrous union is called the *middle*

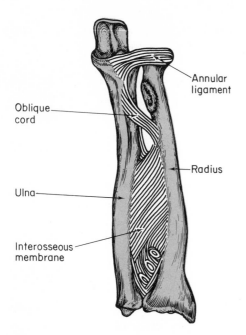

Oblique cord

Annular ligament

Radius

Ulna

Interosseous membrane

Figure 19–7. An anterior view of the interosseous membrane and oblique cord of the forearm.

radioulnar joint (Fig. 19-7). The fibers of the membrane generally course downward and inward from the radius to the ulna. It would appear that this fiber arrangement was suitably situated to check any tendency of the radial head to be displaced upward along the side of the capitulum when the hand and forearm were supporting the body's weight in positions such as those employed when doing push-ups. The membrane is lax in pronation and progressively increases in tension as supination is produced. Some believe the membrane tends to hold the bones together in supination but not to the degree of limiting movement. Possibly its most important function in the forearm is that of increasing significantly the area available for muscle attachments.

The *distal radioulnar* joint is also a pivot joint where the head of the ulna and ulnar notch articulate. Viewed from the anterior, the joint cavity is L-shaped, the horizontal floor of which is provided by the *triangular* articular disk. The disk binds the bones together in conjunction with two transverse capsular thickenings known as the *palmar* and *dorsal radioulnar* ligaments of the distal joint. The entire joint complex is associated with the ligaments of the wrist and must be compliant enough to allow the radial excursions in pronation and supination.

Elbow-Forearm Mobility

With the elbow flexed to 90 deg and the forearm held in the midposition (thumbs up), pronation and supination amount to about 70 and 85 deg, respectively. When the elbow is extended in the pendant position, the range is reduced by about 20%. The axis of these motions runs from the center of the radial head through a point which resides at the junction between the radius and ulna in the distal radioulnar joint. A continuation of this axis carries it very nearly along the long axis of the middle finger.

→ *Demonstrate this by flexing the elbow to 90 deg with the forearm in the midposition. Move up to a wall so that only the tip of the middle finger makes contact. Now supinate and pronate the forearm through its entire range. Note that the finger simply rotates around itself with the rest of the hand and forearm without any marked gyrating. Try the other fingers. What happens when the little finger is employed?*

If the motions of supination and pronation were viewed from beyond the wrist, looking back toward the distal ends of the radius and ulna, the two bones would be seen to rotate about the centrally located axis. The ends of the two bones act to change places with each other to trace the outline of a somewhat flattened circle.

→ *To demonstrate, place a rubber band around your wrist so that it crosses over the radial and ulnar styloid processes. Holding your hand in front of you, fully supinate the forearm and place the end of the index finger of the other hand next to the ulnar styloid process to act as a reference. Now, pronate the segment without moving it or the index finger in any other way. The radial styloid process will very nearly achieve the same position occupied by the ulnar styloid process with respect to the reference finger.*

For this trading of positions to occur, the ulna is abducted to a small degree in a manner which may be associated with the *anconeous* muscle, as suggested by Duchenne.[1]

The *pronator quadratus* is the principal agonist in pronation regardless of limb position, with the *pronator teres* offering assistance under conditions of increased resistance and during rapid pronation. They may act as pure synergists to rule out forearm supination resulting from biceps brachii involvement during heavily resisted elbow flexion. Supination is brought about by the *supinator* alone under most conditions of segment position and velocity. However, when the movement is forcefully resisted or occurs rapidly with the elbow flexed, the biceps brachii assists in the action.

There are two elbow extensors: the triceps brachii and anconeus. The medial head of the triceps appears to be the principal agonist in extension. When forcefully resisted, the remaining heads offer their support. The anconeus is quite active in extension also. They may act as pure synergists in neutralizing the flexion tendency of the biceps brachii when the elbow is extended and strong supination is required against resistance. Under ordinary circumstances no elbow stabilization is required, and the supinator muscle works alone.

Elbow flexion is the result of the activity of three muscles, the brachialis, biceps brachii, and the brachioradialis, with the first listed being the prime contributor under most conditions of position and movement velocity. Because the brachialis inserts into the ulna, it cannot contribute to forearm rotations. In this respect, it performs much like the triceps brachii in extension, bereft of axial rotation functions. The biceps brachii is active in assisting the brachialis in all forearm positions when flexion is heavily resisted. However, when mildly or unresisted in forearm pronation, the biceps brachii activity tends to disappear. The brachioradialis acts most prominently when flexions are rapid or when the movement is resisted in the pronated and midpositions. Under the circumstances given above, it would appear that the natural, midposition is best suited for forceful elbow flexion.

[1]C. B. A. Duchenne, *Physiologie des mouvements*, trans. by E. B. Kaplan (Philadelphia: W. B. Saunders Company, 1959).

Muscle Chart 6: Arm, Elbow Joint, Forearm

Muscle	Origin	Insertion	Innervation
	Attachments		
I. The Arm Muscles			
A. The Anterior Group			
1. Biceps brachii a. Short head	a. Coracoid process of the scapula	Radial tuberosity of the radius	Musculocutaneous nerve
b. Long head	b. Supraglenoid tubercle of the scapula		
2. Brachialis	Distal half of the anterior aspect of the humerus adjacent to the deltoid tuberosity	Tuberosity of the ulna and the anterior surface of the coronoid process	Musculocutaneous nerve
B. The Posterior Group			
1. Triceps brachii a. Long head	a. Infraglenoid tubercle of the scapula	The olecranon of the ulna	Radial nerve
b. Lateral head	b. Posterior surface of the shaft of the humerus proximal to the radial groove		
c. Medial head	c. Posterior surface of the shaft of the humerus distal to the radial groove		

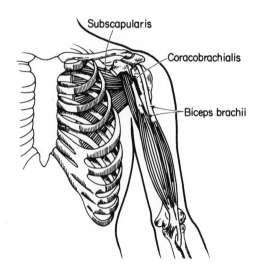

a. and b. Flexion of the elbow
joint; supination of the forearm against resistance; flexion of the shoulder joint
b. Stabilizes the humeral head
in the glenoid fossa

Flexion of the elbow joint

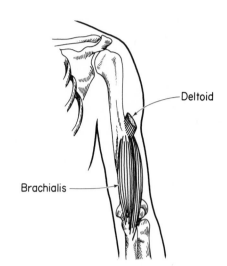
Deltoid

Brachialis

a.–c. Extension of the elbow
joint
a. Extension and adduction of
the shoulder joint

(continued)

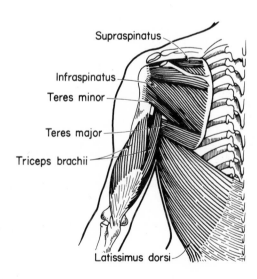
Supraspinatus

Infraspinatus

Teres minor

Teres major

Triceps brachii

Latissimus dorsi

| | Attachments | | |
Muscle	Origin	Insertion	Innervation
II. The Forearm Muscles			
A. The Superficial Anterior Group			
1. Brachioradialis	Proximal two thirds of the lateral supracondylar ridge of the humerus	Styloid process of the radius	Radial nerve

2. Pronator teres
  a. Humeral head
 	
  b. Ulnar head
	a. Medial epicondyle of the humerus
	b. Medial side of the coronoid process of the ulna
		Middle of the lateral surface of the shaft of the radius	Median nerve

3. Flexor carpi radialis	Medial epicondyle of the humerus	Bases of the 2nd and 3rd metacarpals	Median nerve
4. Palmaris longus	Medial epicondyle of the humerus	Central part of the flexor retinaculum and palmar aponeurosis	Median nerve

5. Flexor carpi ulnaris
  a. Humeral head
 	
  b. Ulnar head
	a. Medial epicondyle of the humerus
	b. Medial margin of the olecranon of the ulna
		The pisiform, hamate, and base of the 5th metacarpal	Ulnar nerve

6. Flexor digitorum superficialis
  a. Humeral head
 	
  b. Ulnar head
 	
  c. Radial head
	a. Medial epicondyle of the humerus
	b. Medial side of the coronoid process of the ulna
	c. Oblique line of the radius
		Sides of the shafts of the 2nd phalanges of the four fingers	Median nerve

B. The Deep Anterior Group			
1. Flexor digitorum profundus	Proximal three fourths of the palmar and medial surfaces of the shaft of the ulna	Bases of the distal phalanges of the four fingers	Median nerve
2. Flexor pollicis longus	Palmar surface of the shaft of the radius	Base of the distal phalanx of the thumb	Median nerve
3. Pronator quadratus	Distal fourth of the palmar surface of the ulna	Distal fourth of the palmar surface of the radius	Median nerve

Flexion of the elbow joint

Assists in elbow flexion against resistance; pronation of the forearm

Flexion of the wrist joint; assists in radial flexion of the wrist joint

Assists in flexion of the wrist joint

Flexion of the wrist joint; assists in ulnar flexion of the wrist joint

Assists in flexion of the wrist joint; flexion of the MP and proximal IP joints of the four fingers

May assist in flexion of the wrist joint; flexion of the MP and IP joints of the four fingers

May assist in flexion of the wrist joint; flexion of the MP, proximal, and distal IP joints of the thumb; assists in adduction of the thumb

Pronation of the forearm

(*continued*)

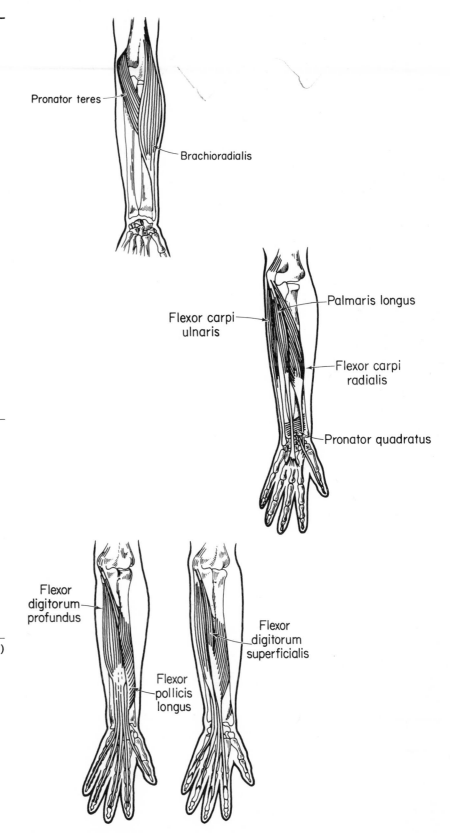

301 *Arm, Elbow Joint, Forearm*

| | Attachments | | |
Muscle	Origin	Insertion	Innervation
C. The Superficial Posterior Group			
1. Anconeus	Posterior surface of the lateral epicondyle of the humerus	Lateral side of the olecranon of the ulna and proximal fourth of the shaft of the ulna	Radial nerve
2. Extensor carpi radialis longus	Distal third of the lateral supracondylar ridge of the humerus	Base of the 2nd metacarpal	Radial nerve
3. Extensor carpi radialis brevis	Lateral epicondyle of the humerus	Base of the 3rd metacarpal	Radial nerve
4. Extensor digitorum	Lateral epicondyle of the humerus	Dorsal surface of the bases of the 2nd phalanges and dorsal expansions of the four fingers	Radial nerve
5. Extensor digiti minimi	Lateral epicondyle by the common extensor tendon	The extensor expansion and tendon of the extensor digitorum at the proximal phalanx of the little finger	Radial nerve
6. Extensor carpi ulnaris	Lateral epicondyle of the humerus by the common extensor tendon	Ulnar side of the base of the 5th metacarpal	Deep radial nerve
D. The Deep Posterior Group			
1. Supinator	Lateral epicondyle of the humerus and adjacent area of the ulna and joint ligaments	Lateral surface of the proximal third of the radius	Deep radial nerve
2. Abductor pollicis longus	Lateral part of the dorsal surface of the shaft of the ulna	Radial side of the base of the first metacarpal	Deep radial nerve
3. Extensor pollicis brevis	Dorsal surface of the shaft of the radius	Base of the first phalanx of the thumb	Deep radial nerve
4. Extensor pollicis longus	Lateral part of the middle third of the dorsal surface of the shaft of the ulna	Base of the distal phalanx of the thumb	Deep radial nerve
5. Extensor indicis	Dorsal surface of the shaft of the ulna	The tendon of the extensor digitorum to the little finger	Deep radial nerve

Extension of the elbow joint

Assists in extension and hyperextension of the wrist joint;
radial flexion of the wrist
joint

Extension, hyperextension, and
radial flexion of the wrist
joint

Extension and hyperextension
of the wrist joint and MP
joints of the four fingers;
extension of the IP joints of
the four fingers

Assists in extension of the wrist
joint; extension and hyperextension of the MP joint of
the little finger; extension
of the IP joints of the little
finger

Extension, hyperextension, and
ulnar flexion of the wrist joint

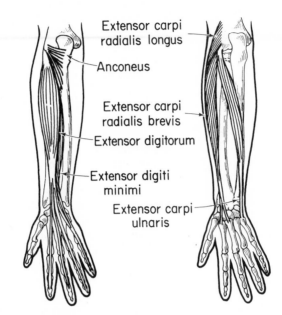

Extensor carpi
radialis longus

Anconeus

Extensor carpi
radialis brevis

Extensor digitorum

Extensor digiti
minimi

Extensor carpi
ulnaris

Supination of the forearm

Assists in flexion and radial
flexion of the wrist joint;
abduction of the CM joint
of the thumb

Assists in radial flexion of the
wrist joint; extension of the
CM and MP joints of the
thumb

Assists in extension and hyperextension of the wrist joint;
extension and adduction of
the CM joint of the thumb;
extension of the MP and IP
joints of the thumb

Assists in extension and hyperextension of the wrist joint;
extension, hyperextension,
and adduction of the MP
joint of the index finger;
extension of the IP joints of
the index finger

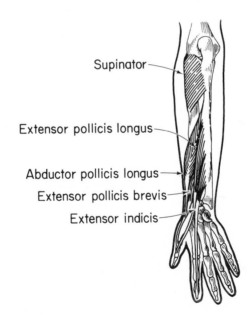

Supinator

Extensor pollicis longus

Abductor pollicis longus

Extensor pollicis brevis

Extensor indicis

REFERENCES

Atkinson, W. B., and Elftman, H. "The Carrying Angle of the Human Arm as a Secondary Sex Character." *Anatomical Record* 91 (1945): 49.

Barnett, C. H.; Davies, D. V.; and MacConaill, M. A. *Synovial Joints: Their Structure and Mechanics*. Springfield, Ill.: Charles C. Thomas, Publisher, 1961.

Basmajian, J. V. *Muscles Alive; Their Function Revealed by Electromyography*. 2d ed. Baltimore: The Williams & Wilkins Company, 1967.

———— "'Spurt' and 'Shunt' Muscles: An Electromyographic Confirmation." *Journal of Anatomy* 93 (1959): 551.

Basmajian, J. V., and Latif, A. "Integrated Actions and Functions of the Chief Flexors of the Elbow." *Journal of Bone and Joint Surgery* 39-A (1957): 1106.

Basmajian, J. V., and Travill, A. "Electromyography of the Pronator Muscles in the Forearm." *Anatomical Record* 139 (1961): 45.

Bassett, David L. *A Stereoscopic Atlas of Human Anatomy*. Portland, Ore.: Sawyer's Inc., 1955.

Bearn, J. G. "An Electromyographic Study of the Trapezius, Deltoid, Pectoralis Major, Biceps and Triceps Muscles, During Static Loading of the Upper Limb." *Anatomical Record* 140 (1961): 103.

Carlsoo, S., and Johansson, O. "Stabilization of and Load on the Elbow Joint in Some Protective Movements." *Acta Anatomica* 48 (1962): 224.

Clarke, H. H.; Irish, E. A.; Trzynka, G. A.; and Popowich, W. "Conditions for Optimum Work Output in Elbow Flexion, Shoulder Flexion, and Grip Ergography." *Archives of Physical Medicine and Rehabilitation* 39 (1958): 475.

Darcus, H. D., and Salter, N. "The Amplitude of Pronation and Supination with the Elbow Flexed to a Right Angle." *Journal of Anatomy* 87 (1953): 169.

DeGoes, H. "The Radio-Humeral 'Meniscus' and its Relation to Tennis Elbow." *Journal of Bone and Joint Surgery* 43-A (1961): 302.

DeSousa, O. M.; DeMoraes, J. L.; and Vieira, F. L. deM. "Electromyographic Study of the Brachioradialis Muscle." *Anatomical Record* 139 (1961): 125.

Doss, W. S., and Karpovich, P. V. "A Comparison of Concentric, Eccentric, and Isometric Strength of Elbow Flexors." *Journal of Applied Physiology* 20 (1965): 351.

Downer, A. H. "Strength of the Elbow Flexor Muscles." *Physical Therapy Review* 33 (1953): 68.

Elftman, H. "The Function of the Arms in Walking." *Human Biology* 11 (1939): 529.

Gardner, Weston D., and Osburn, William A. *Structure of the Human Body*. Philadelphia: W. B. Saunders Company, 1967.

Goss, Charles Mayo, ed. *Gray's Anatomy of the Human Body*. 28th ed. Philadelphia: Lea & Febiger, 1966.

Hall, Michael C. *The Locomotor System: Functional Anatomy*. Springfield, Ill.: Charles C Thomas, Publisher, 1965.

Haxton, H. A. "A Comparison of the Action of Extension of the Knee and Elbow Joints in Man." *Anatomical Record* 93 (1945): 279.

Hermann, G. W. "An Electromyographic Study of Selected Muscles Involved in the Shot Put." *Research Quarterly* 33 (1962): 1.

Hogue, R. E. "Upper-Extremity Muscular Activity at Different Cadences and Inclines During Normal Gait." *Physical Therapy* 49 (1969): 963.

Hubbard, A. W. "Homokinetics." In *Science and Medicine of Exercise and Sports*, edited by W. R. Johnson. New York: Harper & Row, Publishers, 1960.

Kamon, E. "Electromyography of Static and Dynamic Postures of the Body Supported on the Arms." *Journal of Applied Physiology* 21 (1966): 1611.

Klopsteg, Paul E., and Wilson, Philip D., eds. *Human Limbs and Their Substitutes*. New York: McGraw-Hill Book Company, 1954.

Krahl, V. E. "The Torsion of the Humerus. Its Localization, Cause and Duration in Man." *American Journal of Anatomy* 80 (1947): 275.

Little, A. D., and Lehmkuhl, D. "Elbow Extension Force." *Physical Therapy* 46 (1966): 7.

MacConaill, M. A. "The Movements of Bones and Joints: II. Function of the Musculature." *Journal of Bone and Joint Surgery* 31-B (1949): 100.

——— "Some Anatomical Factors Affecting the Stabilizing Functions of Muscles." *Irish Journal of Medical Science* 6 (1946): 160.

Martin, B. F. "The Annular Ligament of the Superior Radio-Ulnar Joint." *Journal of Anatomy* 92 (1958): 473.

——— "The Oblique Cord of the Forearm." *Journal of Anatomy* 92 (1958): 609.

McCraw, L. W. "Effects of Variations of Forearm Positions in Elbow Flexion." *Research Quarterly* 35 (1964): 504.

Nelson, R. C., and Fahrney, R. A. "Relationship Between Strength and Speed of Elbow Flexion." *Research Quarterly* 36 (1965): 455.

Olson, J. K., and Waterland, J. C. "Behavior of Independent Joints Served in Part by Muscles Common to Both: Elbow and Radioulnar Joints." *Perceptual and Motor Skills* 24 (1967): 339.

Pauly, J. E.; Rushing, J. L.; and Scheving, L. E. "An Electromyographic Study of Some Muscles Crossing the Elbow Joint." *Anatomical Record* 159 (1967): 47.

Provins, K. A., and Salter, N. "Maximum Torque Exerted About the Elbow Joint." *Journal of Applied Physiology* 7 (1955): 393.

Quiring, Daniel P., and Warfel, John F. *The Extremities.* Philadelphia: Lea & Febiger, 1967.

Ramsey, R. W.; Norris, A. H.; LeVore, N. W.; Shock, N. W.; Street, S.; Bower, J.; Miller, M. R.; Rosser, R.; and Szumski, A. "An Analysis of Alternating Movements of the Human Arm." *Federation Proceedings* 19 (1960): 254.

Rasch, P. J. "Effect of the Position of Forearm on Strength of Elbow Flexion." *Research Quarterly* 27 (1956): 333.

Ray, R. D.; Johnson, R. J.; and Jameson, R. M. "The Rotation of the Forearm." *Journal of Bone and Joint Surgery* 33-A (1951): 993.

Salter, N., and Darcus, H. D. "The Amplitude of Forearm and of Humeral Rotation." *Journal of Anatomy* 87 (1953): 407.

——— "The Effect of the Degree of Elbow Flexion on the Maximal Torque Developed in Pronation and Supination of the Right Hand." *Journal of Anatomy* 86 (1952): 197.

Scheving, L. E., and Pauly, J. E. "An Electromyographic Study of Some Muscles Acting on the Upper Extremity of Man." *Anatomical Record* 135 (1959): 239.

Sobotta, Johannes. *Atlas of Human Anatomy*, edited by Frank H. J. Figge. Vol. 1. *Skeleton, Ligaments, Joints, and Muscles.* New York: Hafner Publishing Company, Inc., 1968.

Steel, F. L. D., and Tomlinson, J. D. W. "The 'Carrying Angle' in Man." *Journal of Anatomy* 92 (1958): 315.

Steindler, Arthur. *Kinesiology of the Human Body.* Springfield, Ill.: Charles C Thomas, Publisher, 1955.

Sullivan, W. E.; Mortensen, D. A.; Miles, M.; and Green, L. S. "Electromyographic Studies of M. Biceps Brachii During Normal Voluntary Movement at the Elbow." *Anatomical Record* 107 (1950): 243.

Travill, A. A. "Electromyographic Study of the Extensor Apparatus of the Forearm." *Anatomical Record* 144 (1962): 373.

——— "Transmission of Pressures Across the Elbow Joints." *Anatomical Record* 150 (1964): 243.

Travill, A., and Basmajian, J. V. "Electromyography of the Supinators of the Forearm." *Anatomical Record* 139 (1961): 557.

Yashmon, L. J., and Bierman, W. "Kinesiologic Electromyography. III. The Biceps." *Archives of Physical Medicine* 30 (1949): 286.

20

Forearm,
Wrist Joint,
Hand

The distal end of the upper limb is an extraordinary device for manipulation. The multiple movements of the arm and forearm segments are combined to carry the hand through a wide range of positions. As we progress distally in the hand, the segment becomes less massive in conjunction with gaining the facilities of greater internal flexibility and overall mobility. This combination of characteristics is important to the complex dynamics involved in transferring limb forces to external objects so that the desired manipulative outcomes are achieved.

The forearm segment contains many of the muscles which move the hand. Its proximal end is massive in comparison to its distal end as a result of the many muscle bellies which reside in the elbow area. Farther down the forearm, many of these muscles give way to long, slender tendons as they course toward the hand and their distal insertions. Like the leg segment, this organization markedly reduces the mass of the structures crossing the wrist and allows a greater number of muscles to act upon the hand without inordinate bulkiness being the result. Consequently, a number of these muscle tendons may be identified since they are situated superficially under the skin and become prominent when activated to move the hand.

THE WRIST JOINT

The distal end of the radius is somewhat concave to receive the *scaphoid* and *lunate* bones of the hand and angles to face slightly medialward. The distal end of the ulna does not articulate directly with the hand (Fig. 20-1). The *triangular*, articular disk separates it from the *triangular* and *lunate* bones of the hand. The disk's distal surface then continues the dome of the wrist joint on the ulnar side. The proximal row of *carpal* bones (see Fig. 20-3), the scaphoid, lunate, and triangular, form the tightly bound, opposing articular surface. Since the wrist joint joins the radius of the forearm with the carpal area of the hand, it is also known as the *radiocarpal* joint.

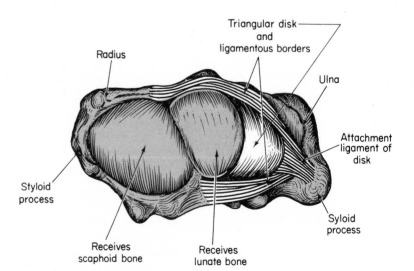

Figure 20–1. Inferior view of the radius and ulna, showing the articular surfaces which enter into the wrist joint.

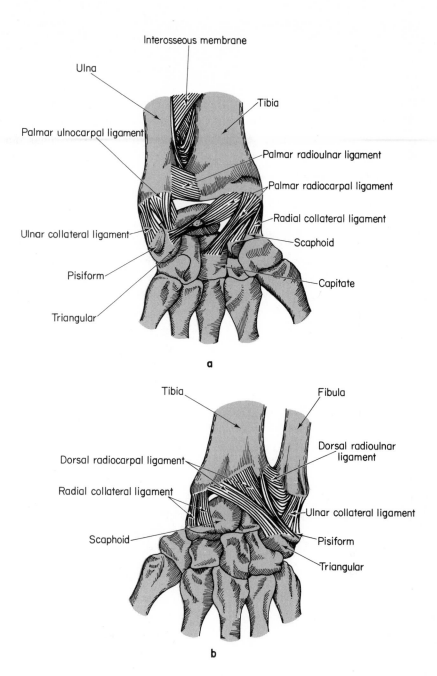

Figure 20–2. (*a*) Palmar and (*b*) dorsal views of the left wrist joint and its important ligaments. Note also the distal, palmar, and dorsal radioulnar ligaments.

Joint Stability

The wrist area is very stable. Although a portion of this stability is due to the movements of the carpal bones to brace one another in various terminal positions, it appears that the predominant stabilizing function is carried by the ligaments of the joint and the numerous muscle tendons that pass over it. Figure 20-2 illustrates the ligaments of the wrist joint. *Palmar* and *dorsal radiocarpal* ligaments and the *palmar ulnocarpal* ligament reinforce the joint capsule, with the palmar ligaments being the more robust. The radiocarpal fiber arrangement is generally downward and toward the ulnar side, and with the ulnocarpal ligament, they ensure that the hand accompanies the forearm in pronation and supination movements. The *radial* (lateral) and *ulnar* (medial) *collateral* ligaments offer bilateral binding, as their names have come to indicate. The former crosses the joint from the tip of the radial styloid process to the scaphoid and *trapezium*. The latter arises from the ulnar styloid process and triangular disk and divides into two parts which attach to the *pisiform* and triangular bones. These ligaments limit excessive ulnar and radial flexions, respectively.

The many muscles which cross the wrist joint (15) are arranged to provide an abundance of stabilizing actions in at least four ways. First, they are situated to produce formidable stabilizing force components because they are generally oriented along the long axes of the forearm and hand segments. Therefore, upon contraction there is a strong tendency to pull the hand upward into the distal concavity of the forearm. Because a number of these muscles motivate movements of structures below the wrist joint, forcible actions such as clenching the hand into a fist also tend to immobilize and stabilize the wrist. A number of the many tendons of these muscles are arranged to produce diagonally directed forces which result in combinations of wrist movements rather than any single, pure movement. Consequently, abundant synergic action takes place to neutralize potential actions, which ultimately results in rather continuous stabilization. Finally, extreme flexions and hyperextensions of the wrist joint are checked by these same muscles owing to the tensions developed in reaching their extended lengths.

Joint Mobility

The wrist joint is an ellipsoid joint whose 2 DF allow flexion-extension, hyperextension, radial and ulnar flexions, and, in combination, circumduction. Active rotations are essentially nonexistent, although the hand may be passively rotated on the forearm to a small degree. The lack of rotation facility is of little consequence, however, inasmuch as the hand may be carried through about 270 deg of rotation resulting from combined arm and forearm rotations. The movements of the hand on the forearm (neglecting movements of the fingers), as observed externally, are not limited to the wrist joint proper. They are the result of combined movements of the wrist and the *intercarpal* joints. Therefore their detailed description is deferred until a more thorough coverage of the hand has been undertaken.

THE HAND SEGMENT

The bones of the hand, numbering 27 in all, are arranged into three groups: the *carpal* or wrist bones, the *metacarpal* or palm bones, and the *phalanges* or finger bones. Figure 20-3 illustrates palmar and dorsal views of the skeleton of the hand, identifying the 8 carpal bones, 5 metacarpal bones, and 14 phalanges. A review of Fig. 14-1 will establish the organizational similarity between the bones of the hand and foot segments.

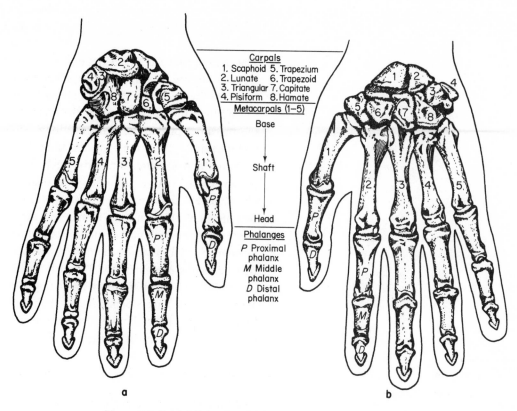

Figure 20–3. (*a*) Palmar and (*b*) dorsal views of the bones of the left hand.

The Bones of the Hand

The wrist area is made up of a proximal row of carpals (1–4 in Fig. 20-3) and a distal row (5–8). The proximal row contains the scaphoid, lunate, triangular, and pisiform bones. The distal row consists of the trapezium, *trapezoid*, *capitate*, and *hamate* bones. As noted earlier, the scaphoid, lunate, and triangular bones enter into the wrist joint with the radius and triangular disk. The junctions between the carpals are known as the inter-carpal (IC) joints, of which there are three sets. The first and third sets consist of the articulations of the bones of the proximal and distal rows, respectively. The second set consists of the articulations between the two rows and is named, collectively, the *midcarpal* (MC) joint. Careful examin-ation of Fig. 20-3 will indicate the transverse curvature of the wrist area, which is convex toward the back of the hand. Note that the trapezoid is more prominent in the dorsal view.

Also articulating with the distal row of carpals are the metacarpals. They are numbered 1 through 5 from the thumb side and constitute the framework for the palm area of the hand. Each metacarpal is somewhat curved along its length. The shortest and longest are the first and second, respectively, the former diverging from the nearly parallel arrangement of the remaining four. All are small, long bones which exhibit a base, shaft, and head.

→ *Palpate them on the dorsal surface of the hand.*

The joints formed between the distal row of carpals and the bases of the metacarpals are known as the *carpometacarpal* (CM) joints. The CM joint cavity of the thumb is separate and complete.

Joining the metacarpals at the *metacarpophalangeal* (MP) joints are the proximal phalanges. They are long bones also. In keeping with the architectural plan of the foot, the thumb includes only two phalanges, a proximal and a distal. Similarly, each of the four fingers contains three phalanges, a proximal, middle, and distal. The joints between adjacent phalanges are called the *interphalangeal* (IP) joints. It is interesting to note that most of the common names for the fingers reflect the descriptive intent of their technical names. Because of its strength, the thumb is technically referred to as the *pollex*. The middle finger is the *medius*, the ring finger the *annularis*, and the little finger the *minimus*. Both common and technical usage refer to an *index* finger because of its use as a pointer. With the other fingers clenched inward toward the palm, the index finger may perform almost limitless services from sampling a cake frosting to dialing a phone number or beckoning someone to come closer.

Mobility of the Wrist Area on the Forearm

The carpal bones are effectively bound together on their palmar and dorsal surfaces. Moreover, interosseous ligaments join the sides of these bones and act as partitions for the intercarpal joints. The movements available at the wrist joint have been listed on p. 308. The midcarpal joint adds to the wrist movements of flexion-extension and hyperextension owing to its hinge joint organization. When the hand is a straight-line extension of the forearm, neither the wrist joint nor the midcarpal joint is in its neutral position. The neutral position in this situation is defined as being the position from which the widest ranges of movement may occur. The neutral position shows the wrist to be slightly hyperextended (about 12 deg) and ulnar-flexed an even smaller amount (about 3 deg). From this position, the hand may be carried through a flexion-extension range of about 85 deg. From the 180-deg position, about 73 deg are available. Hyperextension from the neutral position amounts to about 60 deg; from the 180-deg position, it amounts to approximately 72 deg. Wrist and midcarpal contributions to flexion appear to be similar, while the midcarpal joint offers the greater contribution to hyperextension.

The movement ranges for radial and ulnar flexions are unevenly distributed to favor the latter. These movements are not normally pure but show small amounts of flexion with radial flexion and hyperextension with ulnar flexion. In addition, some gliding occurs during these movements which follows the typical pattern of a convex surface (proximal articular surface of the wrist) rolling over a concave surface (distal articular surface of the forearm).

→ *In what directions does the proximal row of carpals glide during these two movements?*

From either the neutral or 180-deg position, radial and ulnar flexions amount to about 19 and 33 deg, respectively. The magnitudes of these movements vary widely between individuals. The distal row of carpals is pulled along with the proximal row in a pivoting action which is focused near the center of the capitate bone.

→ *Attempt to ulnar- and radial-flex your wrist while it is either fully flexed or hyperextended. What is the outcome and why is it so?*

The muscles of the forearm which cross into the hand are conveniently named for descriptive purposes. Thus, reference to location, size, and movement function is usually indicated; refer to Muscle Chart 7. Those which are situated logically to produce wrist flexion are the *flexor carpi radialis* and *ulnaris* and the relatively weak *palmaris longus*. In addition, several others which course on to more distal locations can assist in flexion. Among the several extensors, the *extensor carpi radialis brevis* and *longus* and the *extensor carpi ulnaris* are the principal motivators. As with flexion, other, more distally inserting muscles may assist, particularly the *extensor digitorum*. Both flexors and extensors become active to synergically produce radial and ulnar flexions. In the former, the extensor carpi radialis longus and brevis join the flexor carpi radialis, whose action appears centered around neutralizing extension tendencies. Ulnar flexion has a larger range and is synergically produced by the concurrent actions of the extensor carpi ulnaris and flexor carpi ulnaris.

→ *What type of synergy is involved? What movement tendencies are neutralized during flexions and extensions?*

Movements Within the Hand

The movements which can take place within the hand depend on the specific articulations involved, both individually and collectively. The locations within the hand which provide the primary mobilities are now discussed.

CARPOMETACARPAL (CM) MOBILITY: The movements available at these joints point up at least one location for differences between the thumb and the remaining four fingers. The bases of the metacarpals arc in the same manner as the distal row of carpals. The CM joints, 2 through 5, exhibit very limited movement ranges, particularly CM 3. Some gliding action between the joint surfaces accompanies the very limited flexions and extensions. The magnitudes increase in CM 4 and 5 to allow some slight rotation of the fifth metacarpal around the base of the fourth. This rotation, in combination with flexion, provides for the limited ability to cup the palm of the hand.

The first carpometacarpal joint is the best example of a saddle joint in the body. The first metacarpal joins only the trapezium in a separate joint capsule. Thus it is set apart from the palm of the hand so that its longitudinal curvature is concave toward the second metacarpal. If the first metacarpal were oriented in the same manner as the other four in the

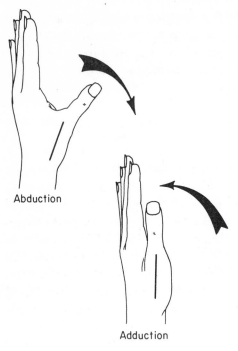

Abduction

Adduction

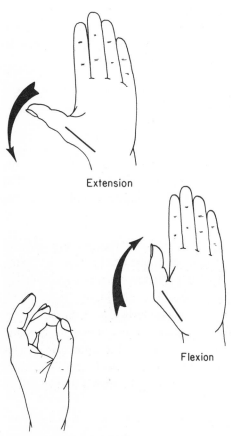

Extension

Flexion

Opposition

Figure 20–4. The movements of the thumb.

anatomical position, about 100 deg of inward rotation about its long axis would be required to place it in its natural position in the relaxed hand. The palmar surface of the thumb itself, as seen in the living, relaxed hand, forms an angle of about 80 deg with the plane of the other fingers.

The movements of the thumb at the CM joint require special consideration because of the thumb's unique position in the hand and versatility of mobility resulting from its saddle-joint architecture. Figure 20-4 illustrates the special movements of the thumb. In demonstrating these movements with your own thumbs, it will be noted that none is a pure movement. All include concurrent axial rotations which may be described as supinations and pronations. Flexion and extension movements are essentially parallel to the plane of the palm of the hand. Abduction and adduction are movements which are perpendicular to the plane of the palm.

→ *Place the back of your relaxed hand on the table in front of you. Position your pencil to cross the palm of the hand bilaterally, with the metal eraser sleeve lying directly below the thumb. Press the thumb downward upon the metal sleeve in adduction. Lift the thumb away from the sleeve in abduction.*

With the convex metacarpal surface moving on the concave trapezium surface in abduction and adduction, the base of the metacarpal tends to glide in the opposite direction of the primary movement.

→ *Palpate the base of the first metacarpal during abduction and adduction and this will become apparent.*

In flexion and extension, however, with the concave metacarpal surface moving on the convex trapezium surface, the gliding is in the same direction as the primary motion.

→ *Demonstrate circumduction of the thumb in both directions and carefully observe the varying position of the thumbnail to indicate the supinations and pronations occurring concurrently.*

The special movement which brings the pad of the thumb into contact with those of the other fingers is named *opposition*. This motion is similar to the first part of the circumduction which you have just demonstrated, if it were clockwise in direction for the left thumb or counterclockwise for the right thumb. The excursion is seen to be a combination of abduction, flexion, and pronation of the first metacarpal, and then some adduction to bring the pad of the thumb into contact with the other fingers. It is also customary for some finger flexion to occur to facilitate the contact. Return from opposition is called *reposition* and is essentially the reversed sequence of movements which occurred in opposition.

Muscular motivation of the thumb is brought about by those muscles carrying the term *pollicis*, referring to the thumb or pollex. Some cross the wrist, while others are intrinsic to the hand and belong to the *thenar eminence*, the fleshy mass overlying the first metacarpal on its palmar surface. The tendons of the *extensor pollicis longus* and *brevis* may be

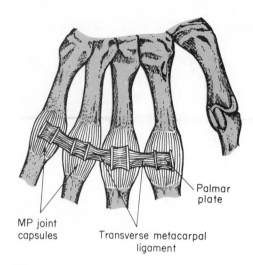

Figure 20–5. The transverse metacarpal ligament.

MP joint capsules

Transverse metacarpal ligament

Palmar plate

identified easily when the thumb is extended and abducted as far as possible and then wiggled back and forth. The former can be followed back to the point above the wrist where it courses around the dorsal radial tubercle. The small triangular indentation between these two tendons is fancifully termed the "anatomical snuffbox." For a more complete description of the intricate thumb mechanism, refer to the recommended readings at the end of this chapter.

METACARPOPHALANGEAL (MP) MOBILITY: These are ellipsoid joints between the bases of the proximal phalanges and the heads of the metacarpals. When the fist is forcibly clenched, the skin over the dorsal surface of these joints is tightened and blanched to show prominent knuckles. In contrast to the CM joints, these show the greatest mobility in the fingers rather than the thumb. The joint capsules are reinforced laterally by collateral ligaments which run diagonally across the joints, providing maximal tautness in flexion. The palmar aspect of these joint capsules exhibits a fibrocartilaginous thickening which is grooved to receive and pad the flexor tendons of the fingers. The MP joints of the fingers are interconnected to their adjacent neighbors by the *transverse metacarpal* ligament (Fig. 20-5), which holds the metacarpal heads together to limit abduction of the fingers. The dorsal surfaces are covered by a fibrous expansion from the extensor tendons, which wrap down and around the joint to the palmar ligaments. The structure is known as the *hood* of the *extensor expansion*; refer to Fig. 20-8.

The MP joint of the fingers allows flexions and extensions through about 90 deg. Hyperextension is available to a limited degree also; some individuals with unusually pliable hands may exhibit it to a very marked extent (Fig. 20-6). Even with very inflexible hands, hyperextension may be produced passively.

→ *Press the distal pads of your four fingers firmly against the table top so that they form an angle of about 30 deg with its surface. With the fingers completely extended, press down harder while lifting the forearm and palm upward.*

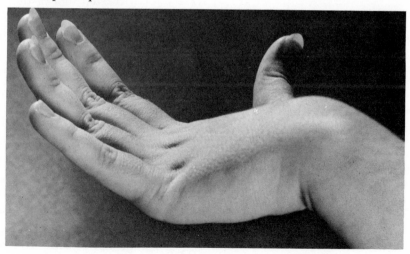

Figure 20–6. A very pliable hand, showing considerable hyperextension at the metacarpophalangeal joints.

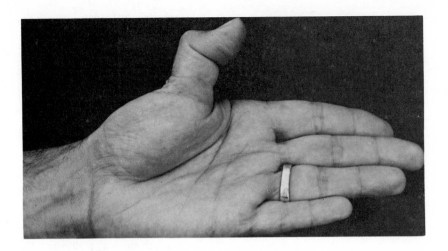

Figure 20–7. A particularly mobile thumb.

You may even note different MP hyperextension mobilities between your own hands which may be due to the amount of heavy work undertaken with respect to handedness. Occasionally, uncommon MP mobility is encountered in the thumb (Fig. 20-7).

→ *How would you explain the attainment of the position shown?*

Abductions and adductions are available depending on the flexion-extension position held and may be accomplished with pairs of fingers as well as individually. In flexion, the collateral ligaments limit abduction and adduction. In extended positions the joints are generally free for these movements. Some limited axial rotation is possible, being most prevalent in the thumb as pronation to complete opposition of the thumb to the fingers.

→ *See if you can circumduct your thumb and each of your fingers at this level.*

INTERPHALANGEAL (IP) MOBILITY: The IP joints are simple hinge joints which are limited to flexion and extensions and some limited hyperextension in pliable hands. Again, hyperextension may be obtained to a greater extent passively in situations like that discussed above. When the IP joints are flexed with the MP joints adducted without calling in MP flexion, the fingertips point along the plane of the palm of the hand. When the MP joints are then flexed maximally, the fingertips point directly into the palm of the hand. If the thumb is then flexed at its MP and IP joints, the distal phalanx may be curled to reside in front of the middle phalanges of the index and middle fingers in the typical fist position of the boxer.

The IP joints are reinforced in a manner similar to the MP joints except that no transverse ligament is possible because of the individuation of each finger beyond the palm. The discussion of IP mobility must, of necessity, wait until a discussion of the *extensor mechanism* of the fingers has been undertaken.

THE EXTENSOR MECHANISM AND FINGER MOVEMENTS: In the discussion of the metacarpophalangeal joints the proximal part of the extensor expansion was mentioned as being the hood. Figure 20-8 illustrates the entire mechanism for one finger from lateral and dorsal views. The hood acts to anchor the entire expansion to the palmar ligament of the MP joint, to enclose the deep tendons of the *interosseous* muscles, and to accept fibrous connections from them. It is a thin aponeurosis, which overlaps the joint in extension and slides downward upon flexion. Distal to the hood, these fibers show three thickenings: one continuing along the dorsal surface of the finger to insert into the base of the middle phalanx and two lateral bands which cross the first IP joint bilaterally somewhat above its center to then converge to a single insertion on the dorsal surface of the base of the distal phalanx. Between these thickenings, the tissue is less dense. The superficial tendons of the interosseous muscles on each side of the finger join the expansion at its lateral bands and send fibers upward to blend with the central band. The *lumbrical* muscle inserts into the expansion from below on the radial side just beyond the insertion of the interosseous tendon. The long flexor tendons are seen to course distally along the

Figure 20–8. (a) Dorsal and (b) lateral views of the extensor mechanism of the finger.

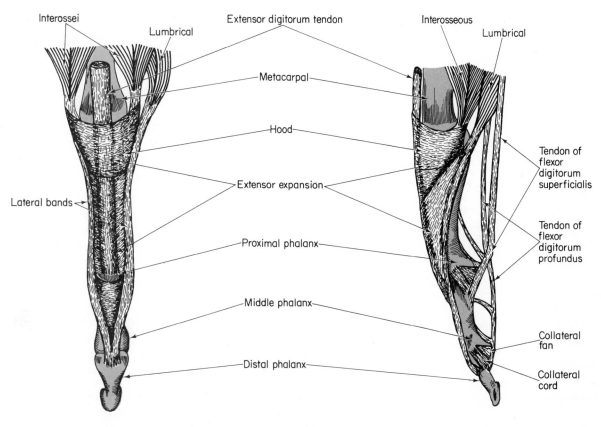

a

b

palmar aspect of the finger to insert across the proximal IP joint (*flexor digitorum superficialis*) and the distal IP joint (*flexor digitorum profundus*). These tendons are shown to be very lax as the result of dissection. In the living, they are compactly held within fibrous tendon sheaths which hold them close to the phalanges.

Because the tendons of the long extensor and flexor muscles cross the wrist joint as well as those of the hand, their actions are rather involved. The *extensor digitorum* appears to be active in both IP and MP extension. Obviously, it is the true contributor to extension and hyperextension of the MP joints. The long flexor tendons are involved in flexing the IP and MP joints simultaneously. The interossei may assist in MP flexion if their primary actions of IP extension are allowed to take place also. Under these conditions, the lumbricales function similarly. In combination, the interossei and lumbricales act to extend the IP joints through the extensor expansion regardless of the position of the MP joint. When the MP joint nears complete extension as the result of extensor digitorum action, the interosseous-lumbrical action at the MP joint appears to be one of antagonism to the tendency to hyperextend that joint, thus adding much to its stability.

→ *You can simulate this antagonism with the use of a bath towel and your own knee joint. Wrap the towel across the front of your leg just below the knee to represent the extensor expansion. While forcefully extending the knee, pull downward and backward on the two ends of the towel. Providing the towel does not slip upward, a near stalemate can be achieved. If the knee extension force is lessened during your active towel pulling, what is the outcome?*

Similarly, it would be expected that the actions of the intrinsic pair could then assist the long flexors in the flexion of the MP joint while holding the IP joints in extension, a most unique example of pure synergy at the IP joints to rule out the flexion tendencies of the long flexors.

If flexions of all the finger joints are desired, the interossei and lumbricales must release their IP holding action to allow the profundus to flex the distal IP joint and the superficialis to flex the proximal IP joint. The extensor digitorum may act as a cocontractor in some flexion movements, in which case it appears to perform as a governor, eccentrically controlling the flexion motivation of the flexor digitorum superficialis. Sufficient action of the flexor profundus may, in some individuals, flex the distal IP joints while the other joints remain extended.

→ *See if you can perform this action. Can you describe how this movement may be isolated from the extension influence exerted by the interosseous-lumbrical pair? To extend your investigations of finger movements, place your pencil across your hand so that it lies between the proximal IP creases of the fingers and the creases where the fingers join the palm on its palmar surface. Now, curl (flex) your fingers around the pencil so that it is encircled by them and then completely close the fist. From this position, extend the MP joints, carrying the pencil through an arc of about 90 deg within the curled fingers. Return the fingers again to their original position. What muscular actions were involved in these movements?*

Extreme wrist positions compromise the degree to which finger movements may be performed. For example, when the wrist is flexed maximally, the tight extensor tendons and extensor expansion act to limit finger flexions. When the wrist is forcefully hyperextended, the fingers naturally tend to curl into flexion owing to the increasing tension developed in the long flexor tendons. Wright has described the actions of the principal wrist flexors in stabilizing the wrist against the tendency of the powerful extensor digitorum to hyperextend the wrist while performing extension or hyperextension of the MP joints.[1] The usual position maintained at the wrist is partial flexion, a position commonly recruited in forceful grasping events in gymnastics and known as a "false grip."

→ *What kind of synergic action is involved?*

Similarly, in clenching the fist, the long flexors of the hand and fingers, crossing the wrist joint as well, would tend to flex the wrist.

→ *How is this avoided?*

[1]Wilhelmine G. Wright, *Muscle Function* (New York: Hafner Publishing Company, 1962), p. 50.

Muscle Chart 7:   Forearm, Wrist Joint, Hand

Muscle	Origin	Insertion	Innervation
	Attachments		

I. The Forearm Muscles

A. The Superficial Anterior Group

Muscle	Origin	Insertion	Innervation
1. Flexor carpi radialis	Medial epicondyle of the humerus	Bases of the 2nd and 3rd metacarpals	Median nerve
2. Palmaris longus	Medial epicondyle of the humerus	Central part of the flexor retinaculum and palmar aponeurosis	Median nerve
3. Flexor carpi ulnaris a. Humeral head b. Ulnar head	a. Medial epicondyle of the humerus b. Medial margin of the olecranon of the ulna	The pisiform, hamate, and base of the 5th metacarpal	Ulnar nerve
4. Flexor digitorum superficialis a. Humeral head b. Ulnar head c. Radial head	a. Medial epicondyle of the humerus b. Medial side of the coronoid process of the ulna c. Oblique line of the radius	Sides of the shafts of the 2nd phalanges of the four fingers	Median nerve

B. The Deep Anterior Group

Muscle	Origin	Insertion	Innervation
1. Flexor digitorum profundus	Proximal three fourths of the palmar and medial surfaces of the shaft of the ulna	Bases of the distal phalanges	Median nerve
2. Flexor pollicis longus	Palmar surface of the shaft of the radius	Base of the distal phalanx of the thumb	Median nerve

C. The Superficial Posterior Group

Muscle	Origin	Insertion	Innervation
1. Extensor carpi radialis longus	Distal third of the lateral supracondylar ridge of the humerus	Base of the 2nd metacarpal	Radial nerve
2. Extensor carpi radialis brevis	Lateral epicondyle of the humerus	Base of the 3rd metacarpal	Radial nerve
3. Extensor digitorum	Lateral epicondyle of the humerus	Dorsal surface of the bases of the 2nd phalanges and dorsal expansions of the four fingers	Radial nerve
4. Extensor digiti minimi	Lateral epicondyle of the humerus by the common extensor tendon	The extensor expansion and tendon of the extensor digitorum at the proximal phalanx of the little finger	Radial nerve
5. Extensor carpi ulnaris	Lateral epicondyle of the humerus by the common extensor tendon	Ulnar side of the base of the 5th metacarpal	Deep radial nerve

Flexion of the wrist joint;
assists in radial flexion of
the wrist joint

Assists in flexion of the wrist
joint

Flexion of the wrist joint;
assists in ulnar flexion of the
wrist joint

Flexion of the MP and IP joints
of the four fingers; assists
in flexion of the wrist joint

Flexion of the MP and IP joints
of the four fingers; may
assist in flexion of the wrist
joint

Flexion of the MP and IP
joints of the thumb; assists
in adduction of the thumb;
may assist in flexion of the
wrist joint

Assists in extension and hyperextension of the wrist joint;
radial flexion of the wrist
joint

Extension, hyperextension, and
radial flexion of the wrist
joint

Extension and hyperextension
of the MP joints of the four
fingers; extension and
hyperextension of the wrist
joint

Extension and hyperextension
of the MP joint of the little
finger; extension of the IP
joints of the little finger;
assists in extension of the
wrist joint

Extension, hyperextension, and
ulnar flexion of the wrist
joint

(continued)

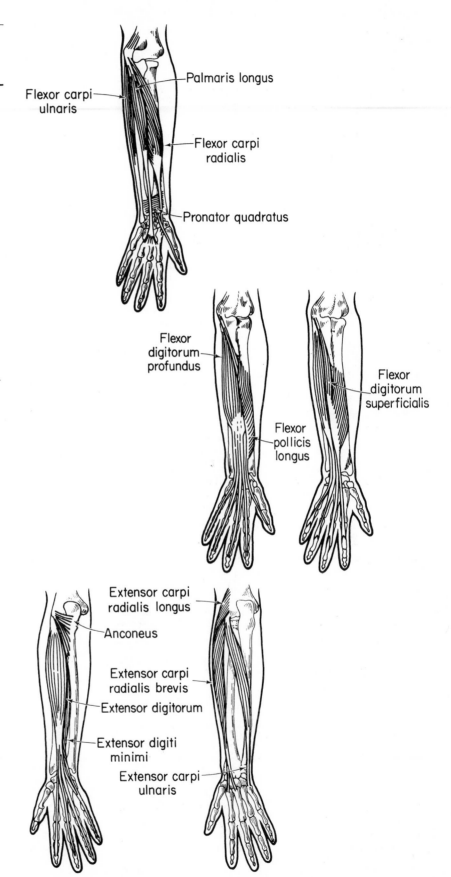

319   Forearm, Wrist Joint, Hand

| Muscle | Attachments | | Innervation |
	Origin	Insertion	
D. The Deep Posterior Group			
1. Abductor pollicis longus	Lateral part of the dorsal surface of the shaft of the ulna	Radial side of the base of the 1st metacarpal	Deep radial nerve
2. Extensor pollicis longus	Lateral part of the middle third of the dorsal surface of the shaft of the ulna	Base of the distal phalanx of the thumb	Deep radial nerve
3. Extensor pollicis brevis	Dorsal surface of the shaft of the radius	Base of the 1st phalanx of the thumb	Deep radial nerve
4. Extensor indicis	Dorsal surface of the shaft of the ulna	The tendon of the extensor digitorum to the little finger	Deep radial nerve
II. The Intrinsic Hand Muscles			
A. The Thenar Group			
1. Abductor pollicis brevis	Transverse carpal ligament, tuberosity of the scaphoid, and the trapezium	Radial side of the base of the proximal phalanx of the thumb	Median nerve
2. Opponens pollicis	Flexor retinaculum and the ridge of the trapezium	Base and shaft of the metacarpal of the thumb	Median nerve
3. Flexor pollicis brevis			
a. Lateral head (superficial)	a. Flexor retinaculum and the ridge of the trapezium	a. Radial side of the base of the proximal phalanx of the thumb	a. Median nerve
b. Medial head (deep)	b. Ulnar side of the first metacarpal	b. Ulnar side of the base of the proximal phalanx of the thumb	b. Ulnar nerve
4. Adductor pollicis			
a. Oblique head	a. Capitate bone and the bases of the 2nd and 3rd metacarpals	Ulnar side of the base of the proximal phalanx of the thumb	Ulnar nerve
b. Transverse head	b. Distal two thirds of the palmar surface of the 3rd metacarpal		
B. The Hypothenar Group			
1. Abductor digiti minimi	Tendon of the flexor carpi ulnaris and the pisiform	Ulnar side of the base of the proximal phalanx of the little finger and the ulnar border of the aponeurosis of the extensor digiti minimi	Ulnar nerve
2. Flexor digiti minimi brevis	Hamulus of the hamate and the flexor retinaculum	Ulnar side of the base of the proximal phalanx of the little finger	Ulnar nerve
3. Opponens digiti minimi	Hamulus of the hamate and the flexor retinaculum	Entire ulnar border of the metacarpal of the little finger	Ulnar nerve

Abduction of the CM joint of the thumb; assists in flexion and radial flexion of the wrist joint

Extension and adduction of the CM joint of the thumb; extension of the MP and IP joints of the thumb; assists in extension and hyper-extension of the wrist joint

Extension of the CM and MP joints of the thumb; assists in radial flexion of the wrist joint

Extension, hyperextension, and adduction of the MP joint of the index finger; extension of the IP joints of the index finger; assists in extension and hyperextension of the wrist joint

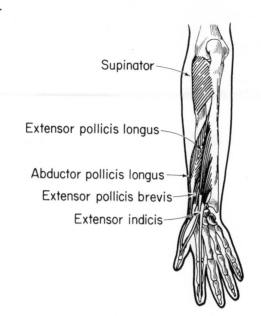

Abduction and flexion of the CM and MP joints of the thumb; opposition of the thumb

Abduction and flexion of the CM joint of the thumb; opposition of the thumb

Flexion and adduction of the CM and MP joints of the thumb; opposition of the thumb

Adduction of the CM and MP joints of the thumb; assists in flexion of the CM and MP joints of the thumb; opposition of the thumb

Flexion and abduction of the MP joint of the little finger; opposition of the little finger

Flexion and adduction of the MP joint of the little finger; opposition of the little finger

Flexion and abduction of the MP joint of the little finger; opposition of the little finger

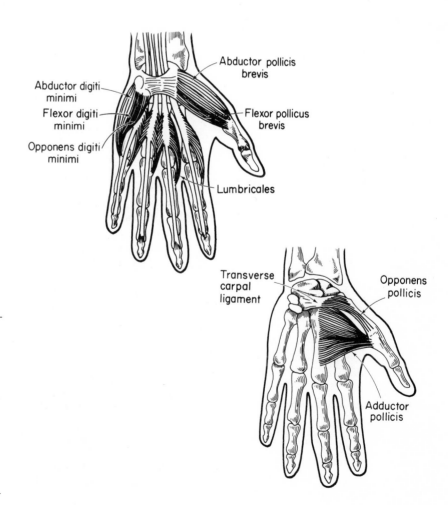

| Muscle | Attachments | | Innervation |
	Origin	Insertion	
C. The Intermediate Group			
1. Lumbricales	Tendons of the flexor digitorum profundus	Radial side of the extensor expansions of the four fingers	Median nerve—1st and 2nd lumbricales Ulnar nerve—3rd and 4th lumbricales
2. Dorsal interossei	Adjacent sides of all the metacarpals	Base of the proximal phalanx and the extensor expansion on both sides of the middle finger, radial side of the index finger, and ulnar side of the ring finger	Ulnar nerve
3. Palmar interossei	Palmar surfaces of the 2nd, 4th, and 5th metacarpals	Origin side of the 1st phalanx and extensor expansion of the index, ring, and little fingers	Ulnar nerve

REFERENCES

Backdahl, M., and Carlsoo, S. "Distribution of Activity in Muscles Acting on the Wrist (An Electromyographic Study)." *Acta Morphologica Neerlando-Scandinavica* 4 (1961): 136.

Backhouse, K. M. "Digital Rotation." *Journal of Anatomy* 94 (1960): 453.

——— and Catton, W. T. "An Experimental Study of the Functions of the Lumbrical Muscles in the Human Hand." *Journal of Anatomy* 88 (1954): 133.

Barnett, C. H.; Davies, D. V.; and MacConaill, M. A. *Synovial Joints, Their Structure and Mechanics.* Springfield, Ill.: Charles C. Thomas, Publisher, 1961.

Basmajian, J. V. *Muscles Alive; Their Function Revealed by Electromyography.* 2d ed. Baltimore: The Williams & Wilkins Company, 1967.

Boivin, G.; Wadsworth, G. E.; Landsmeer, J. M. F.; and Long, C. "Electromyographic Kinesiology of the Hand: Muscles Driving the Index Finger." *Archives of Physical Medicine and Rehabilitation* 50 (1969): 17.

Bradley, K. C., and Sunderland, S. "The Range of Movement at the Wrist Joint." *Anatomical Record* 116 (1953): 139.

Bunnell, Sterling. *Surgery of the Hand.* 3rd ed. Philadelphia: J. B. Lippincott Company, 1956.

Clarke, H. H.; Irish, E. A.; Trzynka, G. A.; and Popowich, W. "Conditions for Optimum Work Output in Elbow Flexion, Shoulder Flexion, and Grip Ergography." *Archives of Physical Medicine and Rehabilitation* 39 (1958): 475.

Close, J. R., and Kidd, C. C. "The Functions of the Muscles of the Thumb, the Index, and Long Fingers." *Journal of Bone and Joint Surgery* 51 (1969): 1601.

Cyriax, E. F. "On the Rotary Movements of the Wrist." *Journal of Anatomy* 60 (1926): 199.

Extension of the IP joints of the four fingers; assists in flexion of the MP joints of those fingers with IP joints in extension

Adduction of the MP joints of the index and ring fingers; radial and ulnar deviation of the middle finger; extension of the IP joints of the four fingers; flexion of the MP joints of the four fingers with IP joints in extension

Adduction of the MP joints of the index, ring, and little fingers; extension of the IP joints of the four fingers; flexion of the MP joints of the four fingers with IP joints in extension

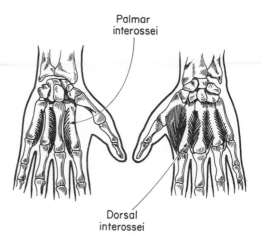

Palmar interossei

Dorsal interossei

Dempster, W. T., and Finerty, J. C. "Relative Activity of Wrist Moving Muscles in Static Support of the Wrist Joint: An Electromyographic Study." *American Journal of Physiology* 150 (1947): 596.

Ebskov, B., and Long, C. "A Method of Electromyographic Kinesiology of the Thumb." *Archives of Physical Medicine and Rehabilitation* 48 (1967): 78.

Eyler, D. L., and Markee, J. E. "The Anatomy and Function of the Intrinsic Musculature of the Fingers." *Journal of Bone and Joint Surgery* 36-A (1954): 1.

Flatt, A. "Kinesiology of the Hand." Instructional Course Lectures. *American Academy of Orthopaedic Surgeons* 18 (1961): 266.

Forrest, W. J., and Basmajian, J. V. "Function of Human Thenar and Hypothenar Muscles: An Electromyographic Study of Twenty-five Hands." *Journal of Bone and Joint Surgery* 47-A (1965): 1585.

Goss, Charles Mayo, ed. *Gray's Anatomy of the Human Body*. 28th ed. Philadelphia: Lea & Febiger, 1966.

Grant, C. Boileau. *An Atlas of Anatomy*. 5th ed. Baltimore: The Williams & Wilkins Company, 1962.

Haines, R. W. "The Mechanism of Rotation at the First Carpo-Metacarpal Joint." *Journal of Anatomy* 85 (1951): 251.

Harris, H., and Joseph, J. "Variation in Extension of the Metacarpophalangeal and Interphalangeal Joints of the Thumb." *Journal of Bone and Joint Surgery* 31 (1949): 547.

Hubay, C. A. "Sesamoid Bones of the Hands and Feet." *American Journal of Roentgenology, Radium Therapy, and Nuclear Medicine* 61 (1949): 493.

Jones, F. W. *The Principles of Anatomy as Seen in the Hand*. 2d ed. London: Bailliere, Tindall & Cox, Ltd., 1944.

Joseph, J. "Further Studies of the Metacarpo-Phalangeal and Interphalangeal Joints of the Thumb." *Journal of Anatomy* 85 (1951): 221.

Kaplan, E. B. "Functional Significance of the Insertions of the Extensor Communis Digitorum in Man." *Anatomical Record* 92 (1945): 293.

Kendall, Henry O., and Kendall, Florence P. *Muscles, Testing and Function*. Baltimore: The Williams & Wilkins Company, 1949.

Landsmeer, J. M. F. "The Anatomy of the Dorsal Aponeurosis of the Human Finger and its Functional Significance." *Anatomical Record* 104 (1949): 31.

——— "The Co-ordination of Finger Joint Motions." *Journal of Bone and Joint Surgery* 45-A (1963): 1654.

Long, C. "Intrinsic-Extrinsic Muscle Control of the Fingers." *Journal of Bone and Joint Surgery* 50-A (1968): 973.

———— and Brown, M. E. "Electromyographic Kinesiology of the Hand: Muscles Moving the Long Finger." *Journal of Bone and Joint Surgery* 46-A (1964): 1683.

———— "Electromyographic Kinesiology of the Hand: Part III. Lumbricalis and Flexor Digitorum Profundus to the Long Finger." *Archives of Physical Medicine and Rehabilitation* 43 (1962): 450.

———— and Weiss, G. "Electromyographic Kinesiology of the Hand: Part II. Third Dorsal Interosseus and Extensor Digitorum of the Long Finger." *Archives of Physical Medicine and Rehabilitation* 42 (1961): 559.

MacConaill, M. A. "The Mechanical Anatomy of the Carpus and its Bearing on Some Surgical Problems." *Journal of Anatomy* 75 (1941): 166.

MacConaill, M. A., and Basmajian, J. V. *Muscles and Movement, A Basis for Human Kinesiology.* Baltimore: The Williams & Wilkins Company, 1969.

McFarland, G. B.; Krusen, V. L.; and Weatherby, H. T. "Kinesiology of Selected Muscles Acting on the Wrist: Electromyographic Study." *Archives of Physical Medicine and Rehabilitation* 43 (1962): 165.

McFarlane, J. M. "Observations on the Functional Anatomy of the Intrinsic Muscles of the Thumb." *Journal of Bone and Joint Surgery* 44-A (1962): 1073.

Mangini, V. "Flexor Pollicis Longus Muscle." *Journal of Bone and Joint Surgery* 42-A (1960): 467.

Mehta, H. J., and Gardner, W. H. "A Study of Lumbrical Muscles in the Human Hand." *American Journal of Anatomy* 109 (1961): 227.

Napier, J. R. "The Form and Function of the Carpo-Metacarpal Joint of the Thumb." *Journal of Anatomy* 89 (1955): 362.

———— "The Prehensile Movements of the Human Hand." *Journal of Bone and Joint Surgery* 38-B (1956): 902.

Roston, J. B., and Haines, R. W. "Cracking in Metacarpo-Phalangeal Joint." *Journal of Anatomy* 81 (1947): 165.

Salisbury, C. R. "The Interosseous Muscles of the Hand." *Journal of Anatomy* 71 (1936): 395.

Schenker, A. W. "Finger Joint Motion: A New, Rapid, Accurate Method of Measurement." *Military Medicine* 131 (1966): 22.

Stack, H. G. "Muscle Function in the Fingers." *Journal of Bone and Joint Surgery* 44-B (1962): 899.

Starr, I. "Units for the Expression of Both Static and Dynamic Work in Similar Terms, and Their Application to Weight Lifting Experiments." *Journal of Applied Physiology* 4 (1951): 26.

Steindler, Arthur. *Kinesiology of the Human Body.* Springfield, Ill.: Charles C Thomas, Publisher, 1955.

Strong, C., and Perry, J. "Function of the Extensor Pollicis Longus and Intrinsic Muscles of the Thumb: An Electromyographic Study During Interphalangeal Joint Extension." *Physical Therapy* 46 (1966): 935.

Sunderland, S. "The Actions of the Extensor Digitorum Communis, Interosseous and Lumbrical Muscles." *American Journal of Anatomy* 77 (1945): 189.

Taylor, C. L., and Schwartz, R. J. "The Anatomy and Mechanics of the Human Hand." *Artificial Limbs* 2 (1955): 22.

Travill, A. A. "Electromyographic Study of the Extensor Apparatus of the Forearm." *Anatomical Record* 144 (1962): 373.

Tuttle, W. W.; Janney, C. D.; and Thompson, C. W. "Relation of Maximum Grip Strength to Grip Strength Endurance." *Journal of Applied Physiology* 2 (1950): 663.

Weathersby, H. T. "Electromyography of the Thenar Muscles." *Anatomical Record* 127 (1957): 386.

Weathersby, H. T.; Sutton, L. R.; and Krusen, U. L. "The Kinesiology of Muscles of the Thumb: An Electromyographic Study." *Archives of Physical Medicine and Rehabilitation* 44 (1963): 321.

Woodburne, Russell T. *Essentials of Human Anatomy.* New York: Oxford University Press, 1965.

Wright, Wilhelmine G. *Muscle Function.* New York: Hafner Publishing Company, 1962.

Appendix A
The Greek Alphabet

alpha A α	*iota* I ι	*rho* P ρ
beta B β	*kappa* K κ	*sigma* Σ σ
gamma Γ γ	*lambda* Λ λ	*tau* T τ
delta Δ δ	*mu* M μ	*upsilon* Υ ν
epsilon E ε	*nu* N ν	*phi* Φ φ
zeta Z ζ	*xi* Ξ ξ	*chi* X χ
eta H η	*omicron* O o	*psi* Ψ ψ
theta Θ θ	*pi* Π π	*omega* Ω ω

Appendix B
Right Triangles and Trigonometric Functions

THE RIGHT TRIANGLE

A right triangle is composed of three angles and three sides as are all triangles. The sum of the three angles, a, b, and c in Fig. 1, equals 180 deg. Since one of the angles is always a right angle ($c = 90°$), the sum of the remaining, acute angles ($a+b$) equals $90°$ also. For this reason, they are called complementary angles.

The name given to the longest side of the right triangle, opposite the right angle, is the *hypotenuse* (H). The names of the remaining sides depend on which of the two complementary angles is under consideration. In Fig. 1a, angle a is chosen for consideration; hence the side of the triangle toward which it opens is called the *opposite side* (O), and the side with which its angle is formed with the hypotenuse is called the *adjacent side* (A). The same triangle is pictured in Fig. 1b where angle b is chosen for consideration. Under these circumstances, opposite (O) and adjacent (A) side designations are reversed.

TRIGONOMETRIC FUNCTIONS

In a mathematical sense, a function is a quantity whose value varies with and depends upon another quantity or other quantities. A trigonometric function is a quantity which varies with and depends upon the values of the two complementary angles and the lengths of the three sides of the right triangle. These functions are simple ratios of side lengths, referred to one of the complementary angles under consideration: the value of one side is divided by the value of another. Although six functions are possible (*sine, cosine, tangent, cotangent, secant, cosecant*), only the first three will be considered in this text as follows:

1. The *sin* (abbreviation for sine) of an angle is the ratio of its opposite side to the hypotenuse. In Fig. 1*a*, $\sin a = O/H$; in Fig. 1*b*, $\sin b = O/H$.

2. The *cos* (cosine) of an angle is the ratio of its adjacent side to the hypotenuse. In Fig. 1*a*, $\cos a = A/H$; in Fig. 1*b*, $\cos b = A/H$.

3. The *tan* (tangent) of an angle is the ratio of its opposite to adjacent sides. In Fig. 1*a*, $\tan a = O/A$; in Fig. 1*b*, $\tan b = O/A$. (Note that sin *a* in Fig. 1*a* equals cos *b* in Fig. 1*b*.)

In the Natural Trigonometric Functions Table which follows, sin, cos, and tan values are given for whole degrees from 0° through 90°. Figure 2*a* illustrates a 30°–60°–90° right triangle. With the 30-deg angle under consideration, the table tells us that $\sin 30° = .5000$. Since the sin function is the ratio, O/H, the length of the opposite side is exactly one-half that of the hypotenuse. Similarly, with $\cos 30° = .8660 = A/H$, the adjacent side is .8660 (nearly 90%) the length of the hypotenuse. If $H = 10$ in., then $O = 5$ in. and $A = 8.66$ in. Note that sin 30° and cos 60° are the same. These side-length relationships remain unchanged for all 30°–60°–90° triangles regardless of their overall size. Figure 2*b* illustrates a 45°–45°–90° right triangle. With complementary angles demonstrating equal magnitudes, opposite and adjacent sides are also equal, measuring just over 70% of the length of the hypotenuse.

→ *What are the* tan *values for the complementary angles in Figs.* 2a *and* 2b *?*

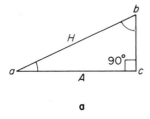

a

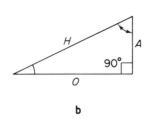

b

Figure 1

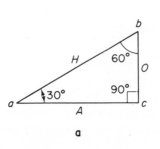

a

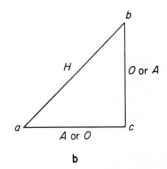

b

Figure 2

ANGLE

Degree	Radian	Sine	Cosine	Tangent
0°	0.000	.0000	1.0000	.0000
1°	0.017	.0175	.9998	.0175
2°	0.035	.0349	.9994	.0349
3°	0.052	.0523	.9986	.0524
4°	0.070	.0698	.9976	.0699
5°	0.087	.0872	.9962	.0875
6°	0.105	.1045	.9945	.1051
7°	0.122	.1219	.9925	.1228
8°	0.140	.1392	.9903	.1405
9°	0.157	.1564	.9877	.1584
10°	0.175	.1736	.9848	.1763
11°	0.192	.1908	.9816	.1944
12°	0.209	.2079	.9781	.2126
13°	0.227	.2250	.9744	.2309
14°	0.244	.2419	.9703	.2493
15°	0.262	.2588	.9659	.2679
16°	0.279	.2756	.9613	.2867
17°	0.297	.2924	.9563	.3057
18°	0.314	.3090	.9511	.3249
19°	0.332	.3256	.9455	.3443
20°	0.349	.3420	.9397	.3640
21°	0.367	.3584	.9336	.3839
22°	0.384	.3746	.9272	.4040
23°	0.401	.3907	.9205	.4245
24°	0.419	.4067	.9135	.4452
25°	0.436	.4226	.9063	.4663
26°	0.454	.4384	.8988	.4877
27°	0.471	.4540	.8910	.5095
28°	0.489	.4695	.8829	.5317
29°	0.506	.4848	.8746	.5543
30°	0.524	.5000	.8660	.5774
31°	0.541	.5150	.8572	.6009
32°	0.559	.5299	.8480	.6249
33°	0.576	.5446	.8387	.6494
34°	0.593	.5592	.8290	.6745
35°	0.611	.5736	.8192	.7002
36°	0.628	.5878	.8090	.7265
37°	0.646	.6018	.7986	.7536
38°	0.663	.6157	.7880	.7813
39°	0.681	.6293	.7771	.8098
40°	0.698	.6428	.7660	.8391
41°	0.716	.6561	.7547	.8693
42°	0.733	.6691	.7431	.9004
43°	0.750	.6820	.7314	.9325
44°	0.768	.6947	.7193	.9657
45°	0.785	.7071	.7071	1.0000
46°	0.803	.7193	.6947	1.0355
47°	0.820	.7314	.6820	1.0724
48°	0.838	.7431	.6691	1.1106
49°	0.855	.7547	.6561	1.1504
50°	0.873	.7660	.6428	1.1918
51°	0.890	.7771	.6293	1.2349
52°	0.908	.7880	.6157	1.2799
53°	0.925	.7986	.6018	1.3270
54°	0.942	.8090	.5878	1.3764
55°	0.960	.8192	.5736	1.4281

ANGLE

Degree	Radian	Sine	Cosine	Tangent
56°	0.977	.8290	.5592	1.4826
57°	0.995	.8387	.5446	1.5399
58°	1.012	.8480	.5299	1.6003
59°	1.030	.8572	.5150	1.6643
60°	1.047	.8660	.5000	1.7321
61°	1.065	.8746	.4848	1.8040
62°	1.082	.8829	.4695	1.8807
63°	1.100	.8910	.4540	1.9626
64°	1.117	.8988	.4384	2.0503
65°	1.134	.9063	.4226	2.1445
66°	1.152	.9135	.4067	2.2460
67°	1.169	.9205	.3907	2.3559
68°	1.187	.9272	.3746	2.4751
69°	1.204	.9336	.3584	2.6051
70°	1.222	.9397	.3420	2.7475
71°	1.239	.9455	.3256	2.9042
72°	1.257	.9511	.3090	3.0777
73°	1.274	.9563	.2924	3.2709
74°	1.292	.9613	.2756	3.4874
75°	1.309	.9659	.2588	3.7321
76°	1.326	.9703	.2419	4.0108
77°	1.344	.9744	.2250	4.3315
78°	1.361	.9781	.2079	4.7046
79°	1.379	.9816	.1908	5.1446
80°	1.396	.9848	.1736	5.6713
81°	1.414	.9877	.1564	6.3138
82°	1.431	.9903	.1392	7.1154
83°	1.449	.9925	.1219	8.1443
84°	1.466	.9945	.1045	9.5144
85°	1.484	.9962	.0872	11.430
86°	1.501	.9976	.0698	14.301
87°	1.518	.9986	.0523	19.081
88°	1.536	.9994	.0349	28.636
89°	1.553	.9998	.0175	57.290
90°	1.571	1.000	.0000	

Index

References to main discussions of body segments are printed in **boldface** type; numbers in *italic* refer to illustrations.

A

Abbott, L. C., 281
Abduction, *74*
    hip mobility and, 235
Abscissa
Acceleration, 30, 36–39
    mass and, 89
    See also Velocity
Acetabular labrum, *232*, 233
Acetabulum, *232*, 233
Acromioclavicular angles, *276*
Acromioclavicular joint, 188, *276*, 277
Acromion, 275–*76*
Action potentials, 162
Adduction, *74*
Adductors, 234
Agonist, 155
Alar ligaments, 254
Amphiarthroses joints, 186
Anatomical neck, of humerus, *290*
Anconeus, 293, 297
Ankle Joint (talocrural), 202–5, 208–11
    balance and, 199
    as first-class lever, *106*
    mobility of, 204–5
    stability of, 202–*3*
Annular ligament, *291*
Annularis, 311
Annulus fibrosus, 254
Antagonist, 156
Anterior arch, of vertebral column, 253
Anterior crest, of tibia, *215*
Anterior cruciate ligament, *219–20*
Anterior inferior iliac spine, *233*, 245
Anterior longitudinal ligament, 255
Anterior lumbosacral angle, *256*
Anterior sacroiliac ligament, *248*, 249
Anterior sternoclavicular ligament, 276–77
Anterior superior iliac spine, 245, 249
Anterior talotibial ligament, 204
Anterior talofibular ligament, 204
Anterior tubercles, 253
Anteroposterior axis (Z axis), 18
Appendicular skeleton, 182
Arcuate line, 246
Arcuate pubic ligament, 247, *248*
Arm, 290–91, 298–303
    appendicular segments, 70
    bone structure of, *290–91*
    circumduction and, *76*
    See also Elbow, Forearm, Hand, Shoulder
Articular cartilage, 182, 187
Articular processes, 252–53
Assistor, 155

Assmussen, E., 172
Atlantoaxial joint, 258
Atlantoöccipital joint, 253, 258
Atlas vertebra, first cervical vertebra, 253–*54*
Auricular surface, 246
Axial skeleton, 182
Axillary borders, of scapula, 275–*76*
Axis vertebra, second cervical vertebra, 253–*54*
Axon, 162, 163

B

Balance, 199–200
Balance point, *109*
Ball and socket joint, 190
Basmajian, J. V., 163
Belly, 144
Bergström, R. M., 166–67
Biceps brachii, 291
    elbow flexor, 294
    electrical activity and, 174
    spurt muscle, 158
    synergist action of, 156
Biceps femoris tendon, 220
Bicipital groove, *290*
Bilateral axis, 65
Bipennate fiber, 146
Body segments, 70–81
    eight components of, *70–71*
    six movement classes of, *71–76*
Bones, 181–93
    of skeleton, 182–*83*, *184*–86; joints, 186–*89*, 190–*92*
    structure of, *181–82*
    See also specific listings
Brachialis, 146
    elbow flexor, 293
    spurt muscle, 158
    synergist action, 156
Brachioradialis
    assistor action, 156
    elbow flexor, 292
    shunt activity, *158*
Brunnstrom, Signe, 203

C

Calcanofibular ligament, 204
Calcaneotibial ligament, 204
Calcaneus, *196–97*
    midtarsal mobility of, 201
Calcium, muscle action and, 163
Capitate bone, 304
Capitulum, 291, 292
Carpal articular surface, 295
Carpal bones, 306, 308–*9*
Carpometacarpal joint, 310
Carpometacarpal mobility, 311–*12*, 313

Cartesian coordinate system, 9
Cartesian rectangular coordinate **axes, 11**
Cartilaginous tissue, 186
Centripetal force, 104–*5*
    vector, 101
Cervical lordosis, *251*, 252
Cervical region, mobility of, 258–59
Cervical vertebrae, 253–*54*
Circular motion, 50–55
    force and, 101–*2*, *103*–4
Circumduction, *76*
Classification, process of, 4–5
Clavicle, *274–75*
Close, J. R., 216
Coccyx, *247*, *251–52*
Collateral ligaments, 292
Components, *110–11*
    vectors, 13–14
Concave-side rotation, 257
Concentric contraction, 153
Concoid ligament, *277*
Condylar joint, 190
Condyles, of tibia, *215*
Contractile component, 151
Contraction, 172–73
    velocity and, 152–53
Convex-side rotation, 257
Coracoacromial ligament, *277*
Coracoclavicular ligament, *277*
Coracohumeral ligament, *280*
Coracoid process, of scapula, 275–*76*
Coronary ligaments, 188, 219
Coronoid fossa, 291
Coronoid process, 295
Cosines, law of, 96
Costal demifacets, 253
Costoclavicular ligament, 276–*77*
Coxa valga, 232
Coxa vara, 232
Cruciate ligaments, 188, *219–20*
Curved motion, 55–56

D

Deltoid ligament (tibial collateral), 188, 204, *219*
Deltoid, 146, 175, *281*
Deltoid tuberosity, 291
Depression, 278
Depressor cuff muscle group, 281
Diaphasis, 182
Diarthroses joints, 186
    classification of, *189*–90
Displacement, 10
    circular motion and, 50
    velocity and, 40–42, 47–48
Distal anterior tibiofibular ligament, 202, *203*
Distal radioulnar joint, 295, 296
Distal tibiofibular joint, 186, 216, *217*
Distensibility, 151–52

Spring ligament, *see* Plantar calcaneonavicular ligament
Spurt, 158
Stabilizer, 157
Steindler, Arthur, 67, 205
Sternoclavicular joint, 188, *277–78*
Sternum, *275*
Styloid process, 296
Subclavius, 280
Subscapular fossa, 276–77
Subscapularis, 276–77, 281, 282
Subtalar mobility, 201–*2*
Superior articular process, 247
Superior border, of scapula, 276–77
Superior capsular ligament, 278
Superior pubic ligaments, 247, *248*
Superior ramus, 245
Supination, rotation and, *75*
Supinator, 155
Supracondylar ridges, 292
Supraspinal ligaments, 255
Supraspinatous fossa, *276–77*
Supraspinatus, 281, *282*
Supratrochlear foramen, 292
Surgical neck, of arm, 292
Symphasis pubis joint, 186, 245
Synathroses joints, 186
Synergist, 156–*57*, 158
Synovial fluid, 187
Synovial membrane, 187

T

Talocalcaneal ligaments, 201
Talocrural joint, *see* Ankle
Talus, *196*–97, 202, 203–*4*
Tarsal bones, *196–97*
Tarsometatarsal joints, 198
Tarsometatarsal mobility, 201
Tendinous action, 236
Tendons, 144
Tension, 172
    force and, *110–11*
    isometrics and, 152
Tensor fascia lata, 220
Teres major, 175
Teres minor, 281, *282*
Thenar eminence, 313
Thigh, 231–33, 236–38
    appendicular segment, 70
    bone structure of, *231–32*, 233
Thoracic region, 252
    mobility of, *257–58*
Thoracic vertebrae, *253*
Thorax, 276
Three-dimensional analysis, 3, 18–20

Tibia, 188, 202–*3*, 215
    knee mobility and, 223
Tibia shaft, *215*
Tibial collateral ligament, *see* Deltoid ligament
Tibial malleolus, 202
Tibialis anterior, 176, 204
Tibialis posterior, 146, 205
Tibiofibular mortise, 202, *203*
Tibionavicular ligament, 204
Tilting
    pelvic mobility and, 249–50
    scapula mobility and, 279
Time, 6
    determination of, 32
    intervals, 33, 34
Tissue
    connective, 144
    soft, 190–91
Toes, *197*–98
    mobility of, 201
Torque, 107–*9*, 114, 132
Translation, 58–63
    animate bodies and, *59*
    circular, 63
    gliding joint motion and, 189
    linear, 58–*61*
    rectilinear, 61–*62*
    rotation and, 66–68
Transverse abduction, 74
Transverse adduction, *74*
Transverse atlantal ligament, 253
Transverse foramen, 253
Transverse metacarpal ligament, *314*
Transverse metatarsal arch, 199
Transverse process, 252
Transverse tarsal curvature, 199
Transverse tarsal joint, 201
Trapezium, 308–*10*
Trapezius, 280
Trapezoid bone, 310
Trapezoid ligament, *278*
Triangular articular disk, 297
Triangular bone, 305
Triceps brachii, *96*, 174–75, 294
Trigonometric functions, 327–29
Trochanters, 232
Trochlea, 292
Trochlear notch, *292*, 296
True effort arm, lever and, *112*
Trunk, 245, 264–69
    axial segment, 70
    circumduction, *76*
    flexion of, *73*
Tubercles, 253
Tuberosity, *215*
Two-dimensional analysis, 3

U

Ulna, 72, 292, *295–96*
Ulna shaft, 296
Ulnar collateral ligament, 293, 307
Ulnar flexion, *72*
Ulnar nerve, 292
Ulnar notch, 296
Unipennate fiber, 146

V

Vasti, 224
Vectors, 10–15, 46, 101
Velocity, 26–55
    average, 26, 46, 50–52, 130
    constant, 27, 35
    displacement and, 40–42
    instantaneous, 33–36, 46
    kinetic energy and, 126–27
    muscular contraction and, 152
    slope, 28–29
    varying, 28
    vector of, 46
    See also Acceleration
Vertebral arch, 252
Vertebral border, of scapula, 276–77
Vertebral Column, 250–59
    mobility of, *256–57*, 258–59; flexion of, *73*
    stability of, 254–*55*
    structure of, 191, *251–52*, *253–54*
Vertebral (neural) foramen, 250

W

Weight, *88*–89
Whole-body, movement of, 80–*81*
Work, 117–41
    angular, 130–41; power and, 130; inertia and, 131–34; rotation and, *141*
    linear, 117–27; gravity and, 118; power and, *118*–20; kinetic energy and, 126–27; potential energy and, 127
    muscles and, 149–50
Wrist, 305–7, 319–24
    bone structure of, *305, 308*
    mobility of, 307, 308, 309
    stability of, *306–7*

X - Y - Z

Y ligament, *see* Iliofemoral ligament